WQ043442

CONTENTS

ACTA NEUROPATHOLOGICA / SUPPLEMENTUM V

SYMPOSIUM ON PATHOLOGY
OF AXONS AND AXONAL FLOW

ORGANIZED BY THE ÖSTERREICHISCHE ARBEITSGEMEINSCHAFT
FÜR NEUROPATHOLOGIE AND THE RESEARCH GROUP
OF NEUROPATHOLOGY OF THE WORLD FEDERATION OF NEUROLOGY

WIEN, SEPTEMBER 10 AND 11, 1970

EDITED BY

R. L. FRIEDE   F. SEITELBERGER
CLEVELAND   WIEN

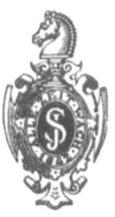

SPRINGER-VERLAG · BERLIN · HEIDELBERG · NEW YORK
SPRINGER-VERLAG · WIEN · NEW YORK

1971

Sponsered by:

Bundesministerium für Wissenschaft und Forschung, Research Committee of WFN,
Firma Brady, Firma CIBA, Firma Geigy, Firma Hoffmann La Roche,
Firma Österreichische Stickstoffwerke, Firma Vedepha

ISBN-13:978-3-540-05433-7   e-ISBN-13:978-3-642-47449-1
DOI: 10.1007/978-3-642-47449-1

Acta neuropath. (Berl.) Suppl. V, 1—2 (1971)

Introduction

The Symposium on Axon Pathology and Axonal Flow was organized by the Österreichische Arbeitsgemeinschaft für Neuropathologie and by the Problem Commission for Neuropathology of the World Federation of Neurology. We wish to thank Dr. Macdonald Critchley, President, World Federation of Neurology, for his encouragement and unfailing support.

One of the foremost goals of the Problem Commission of Neuropathology is to stimulate the advancement of knowledge on selected, current topics in neuropathology; interest is focussed by interdisciplinary discussion among experts who approach the subject from different fields. A similar symposium was held in Vienna in 1965 and provided a timely review of the many interrelated aspects of brain edema.

The plans for the present symposium arose from the urgent need to obtain insight into the relations between the accumulated knowledge on morphologic changes in axons and changes in axonal physiology. Both fields have advanced considerably, although for the most part independently of each other. Axon pathology has come into its rights with the recognition of neuroaxonal dystrophy as a nosological entity involving a primary disease process of the axons, as well as with advancing knowledge of changes in the fine structure and chemistry of normal and diseased axons. Axonal physiology has advanced rapidly in terms of documenting and analyzing the processes of axonal flow—that is, the redistribution of axoplasm along the fiber. It is timely, then, to emphasize the need for correlating morphology with function, as only such correlation will enable us to understand and interpret the changes in diseased axons. Neuropathology, thus, has to be applied in its most advanced and inclusive meaning—that is, as a science aimed at understanding the processes causing morphologic alterations in nerve tissue, including not only the level of the cell but, also, those of fine structure, chemistry and molecular biology. This approach requires communcation and cooperation, of investigators concerned with neurocytology, histochemistry, electron microscopy, neurophysiology and neurochemistry. A gremium of experts was gathered at this symposium in the hope of shedding some light on the derangements in function that cause the morphologic changes in neuroaxonal dystrophy as well as other types of pathologic processes involving axons. Their reports concern the latest development in their respective fields of investigation.

Advances in axon biology are so rapid that every year provides us with a wealth of new facts and observations; hence, this conference cannot reasonable be expected to answer all questions. Rather, its purpose must be to take stock of the available data, to communicate advances and new concepts, and to help us to formulate the goals and approaches for future research. To this end, ample time was allotted during the symposium for discussion, but these exchanges of thoughts cannot, unfortunately, be included in the printed text. We hope that publication of the presentations will provide a valuable source of information on the present state of knowledge on this most important borderland between neuro-pathology, neurophysiology and neurochemistry.

We would like to express our gratitude to all participants of the symposium for contributing their efforts and for their enthusiasm. We are also indebted to Springer Verlag and Bergmann Verlag for publication of the symposium and for their appreciation of the editorial concerns.

Franz Seitelberger   Reinhard L. Friede

Acta neuropath. (Berl.) Suppl. V, 3—16 (1971)
© by Springer-Verlag 1971

Neuroaxonal Dystrophy in Man: Character and Natural History

KURT JELLINGER

Neurological Institute of University of Vienna
(Director: Prof. Dr. F. Seitelberger)

ADAM JIRÁSEK

Hlava's Institute of Pathology I, Charles University Prague
(Director: Prof. Dr. B. Bednář)

Summary. A short correlative review is given of the light and electron microscopical features and histochemical reactions of dystrophic axons in the mature human CNS. Their ultrastructural similarities to axonal changes in the disease entity of the neuroaxonal dystrophies and various experimental conditions are confirmed. The incidence of axonal spheroids in the gracile and cuneate nuclei and in the reticular zone of the substantia nigra was studied in 1450 consecutive autopsies and correlated with age and underlying disease process. Axonal dystrophy of posterior column nuclei and substantia nigra showed a significant age-dependancy without predilection for either sex. The incidence of dystrophic axons in the globus pallidus and other sites was also examined. No clear relationship of the severity and frequency of the involvement of gracile nucleus with any underlying disease was established, while axonal dystrophy in substantia nigra showed significant correlations to alcoholic encephalopathies and Parkinson's syndrome, and a trend to negative relationship with presenile cerebral atrophies. In addition to the natural occurrence of dystrophic axons as a physiological, age-dependant phenomenon, these lesions may arise prematurely and to excess in a variety of natural and experimental disorders. The reported findings suggest that some metabolic factors are involved in the pathogenesis of dystrophic axonal changes. Relations to axonal dying-back processes are discussed.

Key-Words: Dystrophic Axon — Spheroid — Ultrastructure — Topography — Natural Occurrence — Age-Dependance.

Introduction

The occurrence of axonal swellings has been reported in a great variety of conditions, and is thought to reflect a non-specific reaction of the neuron to a variety of noxious stimuli including traumatic, toxic, biochemical and genetic agents. Besides reactive, retrograde-degenerative and regenerative axonal changes *secondary* to a disturbance in the surrounding tissue, a type of axonal enlargement referred to as (neuro)axonal dystrophy (AD) has been described a) as an incidental finding in the CNS of man and various other species, b) in association with various human and experimental diseases, and c) as a characteristic lesion of a group of degenerative diseases of the nervous system which are summarized as "neuroaxonal dystrophies". This type of axonal lesion is assumed to develop *primarily* as the result of some morbid process or disturbance involving the metabolism of axoplasm ("dystrophy"). Dystrophic axons have been shown to present functional and ultrastructural peculiarities which are quite different from the various non-specific axonal lesions secondary to trauma and other lesions [23]. On the other hand, the structural and histochemical similarities of axonal swellings characteristic for the entity of the neuroaxonal dystrophies to axonal lesions in a large variety of natural and experimental diseases has been established [6,11,14—16,23,31,46].

Morphological and Histochemical Aspects

Microscopically, AD is characterized by the presence of round, ovoid or poly-morphic axoplasmic masses of 20 to over 120 μ diameter called "Schollen" [36] or "speroids" [8], which represent focal swellings of the affected axons as demonstrat-ed in longitudinal sections (Fig. 1 A). The appearance of these axoplasmic bodies varies considerably depending upon the stage of development [12]. In the *early* lesions they stain lightly with eosin and are homogenous or finely granular, and occasionally there is a pale periphery and a denser granular central area. Later, they are densely staining acidophilic bodies and may contain one or more dense ambophilic cores within otherwise homogenous or fibrillary axoplasm (Fig. 1 C). The bodies are generally argyrophilic and can be readily demonstrated by various silver methods. In addition to a strongly argyrophilic core, they may contain convoluted or coiled fibrillary masses and concentric lamination (Fig. 2 D). As age advances, the spheroids become more irregular in size, vary in tinctorial properties and tend to become more dense and coarsely granular, sometimes with formation of spiked ball-like structures [30] or "plasmatic chambers" [12]. Later, they un-dergo regressive changes, such as fragmentation of the axoplasmic components with formation of clefts or coarse vacuolation (Fig. 1 B). Microglial cells occasional-ly cluster around dystrophic bodies (Fig. 1 E). Spheroids undergo liquefaction probably due to enzymatic digestion terminating in complete resolution *in situ* with formation of large hollow spaces in the neuropil, often without considerable astroglial reaction (Fig. 1 B). In the gracile nucleus and spinal cord, "old" spheroids are transformed into large amorphous basophilic masses with double-concentric achat-like structures and occasional deposition of calcified, iron-negative material (Fig. 1 D). In the reticular zone of the substantia nigra and in the globus pallidus the bodies are slightly basophilic and finely granulated. They may contain granules of argentaffine lipopigment and small amounts of iron and copper. Intact myelin sheaths cover axons leading into the axoplasmic masses which are only partially or not at all covered by myelin. In general, nerve cells are reduced in severely affected nuclei. Occasional swollen neurons with central chromatolysis or ballooned cytoplasm (Fig. 1 F) and variable degrees of astroglial proliferation are noted.

The light microscopic appearance of the dystrophic axons in mature humans is very similar to that of structures seen in human infantile and late infantile NAD [8, 36, 38], in Hallervorden-Spatz disease [33, 37, 47, 48], in mature apparent-ly normal dogs [27] and other species [30, 39, 42], in rats fed a vitamin E-deficient diet [30, 37] and in various species following administration of various neurotoxic substances [2, 6, 9, 22, 31]. They also resemble reactive and regenerative neurons in peritraumatic regions of the human CNS [35], following experimental transec-tion [13, 25], etc.

Histochemically, the spheroids and eosinophilic bodies in the CNS observed in various conditions are similar in many respects [8, 12, 14, 18, 21, 27, 33, 36, 38, 44, 47, 48]. They are characterized by a complex protein material with variable amounts of lipids and carbohydrates. Some differences in lipid and carbohydrate content are known between the various disease entities associated with AD or are due to the stage of development of the spheroids.

General protein reactions give approximately the same results, indicating a high content of aromatic and alpha-amino acids, of SH- and SS-groups, tyrosine, arginine and histidine,

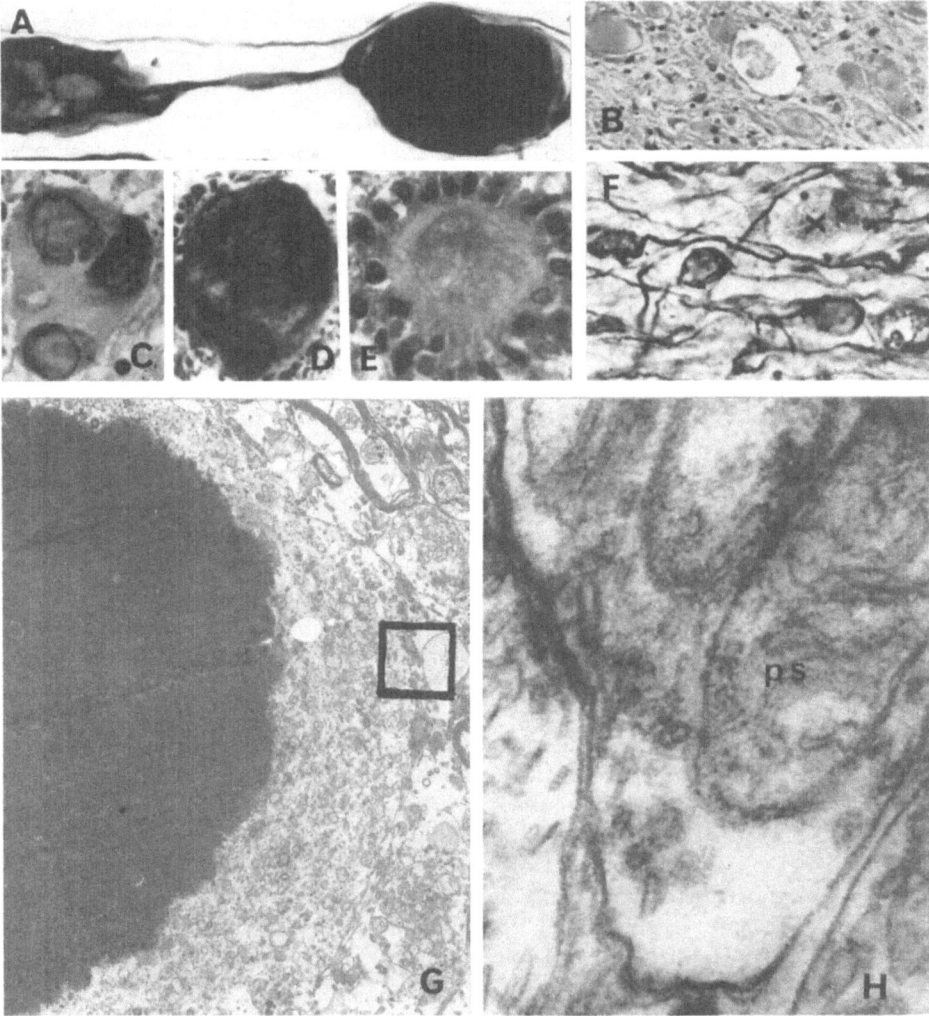

Fig. 1 A—F. Dystrophic axons in human CNS. A Focal axonal enlargement in upper part of gracile tract (male aged 64 years) Bodian ×700; B Presenile AD, grade 3 + in gracile nucleus (male, 36 years), H.-E. ×180; C Spheroid with several dense cores. H.-E. ×700; D Calcified spheroid in gracile nucleus; v. Kossa ×700; E Microglial proliferation around spheroid. H.-E. ×1300; F Multiple terminal axonal swellings in globus pallidus next to swollen nerve cell (x) (male, 66 years), Bodian ×560

Fig. 1 G, H. Dystrophic axon in gracile nucleus of aged human. G Dense homogenous substance in center of "old" axonal spheroid, ×6,000; H Outlining portion of Fig. 1 G from an adjacent section, showing synaptic area with postsynaptic thickening (ps) ×90,000

with constant lack of tryptophane and nucleic acids. In spheroids undergoing vacuolar degeneration, reactions for aromatic amino acids become negative. Variable, usually small quantities of carbohydrates are demonstrated in most of the bodies, while investigation for acid mucopolysaccharides gives inconclusive results except in small spheroids. In mature bodies glycogen granules may be present. Small amounts of complex lipids, probably protein-bound phospholipids, lipoproteins or glycolipids, are demonstrated in some of the small spheroids.

Enzyme-histochemical studies on dystrophic axons in vitamin E-deficient rats and in infantile NAD demonstrated an increase of oxidative enzymes with reduced activity of succinic dehydrogenase [4, 17]. Spheroids in the gracile nucleus of aged humans show strong activity of β-glycerol-phosphate dehydrogenase which disappears in "old" concrement-like axonal bodies (pers. observ.).

Electron microscopic studies performed on autopsy material of the medullary tegmentum of aged humans gave the following results[1]: The spheroids are round, granular bodies with increased density of organels, consisting of varied numbers of normal and enlarged mitochondria, patches of electron dense material, vesicles, granular particles, and multivesicular bodies (Fig. 2 B). The bodies are surrounded by a single unit membrane. The myelin sheaths around the distended axon may be preserved but the ratio of myelin sheath thickness to axon diameter is reduced (Fig. 2 A). Occasional small or large multigranular bodies with accumulation of glycogen-like material are noticed (Figs. 2 B, E). Other spheroids show a variable arrangement of smooth membranes and peculiar tubular structures arranged in orderly bundles (Fig. 2 C). Such enlarged axons filled with irregular branching tubular-membranous structures may correspond to the convoluted fibrillary bodies seen in silver impregnations (Fig. 2 D). The arrangement of the tubular-membranous systems ranges from tightly packed or whorled lamellae to loose aggregates of apparently hollow membranous cisternae (Fig. 2 C). The compactly arranged tubules are composed of smooth membranes which crisscross at all angles in respect to the plane of the section. They are often branched and appear to be a part of continuous sponge-like network, although each tubule appears to form a separate entity. Concentric lamellae (myelin figures) are sometimes present among vesicular-membranous material and granular particles or smooth tubules (Fig. 2 E). A large mass of dense homogenous material in the centre of an axonal body (Fig. 1 G) may correspond to the dense cores in "old" axonal spheroids. A few synapses are seen at the periphery of the dilated axons or axonal bodies (Fig. 1 G). They are recognized by the pre- and postsynaptic thickenings or the boutons (Fig. 1 H), but neither typical "clefts" nor synaptic vesicles could be detected in the postmortem material.

The ultrastructure of these bodies in the gracile nucleus of elderly humans is similar to the axonal swellings found in infantile NAD [14, 15, 34, 46]. in vitamin E-deficient rats [23, 24], in the gracile nucleus of cats with acrylamide neuropathy [31], in the spinal cord of chicken poisoned with tri-ortho-cresyl-phosphate [1], following p-bromophenylacetylurea intoxication in the rat [2], and diethyldithiocarbamate administration to sheep and rabbits [16]. There are also similarities to regenerating axons [13, 23, 24]. The main cytoplasmic component of these dystrophic axonal swellings are tubular-membrane systems very similar in appearance to smooth endoplasmic reticulum associated with increased density of organels, consisting of normal and enlarged mitochondria, dense bodies, microtubules, neurofilaments and small electron dense granules.

---

1 Blocks were taken from the posterior column nuclei 1—2 h after death and were fixed in 1 % buffered osmium acid and embedded in epon or araldite. Sections cut on a Reichert ultramicrotome were stained with lead citrate or uranyl lead and with toluidin blue for light microscopy.

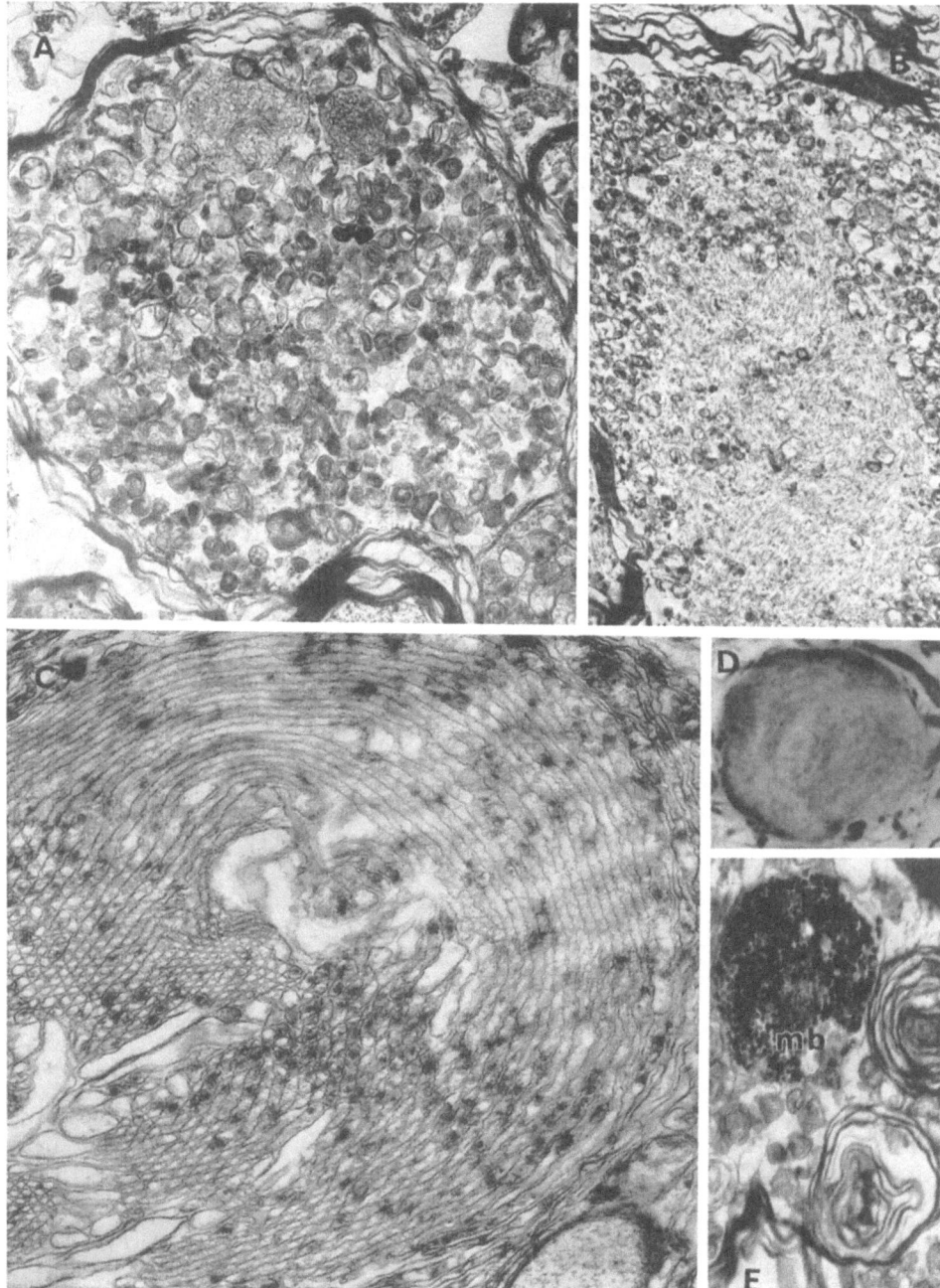

Fig. 2 A—E. Dystrophic Axons in gracile nucleus of aged human. Enlargements reduced by 10%. A Large dystrophic axon showing aggregates of mitochondria, electron dense and multigranulated bodies, vesicles and granular particles. Note the preservation of myelin sheaths. ×10,000; B Axonal body showing aggregates of mitochondria, patchy dense material and some multigranular bodies (×). Neurofilaments and vesicles are abundant. ×8,000; C Large axonal body with whorled arrangement of layered loops, tightly packed interconnected tubular structures and some large membranous cisternae. ×15,000; D Convoluted fibrillary body. Bodian ×1,000; E Multigranular body (mb), degenerating mitochondria and wide concentric membranes (myelin figures) from an adjacent section of Fig. 2 B. ×10,000

Origin of the Axonal Spheroids

It has been variously suggested that these bodies originate in proximal axons, dendrites and neurons [8,10,36,41,42] or in terminal axons [3,7,23,24]. Dystrophic axons, in addition to frequent occurrence in the gracile nucleus, are also noted in the gracile tract close to its termination in the gracile nucleus (Fig. 1 A), in terminal axons in the globus pallidus (Fig. 1 E) and indenting neurons in anterior horn of the spinal cord [17]. Occasionally, however, it is possible to observe an axonal continuation proximal *and* distal to the enlargement and to notice spheroids in proximal parts of axons, e.g. in the ansa lenticularis and arcuate fibres [8,18,36—38].

Electron microscopic findings in infantile NAD, experimental vitamin E-deficiency and NDDC intoxication give evidence to suggest that spheroids predominantly arise in *(pre)terminal axons* of ascending fibres [12a,16,23,24] and *pre-synaptic terminals*, particularly in axodendritic and axoaxonal synaptic complexes [14,15,34,46]. This view is confirmed by demonstration of strong local relationship of axonal bodies to synaptic areas in the gracile nucleus of aged humans. Occasionally, the complex material probably related to an overproduction of the smooth endoplasmic reticulum, and abnormal mitochondria are also present in neuronal perikarya and dendrites [21,46]. In experimental AD, swellings are not limited to the pre-synaptic area, but extend back to the axon. There is an increased density of normal and pathological organelles in the axon proximal to the spheroid [12a, 16] or distal to the swelling [6]. Axonal swelling may develop not only in the pre-synaptic region of the ascending fibres in the gracile nucleus but also at the tip of the viable axon following the "dying-back" of the distal axon [2].

Topographic Distribution of Dystrophic Axons

Apart from a generalized occurrence of dystrophic axons in human infantile and late infantile NAD [8,37,38] and in systemic NAD in sheep [7], axonal spheroids are usually confined to some more or less constantly affected sites in the CNS which show variable intensity and extent of involvement in the various spontaneous and experimental conditions mentioned. The most constantly affected areas are the gracile and cuneate nuclei, the reticular zone of substantia nigra and globus pallidus, other sensory relay nuclei of the brain stem, spinal cord and spinal root ganglia, while peripheral nerve lesions were reported in infantile NAD [9,21] and experimental AD.

In the gracile nucleus and oral parts of the gracile tract, dystrophic axons are observed as random findings in man and animals. Less frequently affected are the cuneate nucleus and other sensory relay nuclei of the medulla, e.g. trigeminal and vestibular nerve nuclei, while occasional spheroids are noticed in the posterior columns, dorsal and anterior grey horns, posterior grey commissure and Clarke's column of the spinal cord [18,42]. Whereas the involvement of the pallido-nigral system has been reported almost exclusively in man, except for occasional spheroids observed in the substantia nigra and pallidum of monkeys [29], all the other sites mentioned are affected in both natural and experimental conditions. In some of the latter, dystrophic axons are also found in the reticular formation, pontine nuclei and motor nuclei of brain stem and spinal cord [6,30].

Natural History of (Neuro-) Axonal Dystrophy

Several reports indicate that the occurrence of dystrophic axons in the gracile nucleus of man is clearly related to age [3,12,40—42]. Increased severity of involvement of this nucleus has been observed in chronic alcoholism [30] and

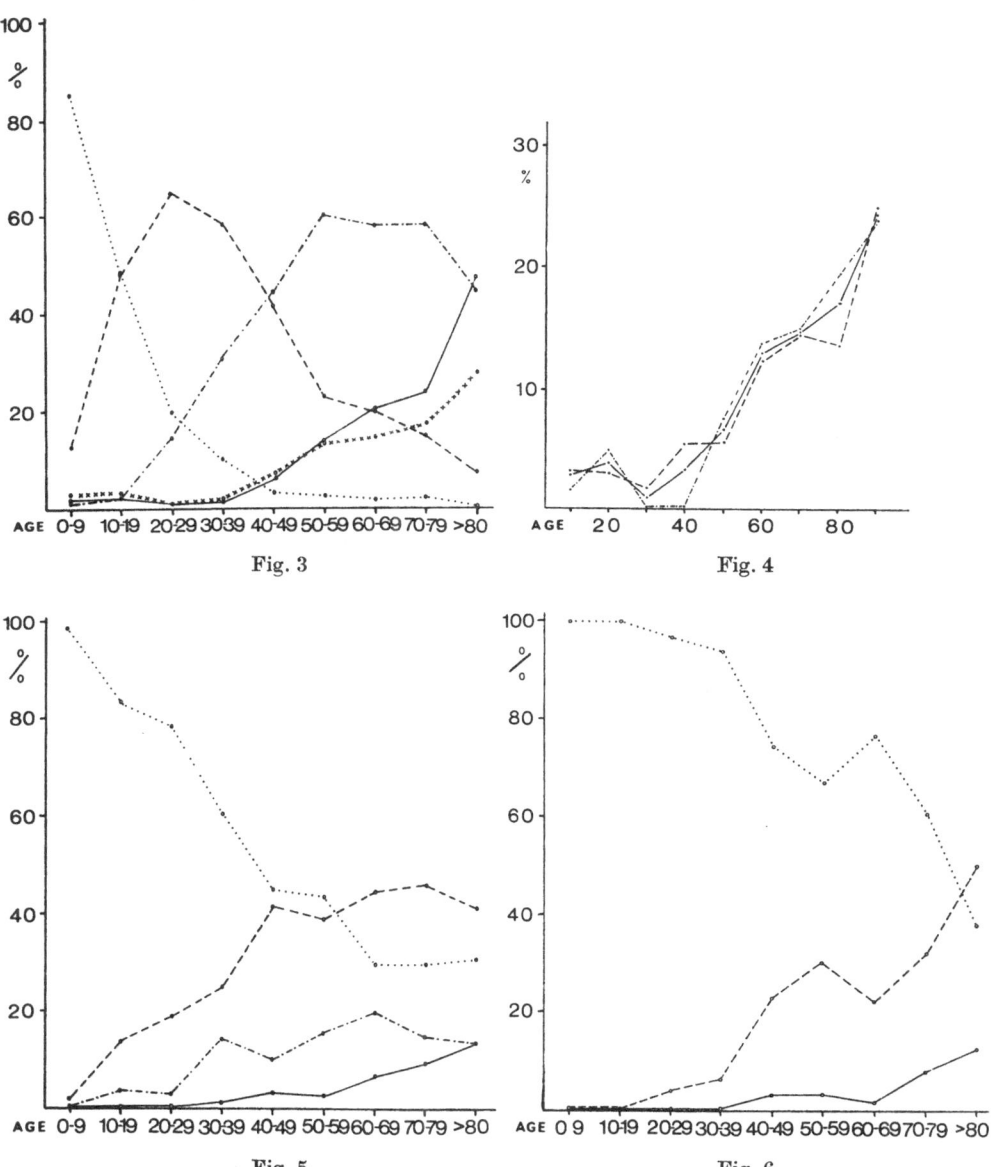

Fig. 3

Fig. 4

Fig. 5

Fig. 6

Fig. 3. Incidence and severity of axonal dystrophy in the posterior column nuclei in relation to age (1470 autopsy cases). ····· = 0; – – – = +; –·–·– = 2 +; ——— = 3 + (Gracile nucleus) × × × Cuneate nucleus (mild degree of AD)

Fig. 4. Age incidence and sex distribution of axonal dystrophy in the cuneate nucleus of man (1470 autopsy cases). – – – Males; –·–·– Females; ——— Total

Fig. 5. Incidence and severity of axonal dystrophy in substantia nigra (reticulata) in relation to age (1430 necropsies). Legends see Fig. 3

Fig. 6. Incidence and severity of axonal dystrophy in globus pallidus in relation to age (240 autopsy cases). ···· = 0; – – – = +; ——— = 2 +

infantile malabsorption syndromes [41,43]. Patients with a history of chronic alcoholism revealed also severe affection of substantia nigra [18,45]. On the other hand, no clear correlation of AD of the gracile nucleus with any underlying disease or previous brain lesion could be established [3,40]. The incidence of axonal bodies in the gracile and cuneate nuclei, substantia nigra, globus pallidus and some other regions was studied in an unselected human autopsy material and correlated with age and underlying disease process. Preliminary results have been published previously [19].

Material and Methods

Sections were cut at 2 to 4 levels from the medulla oblongata and at 2—3 frontal levels from substantia nigra of 1470 and 1430 consecutive autopsy cases, respectively. The number of dystrophic axons was graded using the criteria laid down by Brannon et al. [3]. The globus pallidus of 240 unselected necropsies was examined at 2—3 levels. The number of axonal spheroids was graded using the following criteria: 0 = no axonal changes, 1 + = mild involvement (1—2 axonal bodies after searching several fields), 2 + = moderate involvement (more than one spheroid per low power field). In addition, 100 human spinal cords were studied, using serial sections of 10—30 different segments. For statistical evaluation, the autopsy cases were classified into 11 diagnosis groups according to the underlying letal illness with particular attention to changes of the CNS in chronic alcoholism, diseases of the liver, kidney, and to senile atrophy and Parkinson's disease. The statistical correlation between AD and underlying disease process was evaluated by multiple χ^2 analysis, carried out separately for the involvement of gracile nucleus and substantia nigra.

Results

The *gracile nucleus* was free of dystrophic axons in 85% of the cases up to 10 years of age, and in 48% of the subjects between 10 and 20 years. In the 4th decade this percentage dropped to 10%, while over 40 years of age only a few people—average 2%—were free of axonal changes. The majority of cases of all age groups presented a mild to moderate degree of involvement. Severe AD with progressing increase in frequency was present over 50 years of age (Fig. 3). The absence and the severe degree of axonal changes are clearly related to age without prevalence for either sex [18].

In the *cuneate nucleus* only mild to moderate degrees of AD were noted. The changes encountered up to the age of 40 were minimal and then became gradually more frequent (Fig. 4). There was no clear age-dependency of the severity of affection of this nucleus nor a difference in the affection of either sex or any correlation with the involvement of Goll's nucleus.

In *substantia nigra* (reticulata) dystrophic axons were not found under 10 years of age. The absence of axonal bodies progressively decreased in relation to age, although over age 60 AD was absent in about 30%. The majority of cases of all age groups presented a mild degree of involvement. A moderate degree was present in 10 to 20% of the cases over age 40, while a severe degree occurred in 7 to 14% of the subjects beyond the age of 60 (Fig. 5). There was no clear-cut difference in the affection of either sex [18].

A comparison of axonal changes encountered in the gracile nucleus and in substantia nigra showed a highly significant deviation both in intensity and frequency of the affection in favor of Goll's nucleus ($p < 0.0005$).

Table 1. *Correlation age—neuroaxonal dystrophy*

Disease Process	Nucleus gracilis				Zona reticularis nigrae			
	χ^2	CC_{corr}	n	Sign.	χ^2	CC_{corr}	n	Sign.
Alcoholic Encephalopathy	25,389	0.74	35	N	21,069	0.67	41	N
Hepatic Encephalopathy (without alcoholism)	29,823	0.88	21	N	16,569	0.72	25	N
Parkinsonism (degen.)	6,642	0.63	15	N	7,287	0.42	46	N
Presenile Brain Atrophy	5,449	0.48	25	N	5,478	0.44	32	N
Other System Atrophies	27,803	0.79	31	N	18,980	0.68	35	N
Renal Disease (Coma)	40,058	0.92	23	S	21,285	0.80	23	N
Malignant Tumours, RES-Blood Diseases	55,462	0.68	103	HS	13.250	0.40	96	N
Brain Tumours	165,693	0.80	179	HS	55,355	0.62	136	HS
Cardio-, Cerebrovascular Syndromes	178,609	0.77	219	HS	112,841	0.68	206	HS
Inflammatory, Demyelinating Processes	102,650	0.81	105	HS	61,501	0.66	124	HS
Others (Brain Injuries, Perinatal Lesions etc.)	232,095	0.81	237	HS	91,867	0.61	230	HS
Total	822,920	0.77	993	HS	353,345	0.59	994	HS

$df = 24$ $\chi^2_{0,05} = 36,415$ $\chi^2_{0,01} = 42,980$

$$CC = \sqrt{\frac{\chi^2}{\chi^2 + n}}$$

$$CC_{max} = \sqrt{\frac{r-1}{r}}$$

$$CC_{corr} = \frac{CC}{CC_{max}}$$

r = number of lines or columns

The *globus pallidus* showed only mild to moderate degrees of involvement over 40 years of age with an increase both in severity and frequency of AD after the age of 70 years (Fig. 6).

In the *spinal cord* occasional spheroids were noted in the dorsal and ventral grey horns and posterior columns of various levels after the age of 40 without further age-dependant increase in severity and frequency, the average incidence for the age groups from 40—90 years being 22%.

A data analysis performed on two-thirds of the present material gave the following results (Tables 1 and 2): There are highly significant correlations of AD in the gracile nucleus and in substantia nigra both in frequency and severity with age,

Table 2. *Correlation disease process — neuroaxonal dystrophy*

Age	Nucleus gracilis Goll				Zona reticularis nigrae			
	χ^2	CC_{corr}	n	Sign.	χ^2	CC_{corr}	n	Sign.
			178				148	
0— 9	23,951	0.39		N	0,949	0.09		N
			37				47	
10—19	12,692	0.58		N	17,114	0.59		N
			71				59	
20—29	24,702	0.58		N	7,118	0.37		N
			70				66	
30—39	19,878	0.54		N	30,038	0.64		N
			107				107	
40—49	40,988	0.60		N	22,817	0.48		N
			169				161	
50—59	23,984	0.40		N	43,403	0.53		N
			205				242	
60—69	44,351	0.48		S	58,993	0.51		HS
			134				135	
70—79	30,700	0.49		N	32,337	0.50		N
			22				29	
80—89	11,701	0.68		N	23,949	0.77		N
			993				994	
Total	197,011	0.47		HS	178,149	0.45		HS

$$df = 30 \quad \chi^2_{0,05} = 43,773 \qquad\qquad \chi^2_{0,01} = 50,892$$

irrespective of the underlying disease. In the reticulata nigrae, this stochastic relationship is not so pronounced as in Goll's nucleus (Table 1). Similar clear-cut correlations between axonal changes in both nuclei and advancing age are apparent within each diagnostic group except for presenile brain atrophies. On the other hand, there was also a clear-cut relationship of the basic disease processes to age. There was also a significant correlation between AD in both nuclei and the underlying disease process, but the influence of the latter on the degree of involvement was less than that of age (Table 2). Significant correlation between diagnostic group and axonal changes in Goll's nucleus and particularly in substantia nigra was found only for the age group between 60 and 69 years. The condition responsible for this relationship were alcoholic encephalopathy and Parkinson's disease, where deviations from random occurrence of axonal bodies were seen.

In cases of *alcoholic encephalopathy*, a clear relationship with AD in substantia nigra was established for the age groups over 20 years. This difference from random affection of this nucleus was less prominent in the third to sixth decade ($p < 0.05$) than in the subjects over 50 years of age ($p < 0.001$). However, no statistically significant relationship between AD of the gracile nucleus and alcoholic encephalopathy could be established for these age groups ($p = 0.5$).

A significant correlation of the axonal changes in the reticulata nigrae with *Parkinson's disease* was established for the age groups over 50 years when compared with the remaining sample ($p < 0.05$). This association was more clear-cut in patients between 60 and 69 years of age ($p < 0.01$) than in subjects over 50 years ($p < 0.05$), while in older people with Parkinsonism this difference from random involvement of this nucleus was not statistically significant ($p > 0.05$). No clear relationship between the AD of the gracile nucleus and Parkinsonims was established in the affected age group over 50 by comparison with the random sample ($p > 0.2$).

Severe degrees of involvement of the *gracile nucleus* and of other nuclei of the medullary tegmentum were noted in some children with *mucoviscidosis, congenital liver cirrhosis*, and *Tay-Sachs* disease, while premature affection of the *reticulata nigrae* was observed in cases of *hepatocerebral disease, cerebral lipidosis*, and spongy degeneration of the CNS [20].

In 7 cases of *tabes dorsalis* aged 50—74 years (average 64 years) only mild degrees of involvement of Goll's nucleus were present.

A trend to a negative relationship was noticed between the AD of the substantia nigra and *presenile cerebral atrophies* in patients over 50 years of age. In presenile dementia involvement of this nucleus was less severe than should be expected for this age group, although the difference from random affection was not statistically significant ($p > 0.05$). No clear deviation in the severity of AD in the gracile nucleus from random involvement was detected in cases of presenile brain atrophy.

Conclusions

The reported data confirm the ultrastructural similarities of dystrophic axons in the gracile nucleus of mature humans to axonal changes in the disease entity of the NADs and in various natural and experimental conditions. Further support is given for the view that the axonal spheroids originate in (pre)terminal axons of ascending fibre systems.

AD in the human CNS is observed—in descending order of severity and frequency—in the gracile nucleus, reticular zone of the substantia nigra, cuneate nucleus, globus pallidus, spinal cord, and various sensory relay nuclei of the brain stem. In most of these areas the incidence of dystrophic axons increases progressively with age. The gracile nucleus is significantly more often and more severely involved than all other areas mentioned.

Earlier reports on the age-dependant occurrence of axonal bodies in the gracile nucleus of man [3,12,40—42] are confirmed and a similar clear-cut correlation of axonal changes in the substantia nigra (reticulata) is established. Since no sex-dependant differences in the involvement of both these nuclei and the cuneate nucleus were observed, AD in these areas is considered as an *age-depending phenomenon*. In accordance with previous findings [3,40] no clear relationship between the severity and frequency of the affection of the gracile nucleus with any underlying disease process could be established. The occurrence of dystrophic changes in (pre)-terminal axons and presynaptic terminals of ascending fibre systems might be related to a physiological loss of nerve fibres occurring with age in the peripheral nerves, spinal roots (f. ref. [28]) and in the spinal posterior columns [10,26] which is thought to conform to a "dying-back" process [5]. However, statistical confirmation of this assumption is still lacking. On the other hand, exceedingly mild affection of Goll's nucleus in elderly subjects with tabes dorsalis and complete ascending degeneration of the posterior funiculi suggests that the AD of this nucleus is *not* caused by severe and rather acute Wallerian degeneration of the ascending fibre systems.

While no relationship of axonal changes in the gracile nucleus with any underlying disease process was established, there was a clear-cut *correlation of the involvement of the reticulata nigrae with Parkinsonism*. From recent ultrastructural studies of the normal substantia nigra in the cat it is evident that the pars reticulata contains several types of axonal terminals many of which belong to cells which lie in the pars compacta of this nucleus [32]. Since pathological changes in the zona compacta are the most constant features observed in patients with

Parkinsonism the question arises, whether the increased occurrence of dystrophic axons in the reticulata nigrae might be related to a loss of nerve cells in the pars compacta of the substantia nigra. In *alcoholic encephalopathies*, there was statistical evidence for a *premature affection* of this nucleus, the intensity curve of its involvement being above average. Conversely, a tendency for negative relationship between axonal changes in the substantia nigra and presenile cerebral atrophy was noticed.

In view of the presented findings and the available data on human and experimental axonal pathology one may conclude that the lesion referred to as AD may occur in three nosological forms:

1. as a *physiological ageing phenomenon* in certain, constantly affected areas of the CNS which is probably related to age-dependant dying-back processes of the axon;

2. as a *symptomatic lesion* arising prematurely and to excess at the physiological sites of predilection in a variety of natural and experimental conditions which are supposed to interfere with axonal metabolism or to result in pathological dying-back processes;

3. as a *lesion pathognomonic* for a series of neuropathological syndromes summarized as the disease entity of the "neuroaxonal dystrophies".

The precise nature of the dystrophic axonal changes and the primary site of damage leading to the production of axonal swellings in the above conditions are still unknown. Several possible mechanisms have been discussed: Besides primary affection of the synaptic region [12a, 14], metabolic deficiencies of the axoplasm [24, 37], reduced or slowed axonal flow or "axostasis" [6] which may result from impaired peripheral or intrinsic metabolism of the axon or a failure of the neuronal perikarya to supply the substrate necessary to maintain axonal transport mechanism [31], attempts of axonal regeneration as a sustained response to injury by an unknown agent [15] or resulting from a structural and/or functional loss of axonal contact with the post-synaptic neurone [2] have been suggested as pathogenic factors.

The occurrence of AD as an age-dependant phenomenon in the CNS of man and animals and its premature and excessive production in certain natural and experimental biochemical disorders suggest that some *metabolic factors* are involved in the pathogenesis of dystrophic axonal changes. This type of axonal lesion appears to be closely related to "dying-back" processes of the neurone [2, 5] or, more correctly, of the neuraxon which should be considered as a functional and metabolic entity. Although the distribution of axonal spheroids in the CNS has been related to the location of large polymorphic synapses or terminal axons [14], there is still no satisfactory explanation for the almost constant affection of some particular parts of the CNS under various physiological and pathological conditions. The correlation of dystrophic axonal changes in the pallido-nigral system to some disease processes also needs further elucidation. Until we have a better understanding of the metabolism of axoplasm this particular type of axonal lesion is undetermined and the question concerning the primary site of damage to the neuraxon leading to distal "dystrophic" changes of the axonal unit remains unanswered.

References

1. Bischoff, A.: Ultrastructure of tri-ortho-cresyl phosphate poisoning in the chicken. II. Studies on spinal cord alterations. Acta neuropath. (Berl.) 15, 142—155 (1970).
2. Blakemore, W. F., Cavanagh, J. B.: Neuroaxonal dystrophy occurring in an experimental dying back process in the rat. Brain 92, 789—804 (1969).
3. Brannon, W., McCormick, W., Lampert, P.: Axonal dystrophy in the gracile nucleus of man. Acta neuropath. (Berl.) 9, 1—6 (1967).
4. Carpenter, S.: A histochemical study of oxidative enzymes in the nervous system of vitamin E-deficient rats. Neurology (Minneap.) 15, 328—332 (1965).
5. Cavanagh, J. B.: The significance of the "dying back" process in experimental and human neuronal disease. Int. Rev. exp. Path. 3, 219—267 (1964).
6. Chou, S. M., Hartmann, H. A.: Axonal lesions and waltzing syndrome after IDPN administration in rats. With a concept-"axostasis". Acta neuropath. (Berl.) 3, 428—450 (1964).
7. Cordy, D. R., Richards, W. P., Badford, G. E.: Systemic neuroaxonal dystrophy in Suffolk sheep. Acta neuropath. (Berl.) 8, 133—140 (1967).
8. Cowen, D., Olmstead, E. V.: Infantile neuroaxonal dystrophy. J. Neuropath. exp. Neurol. 22, 175—236 (1963).
9. Duncan, C., Strub, R., McGarry, P., Duncan, D.: Peripheral nerve biopsy as an aid to diagnosis in infantile neuroaxonal dystrophy. Neurology (Minneap.) 20, 1024—1032 (1970).
10. Duncan, D.: The incidence of secondary (Wallerian) degeneration in normal mammals compared to that in certain experimental and disease conditions. J. comp. Neurol. 51, 197—228 (1930).
11. Edington, N., Howell, J. McC.: The neurotoxicity of sodium diethylthicarbamate in the rabbit. Acta neuropath. (Berl.) 12, 339—347 (1969).
12. Fujisawa, K.: An unique type of axonal alteration (so-called axonal dystrophy) as seen in Goll's nucleus of 277 cases of controls. Acta neuropath. (Berl.) 8, 255—275 (1967).
12a. — Shiraki, H., Katsui, G.: Early phase of axonal dystrophy in vitamin E-deficient rats. C. R. VIe Congr. Int. Neuropath., pp. 99—100. Paris: Masson et Cie 1970.
13. Hager, H.: Regenerationsvorgänge am Neuron des zentralen Nervensystems. Verh. dtsch. Ges. Path. 50, 255—275 (1966).
14. Hedley-Whyte, E. T., Gilles, F. H., Uzman, B. G.: Infantile neuroaxonal dystrophy. A diseases characterized by altered terminal axons and synaptic endings. Neurology (Minneap.) 18, 891—906 (1968).
15. Herman, M. M., Huttenlocher, P. R., Bensch, K. G.: Electron microscopic observations in infantile neuroaxonal dystrophy. Arch. Neurol. (Chic.) 20, 19—34 (1969).
16. Howell, J. McC., Ishmael, H., Ewbank, R., Blakemore, W. F.: Changes in the central nervous system of lambs following administration of sodium diethyldithiocarbamate. Acta neuropath. (Berl.) 15, 197—207 (1970).
17. Huttenlocher, P. R., Gilles, F. H.: Infantile neuroaxonal dystrophy. Clinical, pathologic and histochemical findings in a family with 3 affected siblings. Neurology (Minneap.) 17, 1174—1184 (1967).
18. Jellinger, K.: Neuroaxonale Dystrophien. Verh. dtsch. Ges. Path. 52, 92—126 (1968).
19. — Haub, G.: Statistical investigations of the age dependence of neuroaxonal dystrophy. Germ. med. Mth. 13, 341—345 (1968).
20. — Seitelberger, F.: Juvenile form of spongy degeneration of the CNS. Acta neuropath. (Berl.) 13, 276—281 (1969).
21. Kamoshita, S., Neustein, H. B., Landing, B. H.: Infantile neuroaxonal dystrophy with neonatal onset. Neuropathologic and electron microscopic observations. J. Neuropath. exp. Neurol. 27, 300—323 (1968).
22. Koenig, H.: Experimental production of acute neuroaxonal dystrophy. J. Neuropath. exp. Neurol. 28, 173—174 (1969).
23. Lampert, P.: A comparative electron microscopic study of reactive, degenerating, regenerating, and dystrophic axons. J. Neuropath. exp. Neurol. 26, 345—368 (1967).
24. — Blumberg, J. M., Pentschew, A.: A electron microscopic study of dystrophic axons in the gracile and cuneate nuclei of vitamin E-deficient rats. J. Neuropath. exp. Neurol. 23, 60—77 (1964).

25. Lampert, P., Cressmann, M.: Axonal regeneration in the dorsal columns of the spinal cord of adult rat. Lab. Invest. **13**, 825—839 (1964).
26. Morrison, L. R., Cobb, S., Bauer, W.: The effect of advancing age upon the human spinal cord. Cambridge, Mass.: Harvard Univ. Press 1959.
27. Newberne, P. M., Hare, M. V.: Axon dystrophy in clinically normal dogs. Amer. J. Vet. Res. **23**, 403—411 (1962).
28. Ochoa, J., Mair, W. G. P.: The normal sural nerve in man. II. Changes in the axons and Schwann cells during ageing. Acta neuropath. (Berl.) **13**, 217—239 (1969).
29. Pentschew, A.: Person. communication.
30. — Schwarz, K.: Systemic axonal dystrophy in vitamin E-deficient rats. Acta neuropath. (Berl.) **1**, 313—334 (1962).
31. Prineas, J.: The pathogenesis of dying-back polyneuropathies. II. An ultrastructural study of experimental acrylamide intoxication in the cat. J. Neuropath. exp. Neurol. **28**, 598—621 (1969).
32. Rinvik, E., Grofová, I.: Observations on the fine structure of the substantia nigra in the cat. Exp. Brain Res. **11**, 229—248 (1970).
33. Rozdilsky, B., Cumings, J. N., Huston, A. F.: Hallervorden-Spatz disease; late infantile and adult types. Report on two cases. Acta neuropath. (Berl.) **10**, 1—16 (1968).
34. Sandbank, U., Lerman, P., Gefiman, G.: Infantile neuroaxonal dystrophy: cortical axonic and presynaptic changes. Acta neuropath. (Berl.) **16**, 342—352 (1970).
35. Schlote, W.: Morphologische und histochemische Untersuchungen an retrograden Axonveränderungen im Zentralnervensystem. Acta neuropath. (Berl.) **1**, 135—158 (1961).
36. Seitelberger, F.: Zur Morphologie und Histochemie der degenerativen Axonveränderungen im Zentralnervensystem. Rapp. IIIe Congr. Int. Neuropath. Bruxelles: Acta med. belg., pp. 127—147 (1957).
37. — Die Hallervorden-Spatzsche Krankheit. Nervenarzt **37**, 482—493 (1966).
38. — Gootz, M., Gross, H.: Beitrag zur spätinfantilen Hallervorden-Spatzschen Krankheit. Acta neuropath. (Berl.) **3**, 16—28 (1963).
39. Shiraki, H.: Some unusual neuropathologic features in Guam cases in comparison with those in the Japanese, with special reference to Hallervorden-Spatz disease-like lesions. Proc. Vth. Int. Congr. Neuropath., Zürich, Exc. med., I. C. S. Nr. 100, 201—207 (1966).
40. Sroka, Ch., Bornstein, B., Strulovici, N., Sandbank, U.: Neuroaxonal dystrophy: its relation to age and central nervous system lesions. Israel J. med. Sci. **5**, 373—377 (1969).
41. Sung, J. H.: Neuroaxonal dystrophy in mucoviscidosis. J. Neuropath. exp. Neurol. **23**, 567—583 (1964).
42. — Neuroaxonal dystrophy in aging. Proc. Vth. Int. Congr. Neuropath., Exc. Med., I. C. S. Nr. 100, 478—480 (1966).
43. — Stadlan, E. M.: Neuroaxonal dystrophy in congenital biliary artresia. J. Neuropath. exp. Neurol. **25**, 341—361 (1966).
44. Takashima, S., Iwata, Y., Tanaka, K.: An autopsy case of Hallervorden-Spatz disease: Clinicopathological and biochemical study. (Jap.) Advance Neurol. Sci. **13**, 249—259 (1969).
45. Takei, Y., Samuels, S.: Intracytoplasmic hyalin inclusion bodies in the nerve cells of the hypoglossal nucleus in human autopsy material. Acta neuropath. (Berl.) **17**, 14—23 (1971).
46. Toga, M., Bérard-Badier, M., Gambarelli-Dubois, D.: La dystrophie neuroaxonale infantile ou maladie de Seitelberger. Étude clinique, histologique et ultrastructurale de deux observations. Acta neuropath. (Berl.) **15**, 327—350 (1970).
47. Wigboldus, J. M., Bruyn, G. W.: Hallervorden-Spatz disease. In: Handbook of Clinical Neurology, P. J. Vinken and G. W. Bruyn, edts. vol. 6, pp. 604—631. Amsterdam: North Holland Publ. Comp. 1968.
48. Yanagisawa, N., Shiraki, H., Minakawa, M., Narabayashi, N.: Clinicopathological and histochemical studies in Hallervorden-Spatz disease, with torsion dystonia, with special reference to diagnostic criteria of the disease from the clinico-pathological viewpoint. Progr. Brain Res. **21**, 373—425 (1966).

Prof. Dr. Kurt Jellinger
Neurologisches Institut der Universität
A-1090 Wien, Schwarzspanierstraße 17
Österreich

Acta neuropath. (Berl.) Suppl. V, 17—29 (1971)
© by Springer-Verlag 1971

Neuropathological Conditions Related to Neuroaxonal Dystrophy*

Franz Seitelberger

Neurological Institute of the University of Vienna

Summary. Neuroaxonal dystrophy (NAD) is an important autonomic phenomenon in physiological brain ageing as well as the pathognomonic pathological substrate of a group of degenerative processes of the CNS related to normal brain ageing. The pathogenetic analysis of the role of NAD in physiology and pathology opens a wide field of neurobiology and offers a new approach to the general concept of disease in the neurological sciences. Some of the basic problems encountered in this study concern the mechanism of axonal metabolism and transport as well as of ordinary axonal reactions and these problems could be successfully approached by experimental research oriented by those findings in naturally occurring disease.

Key-Words: Neuroaxonal Dystrophy — Spheroid — Infantile Neuroaxonal Dystrophy — Halervorden-Spatz Disease — Neuroaxonal Leucodystrophy — Vitamin E Deficiency.

The term *neuroaxonal dystrophy (NAD)* refers to a dystrophic degenerative process of central nervous neurons characterized by the peculiar dystrophic product of axonal spheroids (Axonschollen) [34,38,40]. In the first and productive phase of this dystrophy, discontinuous swellings along the axis cylinder processes appear. Presumably, terminal parts of the axon are the first to be affected: this is the beginning of NAD. The eventual loss, by necrobiosis, of the neuron, is caused by the later centripetal involvement of the perikaryon.

Histologically, NAD is accompanied by a loss of neurofibrils, homogenisation, and increase in volume of the affected segments of the axon. Then, by discontinuous disintegration of the axon, we have the formation of polymorphic axonal spheroids up to 120 μ which are secondary interstitial formations. By loss of the nucleus and by homogenization and swelling of the cytoplasm, the perikaryon is finally transformed into a spheroid which now cannot be differentiated from an axonal spheroid. It seems that the spheroids may stay for a long time in the tissue whilst they undergo substantial structural alterations. In addition to the homogenous, eosinophilic parts there are also granular and fibrillar structures, and dense, sometimes basophilic condensations as well as vacuoles. Finally the spheroids are degradated by humoral or more rarely by cellular microglial reactions. An incrustation with calcium compounds may also occur, that is the transformation to a calcium-containing but iron-free concrement [19,37,39].

Histochemically, the spheroids consist mainly of protein but nucleoproteins are absent. They contain carbohydrate and lipid in variable amount, and glycogen granules may be found. Histochemically they show a high activity of oxydative

---

* Dedicated to Prof. Dr. G. Peters on the occasion of his 65th birthday.

enzymes except succinic acid dehydrogenase, and some activity of phosphatases. The spheroids of the nucleus gracilis are especially rich in α-glycero-phosphate-dehydrogenase [6,19].

Ultrastructurally the spheroids contain the usual cellular organelles with disorganized mitochondria and numerous neurofilaments. There are also dense granules, microtubules and peculiarily structurized deposits: membrane loops, tubular aggregates and atypical fibrillar material [24,25,27].

By the features described NAD differs significantly from other reactive, degenerative, and regenerative axonal alterations [24,26,45,46] and can be recognized as a distinctive *neuronal dystrophic process* which leads via a productive phase (formation of spheroids) to necrobiosis with loss of the whole affected neuron.

NAD is not a particular pathological state but seems to be a normal tissue phenomenon found in *certain regions of CNS*; those where it commonly occurs are the nuclei of the posterior funiculi of medulla oblongata (nucleus gracilis stronger than nucleus cuneatus), the red zone of the substantia nigra and less constantly the medial part of the pallidum. This physiological NAD is dependent on age but occurs in either sex. Before the 10th year of life NAD is rarely found but after the 50th year it is seldom absent and becomes increasingly common in the following decades. There are structural differences in the NAD from different regions as well as variations in quantity and progression [5,12,19,20,49]. In the substantia nigra and in the pallidum besides NAD there is an age-dependent increase of the glial lipopigment and the concentration of iron. In senile material these regions have a rusty-brown discoloration (status pigmentosus) and many spheroids give a positive reaction for iron.

Among the *ageing processes* of the nervous parenchym, NAD has a special structural, topistic and qualitative form and a particular course. To the atrophying dystrophy, argyrophilic dystrophy and lipopigment dystrophy NAD may be added as a further type of neuronal ageing processes. NAD represents an individual part of the complex process of brain ageing (Table 1). As in other neuronal ageing processes NAD has fluctuations of intensity evident in the amount of abnormal material found. As far as we know these variations occur independently i.e. not related in intensity to other processes e.g. to cerebral atrophy or the number of fibrillary changes and senile plaques but also relatively independent in each of the three main regions of affection. The ordinary quantitative increase in the amount of NAD in senility we call *"senile NAD"* [38,39].

This brings us to the question of the function of NAD in neurological ageing symptoms. This question cannot yet be answered. The physiological NAD of the elderly is integrated into the neurological syndrome of senility with disorder of posterior funiculi sensibility and of motor performance. The senile NAD of the posterior funiculi nuclei can be related in our investigations to senile ataxia and probably to senile impairment of the vibration sensibility. It may be assumed that the senile NAD of the substantia nigra and the pallidum contributes to senile Parkinsonism [43].

So far we have been concerned with NAD as a disturbance of *physiology*. Like other physiological neuronal ageing processes NAD may appear with a *pathologic intensity* and associated with other disturbances may become the substrate of a disease. In this form, NAD represents the pathognomonic morphologic change of

Table 1. *Ageing processes of CNS as related to presenile and degenerative diseases*

Age	Syndrome				
	atrophying dystrophy	argyrophilic dystrophy	neuroaxonal dystrophy (NAD)	lipopigment dystrophy	astroglial dystrophy
Senium	senile dementia; diffuse atrophic changes, regionally accentuated	senile dementia; argyrophilic changes in a regional pattern	Parkinsonism, ataxia; topistic changes: senile NAD	dementia, changes in the lipophilic grisea	dementia, myoclonisms; diffuse corticosubcortical changes: senile glial dystrophy
Presenium	Pick disease	Alzheimer disease	presenile NAD	pigmentary degeneration	presenile glial dystrophy
Mediaevum	Systemic atrophies		Hallervorden-Spatz disease	lipofuscinosis	spongy dystrophies

Table 2. *Neuroaxonal dystrophy (NAD)*

A. *Endogenous Forms*
  I. 1. Physiological NAD
       topistic partial process of brain ageing
     2. Senile NAD
       paraphysiological topistic NAD of senescence

  II. Pathological NAD
     1. Presenile NAD
     2. Hallervorden-Spatz disease
     3. Late infantile Hallervorden-Spatz disease
     4. Infantile NAD: Seitelberger disease
     5. Neuroaxonal Leucoencephalopathy

B. *Symptomatic Forms*
  I. Increased frequency and intensity of physiological NAD in:
     1. Alcoholic encephalopathies
     2. Morbus Parkinson
     3. Morbus Wilson

  II. Excessive, extratopistic NAD in:
     1. Mucoviscidosis
     2. Congenital biliary atresia
     3. Certain Dysmetabolias:
        a) Tay-Sachs disease
        b) Kinky hair disease
        c) Glycogenosis V
        d) Spongy dystrophy

  III. Fe-dependent NAD in:
     Marginal siderosis of CNS

  IV. Experimentally produced NAD

a group of degenerative central nervous diseases called *"neuroaxonal dystrophies"* [2,34,37,49] (Table 2). We can distinguish primary endogenous NADs and secondary symptomatic NADs.

In the *endogenous NADs* the transition from a physiologic to a pathologic manifestation is the dissociation of NAD from a complex of brain ageing processes. NAD does not then remain a part of brain ageing but transgresses its normal chronological and topistic borderlines. It appears earlier, it overlaps the normal regional distribution and it appears in abnormal intensity. In the pathogenetic complex responsible for the NADs the genetic conditions normally regulating NAD seem to be disordered. Among the *endogenous NADs* the following types can be distinguished:

1. *Presenile NAD* is characterized by the precocious and increased appearance of NAD but within the normal anatomical sites. The corresponding clinical picture cannot yet be distinguished from the other presenile neurological syndromes so that we can only speek of a presenile NAD disease with reservation.

2. *Hallervorden-Spatz* disease (HSpD [2,30,37,47,55]). The neuropathological findings of adult as well as juvenile cases are a) NAD in its three usual sites of localisation but in contrast to the physiological NAD, the pallidum is totally affected and not merely in its most medial part, b) an increase of local glial lipopigment and tissue iron in the pallidum and substantia nigra causing a deep red-brown colour of these areas (Figs. 1 A, B). In spite of the striking increase in the iron content of the pallidonigral system demonstrable by histochemical techniques, the chemical analysis discloses only a slight rise of iron in these areas.

The *clinical picture* of HSpD is that of a slowly progressive extrapyramidal disturbance consisting in hyperkinesia of the choreoathetotic type, bulbar disturbances, increased tonus and rigidity accompanied by deterioration of psychic performances leading to complete idiocy. Its duration averages 15 years. The genetic incidence may be that of an autosomal-recessive inheritance. Biochemistry has shown irregularities of the iron and copper balance of the body fluids, but the meaning is obscure and the changes may be secondary. Disorders of total iron metabolism are not present.

A distinction must be made between HSpD and the rare form of cerebral lipidosis in which apart from the neuronal storage process an increase in glial lipopigment is found which extends beyond the globus pallidus and the substantia nigra to all of the grey matter regions. Although the pigment accumulation in the globus pallidus and the substantia nigra is considerable and causes the blackish coloration mentioned above, the axonal changes are completely absent. This is the so-called *pigment variant of cerebral lipidosis* [35].

3. In *late infantile NAD* described by Seitelberger and Gross as late infantile type of HSpD [30,42,41,37] the axonal changes are increased in the usual 3 localisations and also in the whole of the tegmentum of the brain stem, in the thalamus, in the cerebral (Fig.2) and cerebellar cortex, in the cerebellar nuclei and in the posterior horns of the spinal cord. A pathognomonic lesion is the massive appearence of NAD in the cerebellar white matter combined with secondary demyelination (Fig.3). In pallidum and substantia nigra the local accumulation of lipopigment is less apparent and there is an increase of tissue iron: Both grisea show no abnormal discoloration but are increased in volume by the abundant axonal

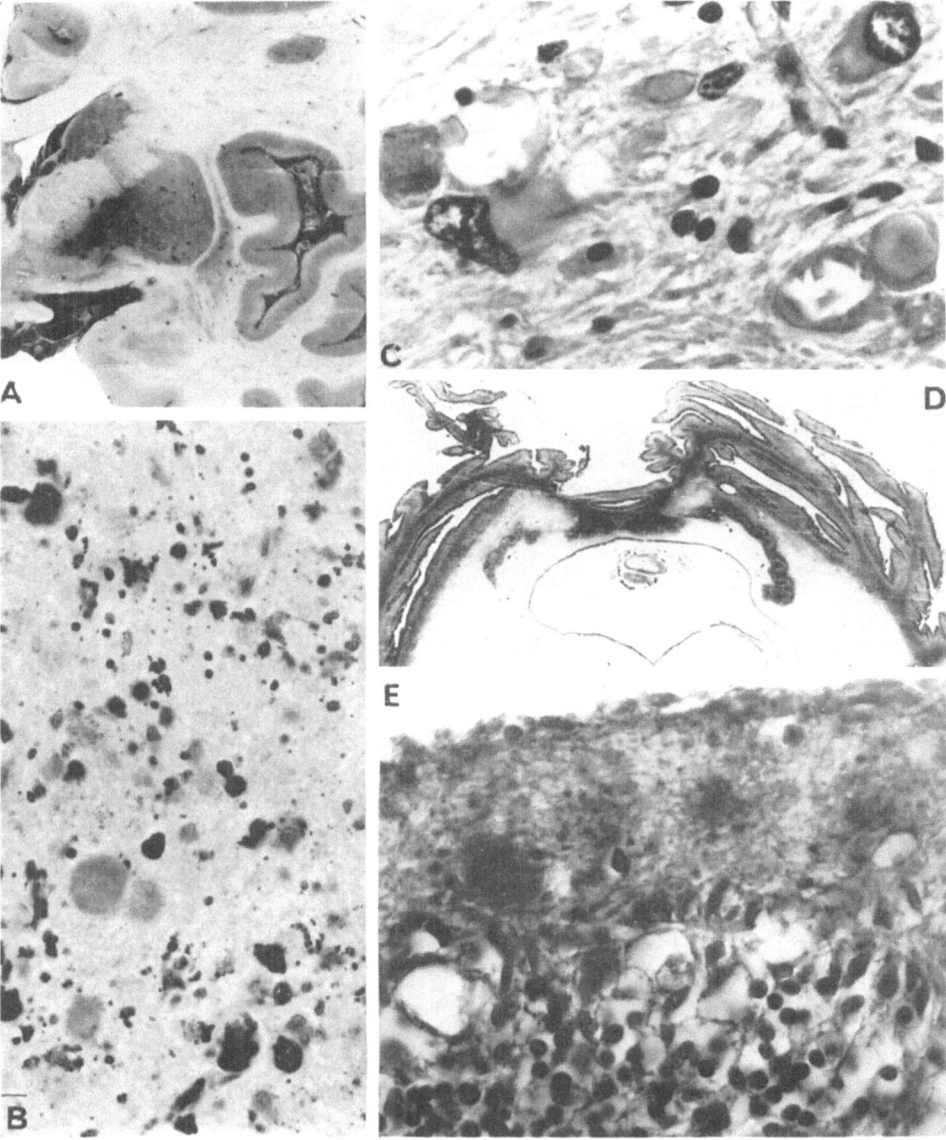

Fig. 1. A Hallervorden-Spatz disease (NI 80/59). Deeply brown discoloration of the pallidum.
B Hallervorden-Spatz disease (Case R.). Substantia nigra, zona reticulata. Fe-reaction, × 325.
Large amounts of Fe-positive material are present. Also some spheroids show positive Fe-
reaction. C Infantile neuroaxonal dystrophy (NI 46/67). Nucleus Goll. H.-E., × 560. Polymor-
phous bodies (spheroids); some with regressive changes. Astroglial reaction with giant nuclei.
D Infantile neuroaxonal dystrophy (NI 46/67). Cerebellum. Holzer. Cerebellar cortical atrophy
and gliofibrillar sclerosis. E Infantile neuroaxonal dystrophy (NI 172/60). Cerebellar cortex.
Sudanblack B, × 600. Atrophy with loss of Purkinje cells; spheroids in the molecular layer;
empty spaces after humoral degradation of spheroids: "neuroaxonogenic spongy state"

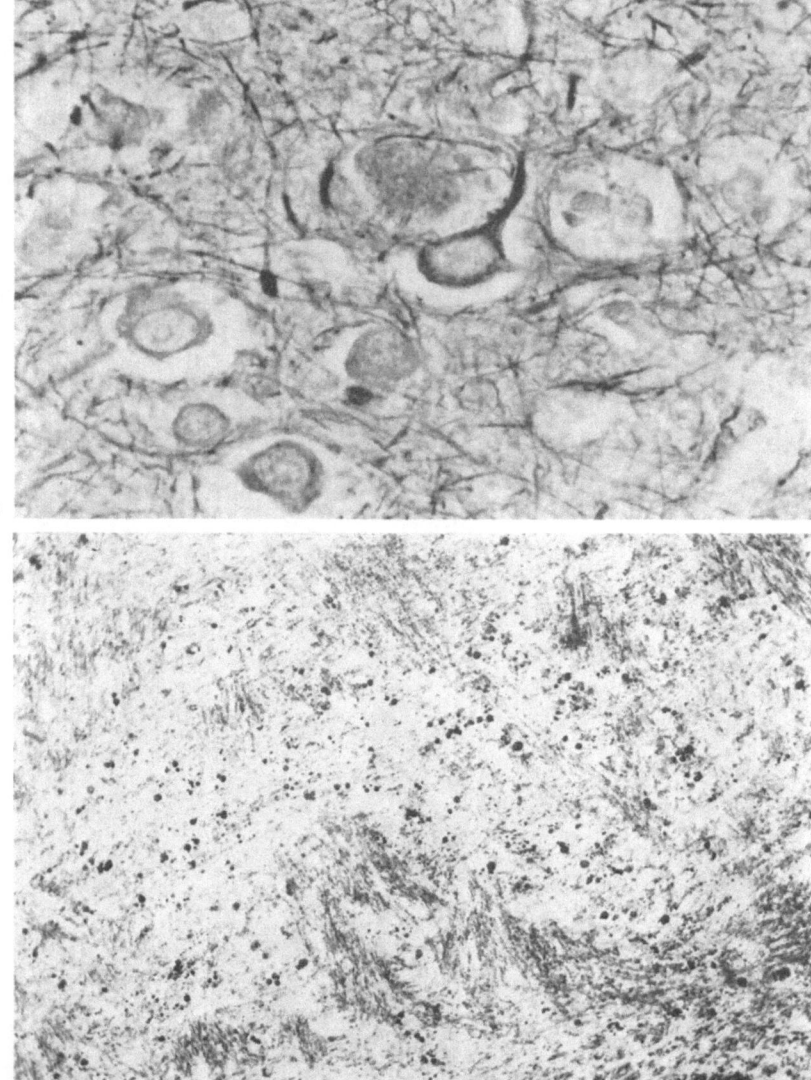

Fig. 2

Fig. 4

Fig. 2. Late infantile Hallervorden-Spatz disease (NI 152/60). Occipital cortex. Bodian, × 560.
Axonal spheroids of various size sometimes attached to more or less intact nerve cell bodies

Fig. 4. Infantile neuroaxonal dystrophy (NI 23/56). Pallidum. Oil red, × 85. Pallidum fat increased; status dysmyelinisatus

spheroids causing a pseudohypertrophy. In these areas due to a massive humoral
disintegration of the spheroids secondary cystic lesions may appear.

Clinically the often familial form has its onset after the second year of life:
the disturbances in the motor and psychic spheres are more severe whereas the

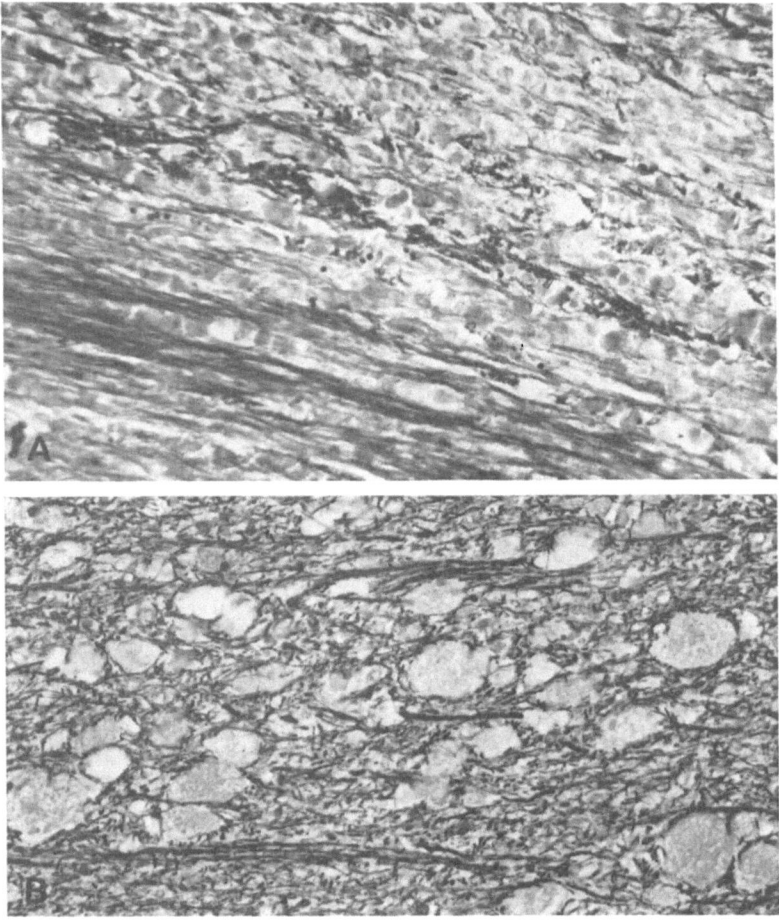

Fig. 3. A Late infantile Hallervorden-Spatz disease (NI 63/53). Ansa lenticularis. Heidenhain, ×180. Numerous axonal spheroids and secondary myelin sheaths degeneration. B Late infantile Hallervorden-Spatz disease (NI 152/60). Cerebellar white matter. Bodian, ×256. Between numerous granular axonal spheroids some intact axons are present: "neuroaxonal leucoencephalopathy"

extrapyramidal motor disturbances are less significant. Death occurs after a duration of only a few years.

4. In *infantile NAD* (Seitelberger's disease [8,9,14,15,17,18,22,23,31,32, 33,34,37,51] there are massive numbers of large axonal spheroids everywhere. These changes are striking in the cerebellum (cortex and nuclei) which seem to be the first site involved, in the tegmentum of the brain stem, in the nucleus lenticularis, in the thalamus, in the cerebral cortex, in the spinal grey column, and in the spinal posterior funiculi (Fig. 1C, D, E). Fasciculus gracilis may be secondarily degenerated. In the pallidum and the substantia nigra, the iron content is increased compared with the normal average for this age. Glial pigment is not present. In

Table 3. *Endogenous neuroaxonal dystrophies*

Form resp. Disease	Age of onset	Topo-chemistry of Pallidum and Nigra	Histo-chemistry of spheroids	Localization of NAD	Other Symptoms
senile NAD	senile	glial lipopig-ment and tissue iron increased	proteins carbo-hydrates	topistic: posterior funiculi nuclei Zona retic. S. nigrae; Pallidum *internum*	*no* status dysmyeli-nisatus of Pallidum; status pigmentosus of Pallidum and Nigra
presenile NAD	presenile				
Hallervorden-Spatz Disease	adult juvenile			topistic: but *total* Pallidum	Status dysmyeli-nisatus of Pallidum; status pigmentosus
	late infantile	under 4 years no glial lipopig-ment; tissue iron increased	proteins; carbol-hydrats *lipids*	topistic and *extratopistic:* cortices, thalamus, brain stem, cerebellar white matter	Status dysmyelini-satus *no* status pigmentosus; Pseudohypertrophy of Pallidum and Nigra; Neutral fat of the Pallidum increased
Seitelberger Disease	infantile			Generalized in CNS (PNS, ANS?)	Status dysmyelini-satus; excessive neutral fat in the Pallidum; degenera-ration of posterior funiculi; Leuco-encephalopathy

the pallidum however, the so-called "pallidum fat" a normal tissue component, is increased and is found in large compound granular corpuscles and as clusters of lipid droplets (Fig. 4). This corresponds to the "status porosus" seen in paraffin slides and causes a "status dysmyelinisatus" because of the poor myelination.

An unique finding in a not yet published case of infantile NAD represents the massive affection of Ammon's horn allocortex by NAD which led to what we may call a "neuroaxonogenic" spongy state of this region.

The *clinical picture* of this disease is that of a hereditary, rapidly progressive and global psychomotor disorganisation with hyperkinesias, flaccid pareses, cranial nerve paralyses, optic atrophy and severe dementia. The disease begins within the first year of life and has a maximal duration of a few years. Biochemistry show elevation of lactic acid dehydrogenase and transaminase in the serum. An intra-vital diagnosis has been verified in two cases by means of cerebral cortical biopsy.

5. In *neuroaxonal leucoencephalopathy* we have an extensive NAD affection of the hemispherical white matter of cerebrum and cerebellum with secondary

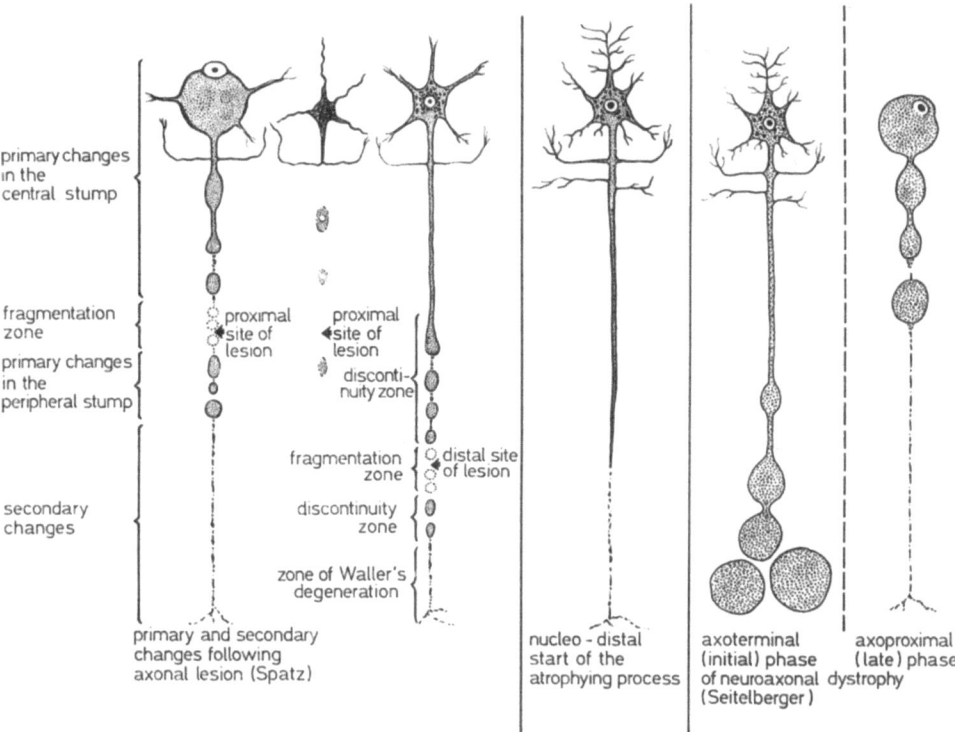

primary changes in the central stump

fragmentation zone

primary changes in the peripheral stump

secondary changes

proximal site of lesion

proximal site of lesion

disconti-nuity zone

fragmentation zone

distal site of lesion

discontinuity zone

zone of Waller's degeneration

primary and secondary changes following axonal lesion (Spatz)

nucleo-distal start of the atrophying process

axoterminal (initial) phase of neuroaxonal dystrophy (Seitelberger)

axoproximal (late) phase

Scheme I. Scheme of physiological axonal reactions as compared with the features of "atro-phying dystrophy" and "neuroaxonal dystrophy"

degeneration of myelin. The type of lesion corresponds to the cerebellar white matter lesion in late infantile NAD. This syndrome has so far been observed only in one Japanese family (observation of Matsuyama and Richardson[1]).

These types of NAD just described show the common main lesion of NAD as an essential part of each disease. However there are transitional forms between the different types and such transitions are particularly common between infantile and late infantile NAD (Table 3). These observations indicate a common patho-genetic basic constellation of the NADs in which there are pathological states arrived at by an intensification of the age dependent physiological NAD. This statement is fundamental for the pathology and pathogenesis of the whole group of degenerative processes of the nervous system which are related to ageing chan-ges. It is also of great importance in general biology and in the definition of the term disease in neurology. Compared with other age-dependent neuronal dystro-phies NAD is associated with atrophying dystrophy above all by its nucleodistal progression. Both dystrophies can be termed "dying back dystrophies of the neuron" and an "atrophying dying back dystrophy" can be differentiated from a "neuroaxonal dying back dystrophy" [40] (Scheme 1). Recent findings in neuro-

---

1 Personal communication by Dr. E. P. Richardson, Boston.

pathies indicate that, in the peripheral nervous system, neuroaxonal dying back dystrophy also can be recognized[2]. The appearance of neuroaxonal dystrophy with spheroid products in the autonomic nervous system is also described, namely in the wall of the rectum [23]. NAD spheroids were found in the nerve cell layer of the retina [53,54].

Finally it must be stressed that NAD which is independent of age may be influenced and triggered in a symptomatic way by certain extracerebral conditions: we may term this *symptomatic NAD*. In this way studies in our institute show that NAD of the substantia nigra is positively correlated with alcoholic encephalo-pathy (in the age group above 20 ys) and with Parkinson's disease (in the group above 50 ys). With these diseases NAD reaches a higher intensity at an earlier age, i.e. shows a steeper curve when intensity is plotted against age [20,21].

Among the symptomatic NADs the type with *mucoviscidosis* and *congenital biliary atresia* is the most important. It was found that in these diseases NAD is increased in number and intensity in the posterior funiculi and may be found also in other regions of the brain stem tegmentum [48,49,50]. Few axon changes are found in other localisations. Histologically the axonal spheroids are similar in every respect to those of endogenous NAD. The appearance of NAD in these diseases is interpreted as a sequel of the protracted vitamin-E deficiency connected with them.

The same structural features present in NAD may be found throughout the brain stem tegmentum in single cases of *infantile lipidoses* (Tay-Sachs disease, Kinky hair disease), in *glycogenoses* (type V) and in *infantile spongy dystrophy*. NAD of the posterior funiculi nuclei and of substantia nigra appears very early and intensely in *Wilson's disease*. The triggering factors in the biochemistry of these diseases are as yet not known. The iron containing axonal spheroids frequent-ly present in *marginal siderosis of CNS* represent a pathogenetic problem [4,36]. Some authors take them for glial degeneration products. As they are present not only in the zone of granular iron storage and of diffuse soaking but also remotely they may be caused not by a direct effect of iron but an indirect induction via intermediary metabolic links.

It should be marked that in degenerations of the posterior funiculi especially in *tabes dorsalis* the number of axonal spheroids in the posterior funiculi nuclei is extremely low. This finding probably is not related to the metabolic cause of NAD but is explained because the terminal axon parts of the posterior funiculi which would be the sites of the spheroid formation are destroyed in the atrophying process of the tabetic posterior funiculi degeneration.

These arguments on human pathology for completion require some remarks on *experimental production of NAD*. Axonal swelling and spheroids can be produced by a variety of toxic substances such as IDPN, sodium-diethylthiocarbamate, p-bromphenylacetylurea, acrylamide, triorthocresylphosphate among other pro-cedures [1,3,7,29]. Axonal swellings, which differ however from the typical NAD were produced by electrophoresis [10,11]. The most important experimental model however is the production of NAD in weaning rats by means of *chronic vitamin-E deficiency* diet [13,28]. This model corresponds to the pathogenesis of

2 See the contribution of Berard-Badier to this symposium pp. 30—39.

the symptomatic types of NAD. A disorder of balance between peroxydation and antioxydation based on the anti-oxydant function of vitamin-E in lipid metabolism was postulated [16].

NAD itself represents, irrespective of its etiology, a disorder of axonal function with a productive character. A protracted regenerative axonal reaction caused by some unknown toxin provides scanty evidence particularly when the reaction products (axonal spheroid formations) are common to several disorders. Other pathogenetic factors to be discussed are axostasis due to axonal or perikaryon metabolism insufficiency [7,29]; further structural and/or functional loss of contact between axon and postsynaptic neuron [3]: This seems to be probably the sequel rather than the cause of NAD. On the other hand due to the slow course of NAD and to the long preservation of vitality of the neuron the features of the spheroid lesion—the products of the metabolic basic disorder—as well as the products of regenerative cellular reactions are present together side by side. Therefore the comparison of NAD with the sequelae of a proximal axonal lesion is a plausible analogy to explain one phase, namely the terminal phase of NAD. From this biological analogy further research in neurobiology of NAD can be directed.

References

1. Bischoff, A.: Ultrastructure of tri-ortho-cresyl phosphate poisoning in the chicken. II. Studies on spinal cord alterations. Acta neuropath. (Berl.) 15, 142—155 (1970).
2. — Regli, F.: Die Hallervorden-Spatzsche Krankheit. Diskussion der pathologisch-anatomischen Befunde anhand eines eigenen autoptisch bestätigten Falles. Arch. Psychiat. Nervenkr. 204, 589—602 (1963).
3. Blakemore, W. F., Cavanagh, J. B.: Neuroaxonal dystrophy occurring in an experimental dying back process in the rat. Brain 92, 789—804 (1969).
4. Blinzinger, K.: Elektronenmikroskopische Beobachtungen bei experimentell erzeugter Randzonensiderose des Kaninchengehirns. Acta neuropath. (Berl.) suppl. IV., 146—157 (1968).
5. Brannon, W., McCormick, W., Lampert, P.: Axonal dystrophy in the gracile nucleus of man. Acta neuropath. (Berl.) 9, 1—6 (1967).
6. Carpenter, S.: A histochemical study of oxidative enzymes in the nervous system of vitamin E-deficient rats. Neurology (Minneap.) 15, 328—332 (1965).
7. Chou, S. M., Hartmann, H. A.: Axonal lesions and waltzing syndrome after IDPN administration in rats. With a concept-"axostasis". Acta neuropath. (Berl.) 3, 428—450 (1964).
8. Cowen, P., Olmstead, E. V.: Infantile neuroaxonal dystrophy. J. Neurpoath. exp. Neurol. 22, 175—236 (1963).
9. Crome, L., Weller, S. D. V.: Infantile neuroaxonal dystrophy. Arch. Dis. Childh. 40, 502—507 (1965).
10. Friede, R. L.: Electrophoretic production of "reactive" axon swellings in vitro and their histochemical properties. Acta neuropath. (Berl.) 3, 217—228 (1964).
11. — Axon swellings produced in vivo in isolated segments of nerves. Acta neuropath. (Berl.) 3, 229—239 (1964).
12. Fujisawa, K.: An unique type of axonal alteration (so-called axonal dystrophy) as seen in Goll's nucleus of 277 cases of controls. A contribution to the pathology of aging process. Acta neuropath. (Berl.) 8, 255—275 (1967).
13. — Shiraki, H., Katsui, G.: Early phase of axonal dystrophy in vitamin E-deficient rats. C. R. VIe congr. Int. Neuropath. pp. 99—100. Paris: Masson et Cie 1970.
14. Hedley-Whyte, E. T., Gilles, F. H., Uzman, B. G.: Infantile neuroaxonal dystrophy. A disease characterized by altered terminal axons and synaptic endings. Neurology (Minneap.) 18, 891—906 (1968).

15. Herman, M. M., Huttenlocher, P. R., Bensch, K. G.: Electron microscopic observations in infantile neuroaxonal dystrophy. Arch. Neurol. (Chic.) 20, 19—34 (1969).

16. Horwitt, M. K.: Interrelations between vitamin E and polyunsaturated fatty acids in adult men. Vitam. and Horm. 20, 541—558 (1962).

17. Huttenlocher, P. R., Gilles, F. H.: Infantile neuroaxonal dystrophy. Clinical, pathologic and histochemical findings in a family with 3 affected siblings. Neurology (Minneap.) 17, 1174—1184 (1967).

18. Indravasu, S., Dexter, R. A.: Infantile neuroaxonal dystrophy and its relationship to Hallervorden-Spatz disease. Neurology (Minneap.) 18, 693—699 (1968).

19. Jellinger, K.: Neuroaxonale Dystrophien. Verh. dtsch. Ges. Path., 52. Tagg. 92—126 (1968).

20. — Haub, G.: Statistical investigations of the age dependence of neuroaxonal dystrophy. Germ. med. Mth. 13, 341—344 (1968).

21. — Jirásek, A.: Acta neuropath. (Berl.) Suppl. V, 3—16 (1971).

22. — Seitelberger, F., Rosenkranz, W.: Infantile neuroaxonale Dystrophie. Frühform mit bevorzugtem Kleinhirnbefall. Acta neuropath. (Berl.) 10, 123—131 (1968).

23. Kamoshita, S., Neustein, H. B., Landing, B. H.: Infantile neuroaxonal dystrophy with neonatal onset. Neuropathologic and electron microscopic observations. J. Neuropath. exp. Neurol. 27, 300—323 (1968).

24. Lampert, P.: A comparative electron microscopic study of reactive, degenerating, regenerating, and dystropic axons. J. Neuropath. exp. Neurol. 26, 345—368 (1967).

25. — Blumberg, J., Pentschew, A.: An electron microscopic study of dystrophic axons in the gracile and cuneate nuclei of vitamin E-deficient rats. J. Neuropath. exp. Neurol. 23, 60—77 (1964).

26. — Cressman, M.: Axonal regeneration in the dorsal colums of the spinal cord of adult rat. Lab. Invest. 13, 825—839 (1964).

27. — Pentschew, A.: An electron microscopic study of spheroid and convoluted bodies in dystrophic terminal axons. Acta neuropath. (Berl.) 4, 158—168 (1964).

28. Pentschew, A., Schwarz, K.: Systemic axonal dystrophy in vitamin E deficient adult rats. Acta neuropath. (Berl.) 1, 313—334 (1962).

29. Prineas, J.: The pathogenesis of dying-back polyneuropathies. II. An ultrastructural study of experimental acrylamide intoxication in the cat. J. Neuropath. exp. Neurol. 28, 598—621 (1969).

30. Rozdilsky, B., Cumings, J. N., Ruston, A. F.: Hallervorden-Spatz disease; late infantile and adult types. Report on two cases. Acta neuropath. (Berl.) 10, 1—16 (1968).

31. Sandbank, U.: Infantile neuroaxonal dystrophy. Arch. Neurol. (Chic.) 12, 155—159 (1965).

32. Seitelberger, F.: Eine unbekannte Form von infantiler Lipoid-Speicher-Krankheit des Gehirns. Proc. 1st Internat. Congr. Neuropath. Rome, vol. 3, pp. 323—333. Torino: Rosenberg & Sellier 1952.

33. — Une affection spéciale du métabolisme des cellules ganglionaires du système nerveux. (Lipoidose infantile tardive atypique du type tronco-cerebello-spinal). Proc. 5e Congrès Neurologique International à Lisbonne, vol. 3, pp. 484—491. Lisbon: Comptes Rendues 1954.

34. — Zur Morphologie und Histochemie der degenerativen Axonveränderungen im Zentralnervensystem. 1er Congrès International des Sciences Neurologiques, Bruxelles 1957: IIIe Congrès International de Neuropath. Rapports, p. 127—147.

35. — Sonderformen zerebraler Lipoidosen. Histochemische und histologische Befunde. Proc. IIIrd Int. Congr. Neuropath. München, pp. 127—147. Stuttgart: G. Thieme 1962.

36. — Eisenstoffwechselstörungen des Zentralnervensystems. Wien. Z. inn. Med. 45, 420—429 (1964).

37. — Die Hallervorden-Spatzsche Krankheit. Nervenarzt 37, 482—493 (1966).

38. — Die neuro-axonale Dystrophie. Ein neues Syndrom der Alternsveränderungen des Gehirns. Proc. VIIth Int. Congr. Geront., Wien, Vol. II, pp. 169—173 (1966).

39. Allgemeine Neuropathologie des Alterns- und Aufbrauchkrankheiten des Gehirns. Verh. dtsch. Ges. Path., 52, 32—61 (1968).

40. — General Neuropathology of degenerative processes of the nervous system. Neurosci. Res. 2, 253—299 (1969).

41. Seitelberger, F., Gootz, M., Gross, H.: Beitrag zur spätinfantilen Hallervorden-Spatz-schen Krankheit. Acta neuropath. (Berl.) 3, 16—28 (1963).
42. — Gross, H.: Über eine spätinfantile Form der Hallervorden-Spatzschen Krankheit. II. Mitteilung. Histochemische Befunde, Erörterung der Nosologie. Dtsch. Z. Nerven-heilk. 176, 104—125 (1957).
43. — Hornykiewicz, O., Bernheimer, H., Jellinger, K., Birkmayer, W.: In Vorbereitung.
44. — Simma, K.: On the pigment variant of amaurotic idiocy. In: Cerebral Shingolipidoses, pp. 29—47. New York: Academic Press Inc. 1962.
45. Schlote, W.: Morphologische und histochemische Untersuchungen an retrograden Axon-veränderungen im Zentralnervensystem. Acta neuropath. (Berl.) 1, 135—158 (1961).
46. — Die läsionsbedingten primär-retrograden Veränderungen der Axone zentraler Nerven-fasern im elektronenmikroskopischen Bild. Acta neuropath. (Berl.) 4, 138—157 (1964).
47. Shiraki, H.: Some unusual neuropathologic features in Guam cases in comparison with those in the Japanese, with special reference to Hallervorden-Spatz disease-like lesions. Proc. Vth Int. Congr. Neuropath. I. C. S., Nr. 100, pp. 201—207. Amsterdam-New York: Excerpta Med. Found. 1966.
48. Sung, J. H.: Neuroaxonal dystrophy in mucoviscidosis. J. Neuropath. exp. Neurol. 23, 567—583 (1964).
49. — Neuroaxonal dystrophy in aging. Proc. Vth Int. Congr. Neuropath., I. C. S. Nr. 100, pp. 478—480. Amsterdam-New York: Excerpta Med. Found. 1966.
50. — Stadlan, E. N.: Neuroaxonal dystrophy in congenital biliary atresia. J. Neuropath. exp. Neurol. 25, 341—361 (1966).
51. Takei, Y.: Infantile neuroaxonal dystrophy (Seitelberger's disease). Report of an autopsy case. Acta neuropath. (Berl.) 5, 1—15 (1965).
52. Toga, M., Bérard-Badier, M., Gambarelli-Dubois, D.: La dystrophie neuroaxonale infantile ou maladie de Seitelberger. Etude clinique, histologique et ultrastructurale de deux observations. Acta neuropath. (Berl.) 15, 327—350 (1970).
53. Vrabec, F.: Spherical swelling of retinal axons in the aged. Brit. J. Ophthal. 49, 113—119 (1965).
54. Wolter, J. R.: Axonal enlargements in the nerve-fiber layer of the human retina. Amer. J. Ophthal. 51, 1—21 (1968).
55. Yanagisawa, N., Shiraki, H., Minakawa, M., Narabayashi, H.: Clinicopathological and histochemical studies in Hallervorden-Spatz disease, with torsion dystonia, with special reference to diagnostic criteria of the disease from the clinico-pathological viewpoint. Progr. Brain Res. 21, 373—425 (1966).

Prof. Dr. F. Seitelberger
Neurologisches Institut der Univ. Wien
A-1090 Wien, Schwarzspanierstraße 17
Österreich

Acta neuropath. (Berl.) Suppl. V 30—39 (1971)

Infantile Neuroaxonal Dystrophy or Seitelberger's Disease

II. Peripheral Nerve Involvement: Electron Microscopic Study in one Case

Magdeleine Berard-Badier, Danielle Gambarelli, Nicole Pinsard, Jacques Hassoun, and Maurice Toga

Laboratoire de Neuropathologie, U.E.R. — Médecine Nord
et Unité de Recherches Neurobiologiques de l'INSERM, Marseille

Summary. Changes in the fine structure of peripheral nerves are reported for a case of infantile neuroaxonal dystrophy (INAD) previously diagnosed from a cortical biopsy, and by autopsy. The axons of peripheral nerves showed accumulations of smooth membranes, tubular and cisternal profiles of agranular endoplasmic reticulum, associated with abnormal mitochondria and other types of deposits. There were no signs of marked myelin degeneration. These observations were compared with findings in the central nervous system for the same case, and other cases reported in the literature, as well as with the fine structure of swollen axons in other human and animal diseases, intoxications, and nutritional disorders.

Key-Words: Neuroaxonal Dystrophy — Neuroaxonal Neuropathy — Electron Microscopy — Biopsies — Cortex — Nerve.

Introduction

Swelling of axons may be observed in numerous degenerative diseases and experimentally induced conditions in the central and/or peripheral nervous system. This histopathological change is one of the most characteristic feature of a familial disorder discovered by Seitelberger (1952) and described by Cowen and Olmstead (1963) as an infantile neuroaxonal dystrophy (INAD).

In recent papers we reported the clinical history and pathological findings by light and electron microscopy in the central nervous system in two cases of this disease. The present ultrastructural study deals with the involvement of peripheral nerves in one of these patients (Toga *et al.*, 1970a, cf.: case I; Berard-Badier, 1970; Berard-Badier *et al.*, 1970).

Material and Methods

A peripheral nerve (N. cutan. femoralis) biopsy was obtained 3 months before death. Specimens of sciatic nerve and abdominal muscles were removed immediately after death. Fixation was in glutaraldehyde buffered with Sorensen's solution at pH 6.4. Specimens were post-fixed in osmium tetroxyde buffered with Sorensen's solution and dehydrated in alcohols. Blocks were embedded in araldite. Sections were cut on a Reichert ultramicrotome and stained with uranyl acetate and lead hydroxide. They were examined with a Philips EM 300 electron microscope.

Results

1. Peripheral and Intramuscular Nerves

By low magnification, in some fascicles (Fig. 1—2), especially in intramuscular nerves containing 10 to 16 fibers averaging 10 microns in diameter, there were one, two or more myelinated or nonmyelinated abnormal fibers. Among these, some

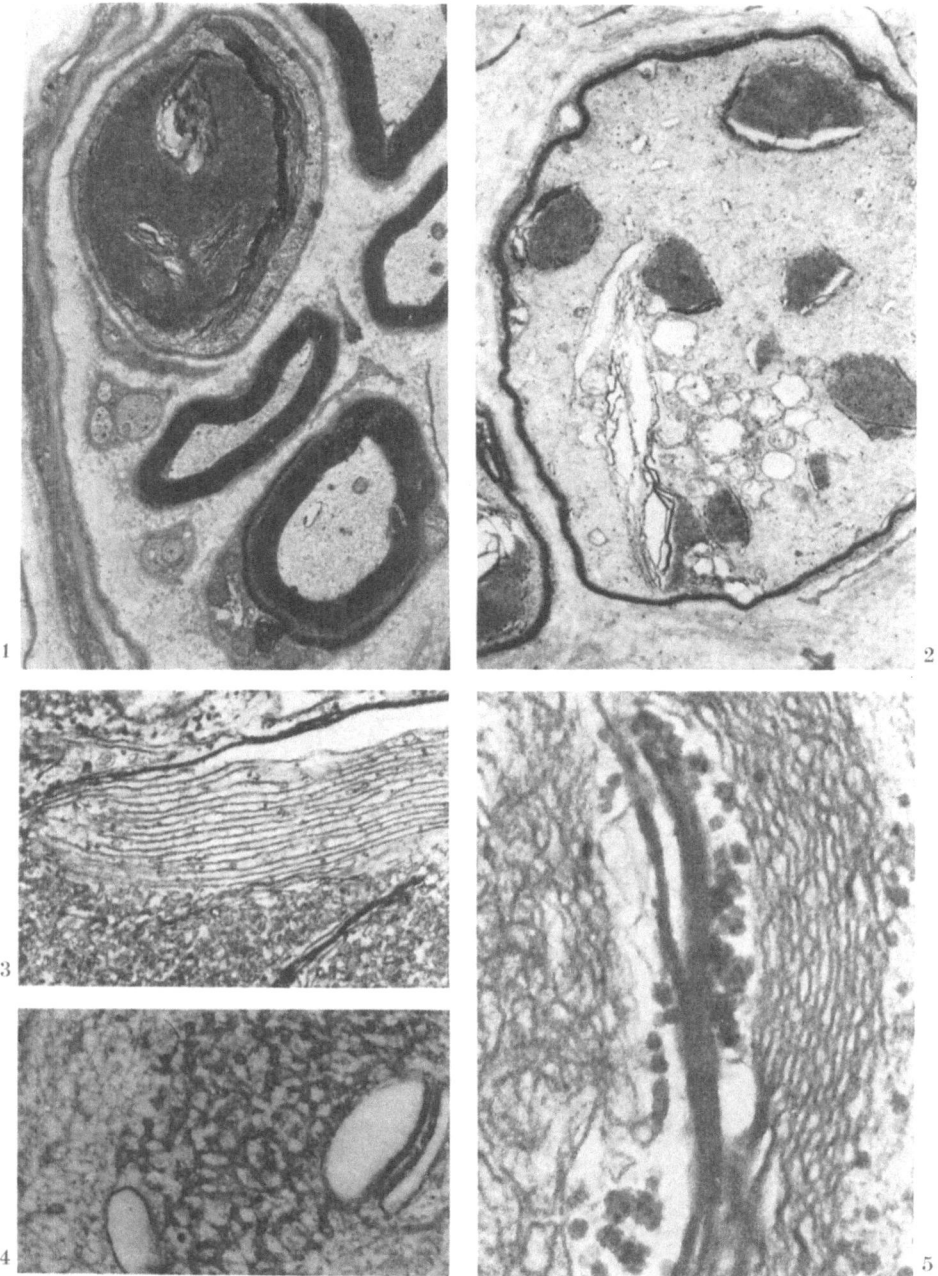

Fig. 1. Peripheral nerve fascicle with an enlarged non-myelinated dystrophic axon. ×9000

Fig. 2. Axonal swelling in two myelinated fibers with myelin sheath thinner than normal. ×5000

Fig. 3. Membranous and branched tubular profiles, layered loops of membranes, myelin-like bundles of membranes and a cleft. ×24,000

Fig. 4. Tubular and branched vesicular profiles. ×48,000

Fig. 5. Membranous networks, electron dense myelin-like bundles of compressed membranes, numerous free glycogen granules. ×80,000

3*

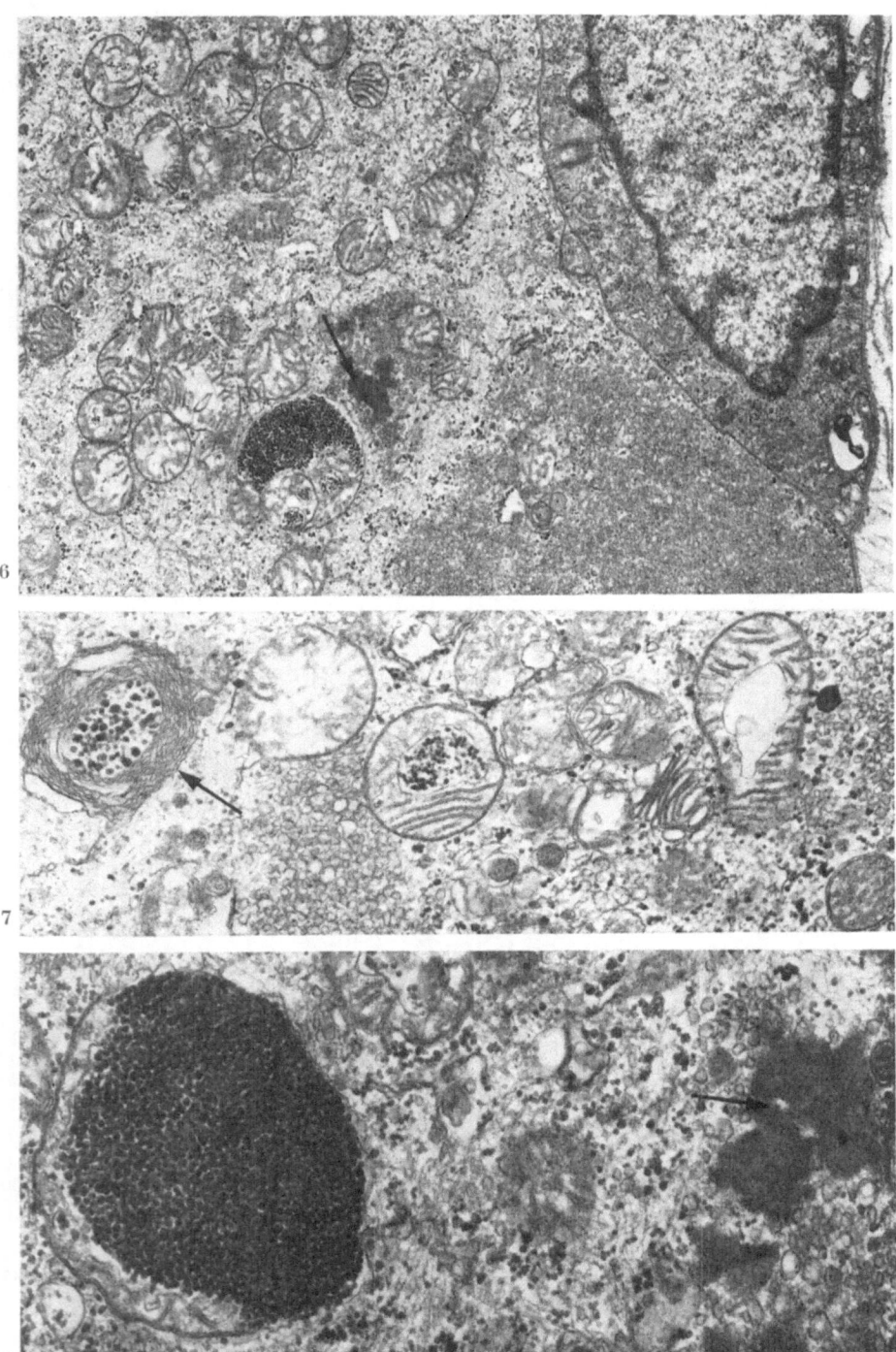

were not increased in size, others were markedly enlarged in longitudinal as well as in cross sections. The myelin sheaths of swelling axons appeared thinner than normal. In their proximity a few whorls or ovoids of collapsed myelin were observed. However, there were no other signs of myelin breakdown. No modification of the nodes of Ranvier were detected. Axolems were generally normal, even if pathological changes had occured in axoplasms.

By high magnification, the most striking feature was the presence in swelling axons of numerous smooth membranes and branched tubulo-vesicular profiles randomly disposed in dense networks. Bundles of parallel or collapsed membranes, producing myelin-like figures, were very frequent as well as layered loops of smooth membranes (Fig. 1 to 5). There were often hundreds of small vesicles, between 300 and 500 Å in diameter (Fig. 6 to 8). Several clefts were noticed within these various components. Compact aggregates of mitochondria from 2 to 3 microns in diameter (Fig. 6 to 8) were associated with smooth membranes in almost all of the sections. Some of these organelles showed various alterations such as ruptured cristae, vesicular changes, glycogen-like deposits. Membrane bound microgranular bodies, produced by accumulation of small, coarse, dense glycogen-like granules within enlarged mitochondria (Fig. 8) were very numerous. In some cases, glycogen-like granules were dispersed in axoplasm following the rupture of the outer membrane of the mitochondrion. Other alterations consisted of abnormal mitochondria, filled with glycogen-like granules and encompassed by fine membranous networks (Fig. 7). Multilamellar bodies and electron dense bodies were relatively infrequent. Less rare were irregular patches of homogeneous and lightly electron dense material, without limiting membranes, scattered among the other components described above (Fig. 6, 7).

The distribution of smooth membranes, branched tubules, mitochondria, various inclusions and deposits was very irregular in longitudinal and in cross sections. All these components tended to be associated, but in some fibers, anyone of them was predominant.

In almost all of the dystrophic axons, microtubules disappeared and neurofilaments were very rare.

2. Neuromuscular Junctions

In enlarged axoplasmic expansions, 1.5 to 6 microns in diameter (Fig. 9) branched tubular and vesicular profiles were occasionally observed in close association with abnormal mitochondria; electron dense bodies occurred rarely. Synaptic

Fig. 6. Normal Schwann cell close to a dystrophic axon filled with organelles including vesicles, mitochondria with glycogen-like granules and patches (arrow) of electron dense lipid-like or protein-like amorphous deposits without limiting membrane. × 12,000

Fig. 7. Numerous altered mitochondria with ruptured cristae and glycogen-like, coarse, dense granules. Accumulations of vesicles. Electron dense bodies. Free glycogen-like deposits. Membranous networks (arrow) around glycogen-like granule deposits probably within mitochondrion. × 30,000

Fig. 8. Enlarged mitochondrion filled with glycogen-like granules. Accumulations of vesicles and patches (arrow) of amorphous lipid-like or protein-like deposits without limiting membrane. × 38,000

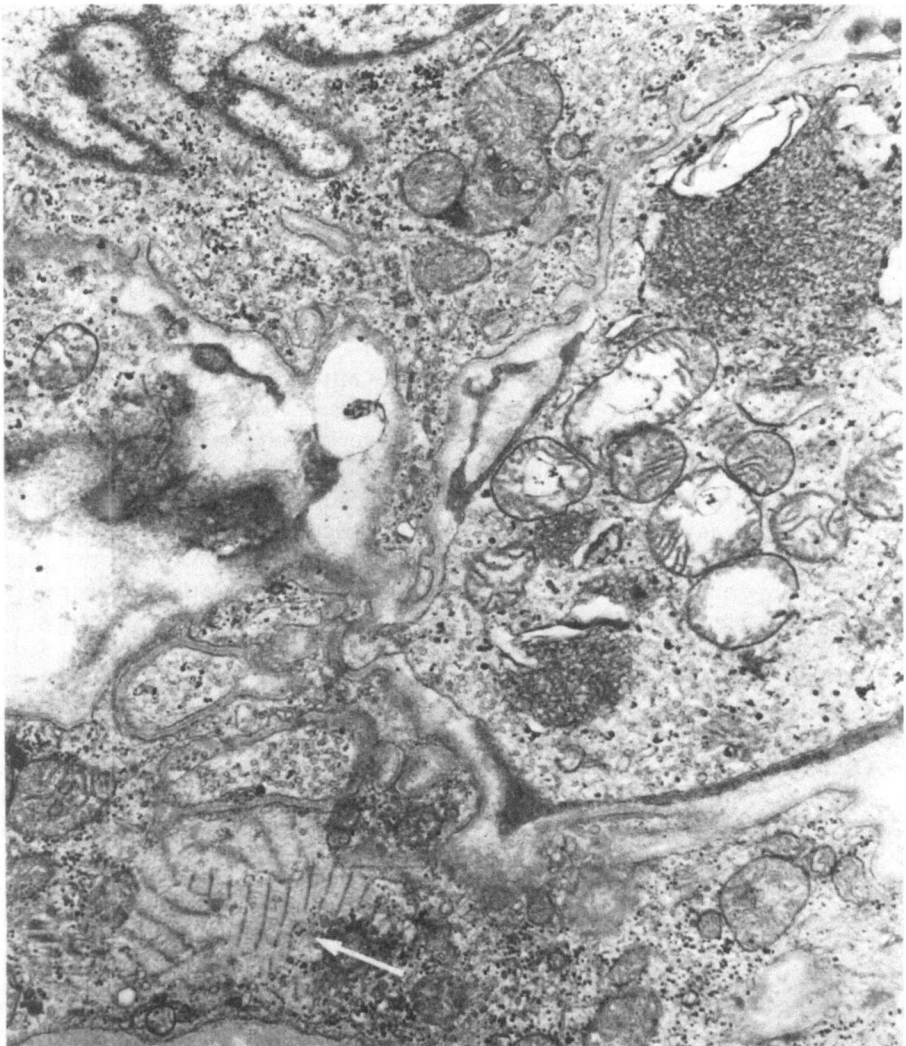

Fig. 9. Neuromuscular junction: enlarged terminal axoplasmic expansion filled with abnormal aggregates of membranous and tubular profiles associated with altered mitochondria. Irregular infoldings of primary and secondary synaptic clefts. Lambda fibrils (arrow) are noticed in underlying muscle cell. × 20,000

vesicles were decreased in number. The primary synaptic clefts appeared of normal size. Rare and irregular infoldings and abnormal widenings of secondary synaptic clefts were noticed.

Adjacent muscle fibers[1] showed various changes; in some of them, lambda fibrils (Gruner, 1961) were very numerous.

---

1 Electron microscopic study of muscle fiber in the same patient will be published later.

Comments

As far as we know, there are no previous electron microscopic studies of peripheral nerves of patients affected by INAD. Thus, our ultrastructural findings may be compared only to the changes in the central nervous system:

The abnormal components observed in myelinated and nonmyelinated fibers of peripheral nerves were very similar to those described recently for a cortical biopsy of the same patient (Toga et al., 1970a, cf.: case 1; Berard-Badier, 1970; Berard-Badier et al., 1970) and in other reports on the central nervous system in INAD (Kamoshita et al., 1968; Hedley-Whyte et al., 1968; Herman et al., 1969; Toga et al., 1970a, cf.: case 2; Sandbank et al., 1970, Rozdilsky et al., 1971).

Comparing our findings in the central nervous system with those in peripheral nerves of the same patient, we specified below some observations concerning the fine structure of myelin sheaths and axoplasms:

— Axonal swellings in both central and peripheral nervous system were characterized by accumulation of smooth endoplasmic reticulum associated with an overproduction of abnormal mitochondria and various types of deposits. They were identified as Lampert's (1967) "dystrophic" axonal changes, whereas "regenerative" and "degenerative" axonal changes were not found.

— Neuromuscular junctions were involved, as well as presynaptic endings in the cerebral cortex: axoplasmic expansions showed the same dystrophic changes in central and peripheral nerve fibers.

— Degenerated mitochondria filled with glycogen-like granules and multigranular bodies were more frequent in peripheral than in cerebral swollen axons. Membranous networks encompassing abnormal mitochondria were found only in peripheral nerve axoplasms. In our opinion, they were not related to tissue fixation.

— Cristalline-like bodies never occurred in peripheral nerve fibers whereas they appeared frequently in cerebral swollen axons.

— No severe myelin breakdown was found in peripheral nerve fibers as it was found frequently in the cerebral white matter: Wallerian degeneration was extremely rare in peripheral nerves.

Aside from these differences, it should be emphasized that INAD swollen axons showed the same basic changes in the peripheral nerves as in the central nervous system, although to a lesser extent: dystrophic axons were extremely numerous in the cerebral biopsy of the same patient, whereas not all nerve fibers were dystrophic in the peripheral and intramuscular nerves.

However, an increased amount of smooth endoplasmic reticulum with or without collections of abnormal mitochondria and various types of deposits, very similar to those noticed in INAD, has been already described for various other conditions involving the central or the peripheral nervous system, or both: in *normal animals*, such changes were observed in mature and growing cells; they were interpreted as remodeling of synaptic endings (Mugnaini and Forstrønen, 1967; Sotelo and Palay, 1970). In *human diseases*, similar changes were found in children with mental retardation (Gonatas and Goldensohn, 1965; Gonatas, 1966; Gonatas et al., 1967; Zeman and Watanabe, 1970), and in Alzheimer's presenile dementia (Toga et al., 1970b). They appeared in *animal diseases*, such as congenital ataxia of lambs (Cordy *et al.*, 1967; Cancilla and Barlow, 1969) and in jimpy mice (Hirano *et al.*, 1969). Many *experimentally induced conditions* led to a marked increase in smooth endoplasmic reticulum associated with mitochondria and abnormal deposits in the central and/or the peripheral nervous system. The following types of *intoxications* produced dystrophic axons. :

Imino-dipropionitrile	Chou and Hartman	1964;	1965
Organophosphorus	Cavanagh		1964
Tri-ortho-cresyl-phosphate	Cavanagh and Patangia		1965
	Bischoff	1967;	1970
	Prineas		1969a
Diethyl-dithiocarbamate	Edington and Howell		1966
	Howell *et al.*		1970
Bromophenylacetylurea	Cavanagh *et al.*		1968
	Blakemore and Cavanagh		1969
Acrylamide	Prineas		1969b
Methamphetamine	Miyakawa *et al.*		1969

In liver cells, hypertrophy of smooth endoplasmic reticulum was induced by phenobarbital (Jones and Fawcett, 1966) and by carbon-tetrachloride in rats (Stenger, 1966). *Nutritionally deficient diets* produced axon swellings: an overproduction of agranular endoplasmic reticulum associated with mitochondria and all the materials described in INAD were very similar to those noticed in vitamin-E deficient rats (Lampert *et al.*, 1964; Lampert and Pentschew, 1964; Lampert and Cressman, 1966; Lampert, 1967); whereas such changes were very rare in thiamine deficient rats (Tellez and Terry, 1968).

Free and membrane bound accumulations of glycogen-like granules were found in the present study of INAD in large amounts in the peripheral nervous system as well as in the central nervous system. They were also noticed in another case of INAD (Toga *et al.*, 1970a, cf.: case 2), in sympathetic neurons following X-irradiation in frogs (Pick, 1965), in tetanus toxin poisoned rats (Perrochia, 1966), in vitamin-E deficient rats (Lampert, 1967), in lead neuropathy (Schlaepfer, 1969) and in bilirubin encephalopathy (Schutta *et al.*, 1970). These granules correspond to an abnormal glycogen storage within altered mitochondria. Their presence suggests a nonspecific disorder of mitochondria metabolism.

Patches of homogeneous light electron dense material without limiting membranes consist of lipid or protein deposits.

Conclusions

In the present paper, ultrastructural findings were reported, to our knowledge, for the first time, for the peripheral nervous system in one case of INAD.

From a *pathological* point of view, all the changes described resembled those found in the central nervous system of the same patient and in other cases of INAD as well as in a variety of experimental intoxications, and nutritional disorders. Hence, these changes were non specific. Nevertheless, they occured with an extremely high frequency and with a very wide distribution only in INAD.

From a *clinical* point of view, one may suggest that electron microscopic diagnosis of INAD might be attempted first by peripheral nerve biopsy, followed, only when necessary, by cerebral cortical biopsy.

From a *pathogenetic* point of view, in spite of numerous explanations suggested for the various pathological and normal conditions decribed above, it was impossible to resolve the problem of axon swellings in INAD and to explain the presence of axostasis of axoplasmic flow (Chou and Hartmann, 1964, 1965). A dying-back process is conceivable but we emphasized that myelin sheath degeneration was rarely found in the peripheral nerves in our patient, whereas it always occurred in dying-back polyneuropathy (Cavanagh, 1964; Blakemore and Cavanagh, 1969; Prineas, 1969 a, b). In the same way, it was impossible to determine the precise classification of INAD: The disease does not fit the category of storage disorders as lipidosis for instance; the large amount of glycolipoproteins noticed by light microscopic histochemical staining reactions in all cases of INAD and in experimentally induced axon dystrophies, was due to the presence in the axoplasm of various types of materials described above. Neither intoxications nor nutritional disorders were apparent in our patient as in other reported cases of INAD. Whether or not the disease may be identified as infantile type of Hallervorden-Spatz's disease (Seitelberger *et al.*, 1963) is not resolved but a recent electron microscopy report on this degenerative disorder (Schoene *et al.*, 1970) has to be taken into consideration.

Nevertheless, dystrophic axons in INAD may be considered an adaptive neuronal response to an unknown noxious agent. The occurrence of several cases in siblings may suggest a metabolic defect (Jellinger, 1968) with overproduction of smooth endoplasmic reticulum and abnormal mitochondria, supposedly related to a genetic disorder. Further investigations are necessary to define the nature of INAD, a familial degenerative disease of the central and peripheral nervous system.

Acknowledgments. We are grateful to Professor René Bernard (Pediatric Department) and to Professor Pierre Laffargue (General Pathology Department) CHU-Nord, Marseille, for providing the clinical and pathological case reports.

We wish to thank J.-P. Ripert, J. Planche, F. Finidori, F. Tagliarini and Y. Mourayre for their careful technical assistance.

References

Berard-Badier, M.: Dystrophie neuroaxonale infantile. I.Ultrastructure des sphéroides. Rapports du 6me Congr. Internat. de Neuropathol., pp. 101—102. Paris: Masson 1970.
— Tripier, M.-F., Pinsard, N., Bernard, R.: A case of infantile neuroaxonal dystrophy. Strabismus '69, pp. 82—85. London: Kimpton 1970.
Bischoff, A.: The ultrastructure of tri-ortho-cresyl phosphate poisoning. I. Studies on myelin and axonal alterations in the sciatic nerve. Acta neuropath. (Berl.) 9, 158—174 (1967).
— II. Studies on spinal cord alterations. Acta neuropath. (Berl.) 15, 142—155 (1970).
Blakemore, W. F., Cavanagh, J. B.: Neuroaxonal dystrophy occurring in an experimental dying-back process in the rat. Brain 92, 789—804 (1969).
Cancilla, P. A., Barlow, R. M.: Structural changes on the central nervous system in swayback of lambs. Acta neuropath. (Berl.) 12, 307—313 (1969).
Cavanagh, J. B.: The significance of the "dying-back" process in experimental and human. neurological disease. Int. Rev. exp. Path. 3, 219—267 (1964).

Cavanagh, J. B., Chen, F. C. K., Kyu, M. H., Ridley, A.: The experimental neuropathology in rats caused by p-bromophenylacetylurea. J. Neurol. Neurosurg. Psychiat. **31**, 471—478 (1968).
— Patangia, G. N.: Changes in the central nervous system in the cat as the result of tri-O-cresyl-phosphate poisoning. Brain **88**, 165—180 (1965).
Chou, S. M., Hartmann, H. A.: Axonal lesions and waltzing syndrome after IDPN administration in rats.With a concept "axostasis". Acta neuropath.(Berl.)**3**, 428—450 (1964).
— — Electron microscopy of focal neuroaxonal lesions produced by B-B'-Iminodipropionitrile (IDPN) in rats. Acta neuropath. (Berl.) **4**, 590—603 (1965).
Cordy, D. R., Richards, W. P. C.: Bradford, G. E.: Systemic neuroaxonal dystrophy in Suffolk sheep. Acta neuropath. (Berl.) **8**, 133—140 (1967).
Cowen, D., Olmstead, E. V.: Infantile neuroaxonal dystrophy. J. Neuropath. exp. Neurol. **22**, 175—236 (1963).
Edington, N., Howell, J. McC.: Changes in the nervous system of rabbits following the administration of sodium diethyldithiocarbamate. Nature (Lond.) **210**, 1060—1062 (1966).
Gonatas, N. K.: Mental retardation, cortical blindness and convulsions associated with neocortical presynaptic terminals. J. Neuropath exp. Neurol. **25**, 144—145 (1966).
— Goldensohn, E. S.: Unusual neocortical presynaptic terminals in a patient with convulsions, mental retardation and cortical blindness. An electron microscopic study. J. Neuropath. exp. Neurol. **24**, 539—562 (1965).
— Evangelista, I., Welsh, G. O.: Axonic and synaptic changes in a case of psychomotor retardation. An electron microscopic study. J. Neuropath. exp. Neurol. **26**, 179—199 (1967).
Gruner, J. E.: La structure fine du fuseau neuromusculaire humain. Rev. neurol. **104**, 490—507 (1961).
Hedley-Whyte, E. T., Floyd, M. B., Gilles, H., Uzman, B. G.: Infantile neuroaxonal dystrophy. A disease characterized by altered terminal axons and synaptic endings. Neurology (Minneap.) **18**, 891—906 (1968).
Herman, M. M., Huttenlocher, P. R., Bensch, K. G.: Electron microscopic observations in infantile neuroaxonal dystrophy. Arch. Neurol. (Chic.) **20**, 19—34 (1969).
Hirano, A., Sax, D. S., Zimmerman, H. M.: The fine structure of the cerebella of jimpy mice and their normal litter mates. J. Neuropath. exp. Neurol. **28**, 388—400 (1969).
Howell, J. McC., Ishmael, J., Ewbank, R., Blakemore, W. F.: Changes in the central nervous system of lambs following the administration of sodium-diethyldithiocarbamate. Acta neuropath. (Berl.) **15**, 197—207 (1970).
Jellinger, K.: Neuroaxonale Dystrophien. Verh. dtsch. Ges. Path. **52**, 92—126. Stuttgart: G. Fischer 1968.
Jones, A. L., Fawcett, D. W.: Hypertrophy of the agranular endoplasmic reticulum in hamster liver induced by phenobarbital. J. Histochem. Cytochem. **14**, 215—232 (1966).
Kamoshita, S., Neustein, H. B., Landing, B. H.: Infantile neuroaxonal dystrophy with neonatal onset. J. Neuropath. exp. Neurol. **27**, 300—323 (1968).
Lampert, P.: A comparative electron microscopy study of reactive, degenerating, regenerating and dystrophic axons. J. Neuropath. exp. Neurol. **26**, 345—368 (1967).
— Blumberg, J. M., Pentschew, A.: An electron microscopic study of dystrophic axons in the gracile and cuneate nuclei of vitamin-E deficient rats (axonal dystrophy in vitamin E deficiency). J. Neuropath. exp. Neurol. **23**, 60—77 (1964).
— Cressman, M. R.: Fine structural changes of myelin sheaths after axonal degeneration in the spinal cord of rats. Amer. J. Path. **49**, 1139—1155 (1966).
— Pentschew, A.: An electron microscopic study of spheroid and convoluted bodies in dystrophic terminal axons. Acta neuropath. (Berl.) **4**, 158—168 (1964).
Mugnaini, E., Forstrønen, P. F.: Ultrastructural studies on the cerebellar histogenesis. I. Differentiation of granule cells and development of glomeruli in the chick embryo. Z. Zellforsch. **77**, 115—143 (1967).
Miyakawa, T., Sumiyoshi, S., Deshimaru, M., Murayama, E., Tatetsu, S.: Electron microscopic studies concerning the structural mechanism of the development of mental disturbance in experimental chronic methamphetamine poisoning. Acta neuropath. (Berl.) **14**, 215—225 (1969).

Perocchia, C.: Ultrastructure of the spinal cord and the sciatic nerve of rats with tetanus toxin poisoning. Lab. Invest. **15**, 479 (1966).

Pick, J.: The fine structure of sympathetic neurons in X-irradiated frogs. J. Cell Biol. **26**, 335—351 (1965).

Prineas, M. B.: The pathogenesis of dying-back polyneuropathy. Part I. An ultrastructural study of experimental tri-ortho-cresyl-phosphate intoxication in the cat. J. Neuropath. exp. Neurol. **28**, 571—597 (1969a).

— Part II. An ultrastructural study of experimental acrylamide intoxication in the cat. J. Neuropath. exp. Neurol. **28**, 598—621 (1969b).

Rozdilsky, B., Bolton, C. F., Takeda, M.: Neuroaxonal dystrophy. Acta neuropath. (Berl.) **17**, 331—340 (1971).

Sandbank, U., Lerman, P., Geifman, M.: Infantile neuroaxonal dystrophy: cortical axonic and presynaptic changes. Acta neuropath. (Berl.) **16**, 342—352 (1970).

Schlaepfer, W. W.: Experimental lead neuropathy: a disease of the supporting cells in the peripheral nervous system. J. Neuropath. exp. Neurol. **28**, 401—418 (1969).

Schoene, W. C., Dooling, E. C., Steiner, M., Richardson, E. P.: Hallervorden-Spatz disease. Rapports du VIme Congr. Internat. de Neuropathol., pp. 1134—1135. Paris: Masson 1970.

Schutta, H. S., Johnson, L., Neville, H. E.: Mitochondrial abnormalities in bilirubin encephalopathy. J. Neuropath. exp. Neurol. **29**, 296—305 (1970).

Seitelberger, F.: Eine unbekannte Form von infantiler Lipoidspeicher-Krankheit des Gehirns. Proc. Ist Congr. Neuropath., Vol. 3, pp. 323—333. Turin: Rosenberg et Sellier 1952.

— Gootz, M., Gros, H.: Beitrag zur spätinfantilen Hallervorden-Spatzschen Krankheit. Acta neuropath. (Berl.) **3**, 16—28 (1963).

Sotelo, C., Palay, S. L.: communication personelle (1970).

Stenger, R. J.: Concentric lamellar formations in hepatic parenchymal cells of carbon-tetrachloride treated rats J. Ultrastruct. Res. **14**, 240—253 (1966).

Tellez, I., Terry, R. D.: Fine structure of the early changes in the vestibular nuclei of the thiamine-deficient rat. Amer. J. Path. **52**, 777—793 (1968).

Toga,.M., Berard-Badier, M., Gambarelli-Dubois, D.: La dystrophie neuroaxonale infantile ou maladie de Seitelberger. Etude clinique, histologique et ultrastructurale de deux observations. Acta neuropath. (Berl.) **15**, 327—350 (1970a).

— Tripier, M.-F., Gambarelli-Dubois, D.: communication personnelle (1970b).

Zeman, W., Watanabe, I.: communication personnelle (1970).

Dr. Magdeleine Berard-Badier
Laboratoire de Neuropathologie,
Faculté de Médecine-Nord
Bd. P. Dramard
F-13 Marseille 15me
France

Acta neuropath. (Berl.) Suppl. V 40—48 (1971)

How Long Can Degenerating Axons in the Central Nervous System Produce Reactive Changes?

An Electron Microscopic Investigation

Wolfgang Schlote

Institut für Hirnforschung der Universität Tübingen

Summary. The response of previously severed rat optic fibers to a second transection after various time intervals was studied by light and electron microscopy. The optic nerve of adult animals was crushed retrobulbar and, after 6, 12, 28 or 48 h recrushed 2 mm distant from the first lesion. The changes in the axoplasm of myelinated fibers in the stumps distal to the two lesions, in reference to the perikarya of the cells (i.e. on the cerebral side of each lesion) were studied 6 or 12 h after the second lesion. In the nerves that had been severed 6 h after the first retrobulbar lesion, mitochondria, dense bodies, neurofilaments and endoplasmic reticulum accumulated in the axoplasm distal to the second lesion 6—12 h after the operation. These changes were identical to those seen in the corresponding distal stump of the primary lesion; they may represent a peritraumatic reactive change preceeding the process of Wallerian degeneration.

In nerves severed for 12 h, the axon stumps distal to the second lesion contained, 12 h after this lesion, enlarged mitochondria with scattered equivalents of cristae, and large empty vacuoles of mitochondrial origin. In addition, focal clear axonal swellings nearly devoid of organelles appeared in fiber portions distal to the second lesion; these were less frequently in the fibers distal to the first lesion. They are probably the result of decreasing energy supply required for the axonal sodium pump.

In nerves severed for 28 h the second lesion evoked only a redistribution of axoplasm of distal axon segments towards the stump end indicated by whorls of neurofilaments.

These observations demonstrate a gradually decreasing reactivity of the separated axon to a second traumatic lesion during the early phase of Wallerian degeneration.

Key-Words: Optic Nerve — Transsection of Nerve Fibers — Axonal Reaction — Wallerian Degeneration.

The axoplasm of rat optic nerve fibers severed from the retinal ganglion cells shows no striking alteration of fine structure in electron micrographs up to 40 h after the lesion. The question as to the events during this morphologically stable period before the onset of Wallerian degeneration is only partially answered. We were interested in studying posttraumatic responses of the axon during the early phase of the degenerative process. The organelle-rich axon swellings that form at both ends of a severed fiber are reactive phenomena, which may be based on a redistribution of preexisting organelles (Martinez and Friede, 1970), on microtubule-mediated plasma streaming (Kreutzberg, 1969), on *de novo* synthesis of structural elements, or—in our opinion—on a superposition of these mechanisms (Schlote, 1970). Are these swellings also evoked in degenerating fibers? Does their composition provide some information as to the phase of the degenerative process? I like to report briefly on an investigation concerned with these questions.

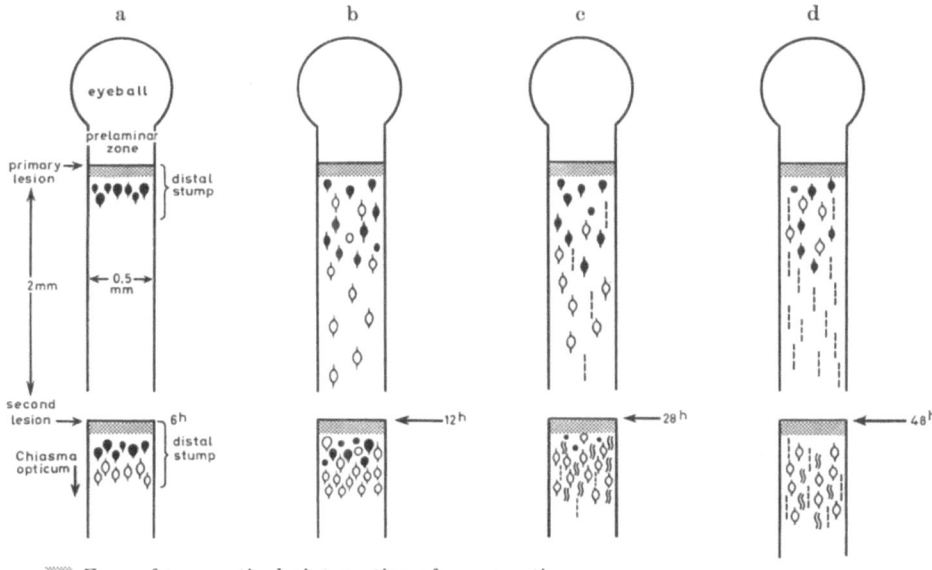

Fig. 1 a—d. Schematic representation of submicroscopic changes in the distal axon stumps of optic fibers 12 h after being recrushed. a Second lesion was performed 6 h after first lesion. b Second lesion was performed 12 h after first lesion. c Second lesion was performed 28 h after first lesion. d Second lesion was performed 48 h after first lesion

Method

   The optic nerve of adult white rats (diameter: 0.5 mm) was crushed retrobulbar, 0.5 mm distal from the eyeball, by slight pressure with watchmaker's tweezers. Six, 12, 28 or 48 h later the wound was reopened and the nerve was crushed again 2 mm distant from the first lesion (Fig. 1 a). Twelve hours, or, in some experiments, 6 h after the second operation the entire nerve was fixed in Veronal acetate buffered (pH 7.4) $1^0/_0$ osmium tetroxide solution, and embedded in Vestopal W. In each case, the complete interruption of nervous tissue at the site of the primary lesion was confirmed in semithin sections; only the meningeal tissue surrounding the nerve remained intact. This proved that the second lesion had been performed on a degenerating nerve. Semi-thin sections of the entire nerve between the eye-ball and the chiasma opticum were made for light microscopic investigation. The electron microscopic study was confined to the two distal stumps, in reference to the perikaryon of the cells, i.e. to approximately 0.5 mm long segments of the optic nerve distal to the two lesions (Fig. 1).

Results

   The optic nerve recrushed (second lesion) after having been severed *6 h* earlier (first lesion), showed, 6 h after the second lesion, organelle-filled axon swellings at the stump distal to the second lesion. These axon swellings were

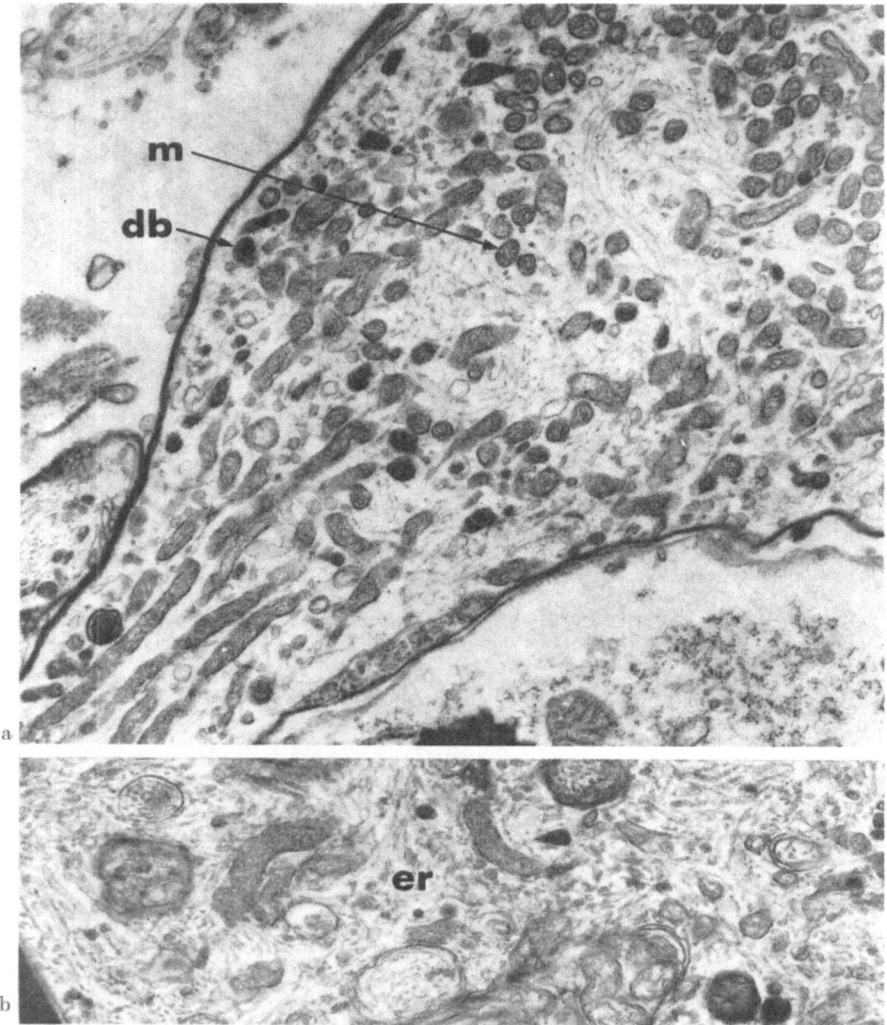

Fig. 2a and b. Optic nerve recrushed after having been severed for *6 h*. a Accumulation of elongated and small spherical mitochondria (*m*) and of dense bodies (*db*) in the axoplasm of a myelinated fiber distal to the second lesion, 6 h after this lesion. b Mitochondria and proliferated smooth endoplasmic reticulum (*er*) in the axoplasm of a myelinated fiber distal to the second lesion, 12 h after this lesion (corresponding to Fig. 1a). a 22050:1; b 24300:1

morphologically identical to those seen at the stump distal to the first lesion. Numerous elongated besides small, round mitochondria and numerous dense bodies accumulated in the axoplasm; the spaces between them were filled with neurofilaments (Fig. 2a). If the nerve, in the same experiment, was studied 12 rather than 6 h after the second lesion, the axon swellings distal to the site of the

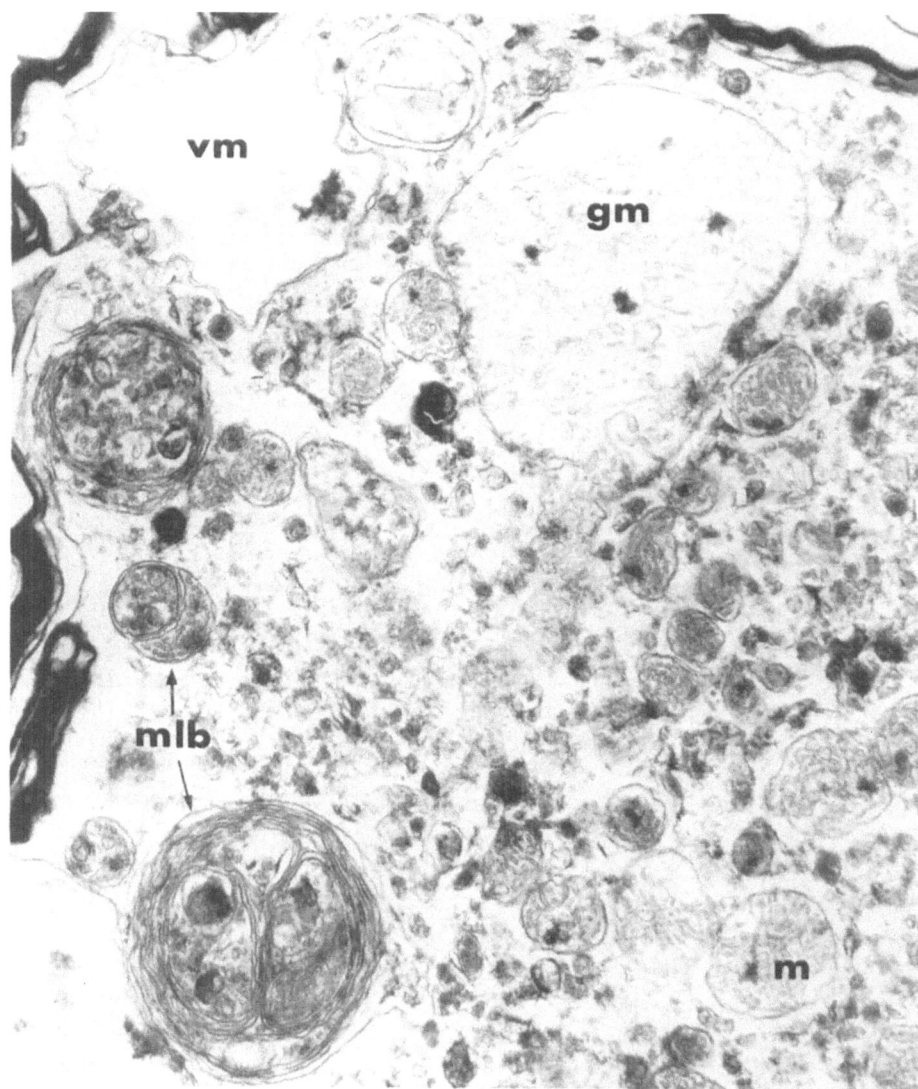

Fig. 3. Optic nerve recrushed after having been severed for *12 h* (corresponding to Fig. 1 b). The axoplasm of a myelinated fiber distal to the second lesion shows, 12 h after this lesion, enlarged mitochondria (*m*) with tubular cristae, giant mitochondria (*gm*) with vesicular elements replacing cristae, vacuolated mitochondria (*vm*) and multilamellated bodies (*mlb*). 22050:1

second lesion contained, in addition, vesicular and tubular elements of a dense endoplasmic reticulum (Fig. 2 b). Between the organelle-filled axon enlargements, there were many focal clear axon swellings which were rarely seen in the stump distal to the primary lesion (Fig. 1 a). In these focal axon dilatations, the entire axoplasm was swollen, the neurofilaments disintegrated; no swollen elements of

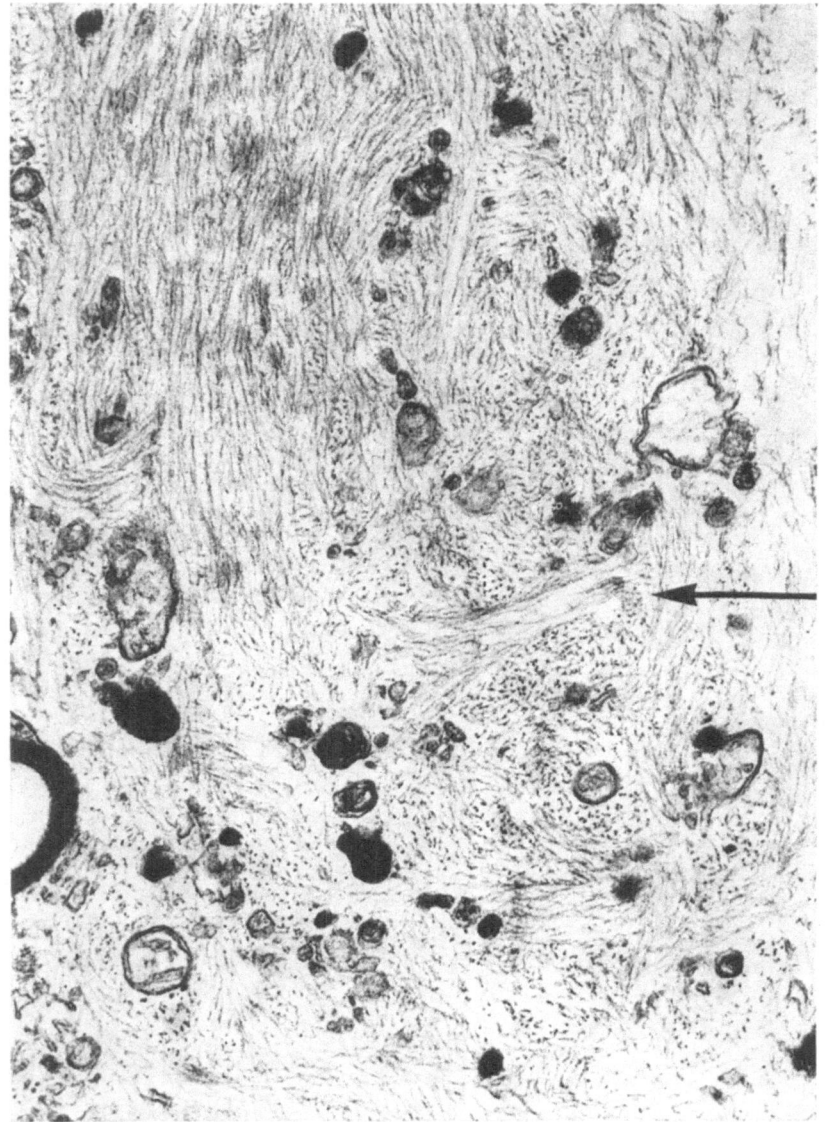

Fig. 4. Optic nerve recrushed after having been severed for *28 h* (corresponding to Fig. 1 c).
Whorls of neurofilaments and scattered organelles (dense bodies and degenerating mitochondria) in the axoplasm of a myelinated fiber distal to the second lesion, 12 h after this lesion
had been performed. 24500:1

endoplasmic reticulum occurred (Fig. 5). The myelin sheaths of the focal clear
swellings as well as those of the organelle-filled axon enlargements were preserved,
but thinned.

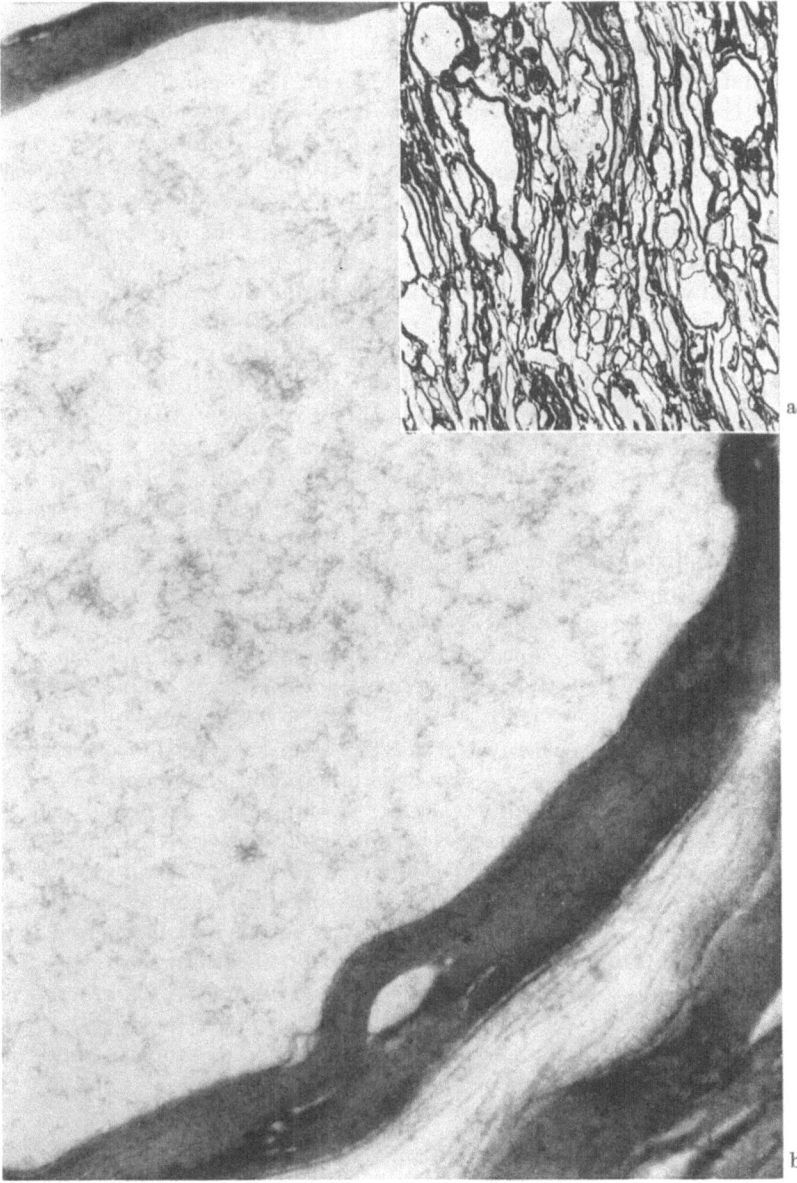

Fig. 5 a and b. Optic nerve recrushed after having been severed for *28 h*. a Portion of the stump distal to the second lesion, 12 h after this lesion. Focal clear swellings of axons and longer, enlarged axon segments (corresponding to Fig. 1 c). Myelinated sheaths are preserved. Semithin section. Giemsa staining. 480:1. b Higher magnification of part of a. Focal axon swellings with irregularly distributed disintegrating neurofilaments. Compare the intact neurofilaments in a non-dilated axon in the lower right of the micrograph. 24500:1

The optic nerve recrushed after having been severed *12 h* earlier had developed, 12 h after the second lesion, as many but larger organelle-filled axon enlargements at the stump distal to the second lesion (Fig. 1 b). The organelles were more loosely arranged. Most of the mitochondria were swollen and displayed a tubular or vesicular transformation of cristae, others were greatly enlarged, contained scattered tubular elements or were of vacuolar appearance, and could be identified as mitochondria only by their double envelope (Fig. 2b). The zone of additional focal clear axon swellings was wider though sharply delineated from the adjacent distal portion of the nerve (Fig. 1 b). At the stump distal to the first lesion organelle-filled axon enlargements were found at greater distance from the lesion, but the organelles were of the same type as in the 6-h-experiment. No altered mitochondria were found.

In the optic nerve recrushed after having been severed *28 h* earlier only a few axon swellings appeared in the stump distal to the second lesion 12 h after this lesion. They contained small vacuolated or degenerating mitochondria and dense bodies near the axolemm or scattered between prominent whorls of neurofilaments (Fig. 4). Dilated axons of this type were found only in the terminal portion of the stump (Fig. 1 c). The adjacent portion of the nerve contained numerous focal, clear axon swellings (Fig. 5). In addition, there were enlarged longer axon segments with curled outlines filled with neurofilaments and few mitochondria. Some fibers had precipitated, electron dense axoplasm and distorted myelin sheaths. Between fibers altered in one of these ways, many fibers appeared normal. The zone of the focal clear axon swellings and of the enlarged longer axon segments was sharply delineated from the adjacent distal portion of the nerve (Fig. 1 c).

The optic nerve recrushed after having been severed *48 h* earlier revealed, 12 h after the second lesion, no organelle-filled axon enlargements distal to the second lesion. The number of focal clear swellings had decreased and the zone in which these swellings occurred was not as circumscribed as in the previous experiments (Fig. 1 d). The number of longer, enlarged axon segments with curled outlines filled with neurofilaments and with some mitochondria was unchanged. The number of fibers with dark, precipitated, condensed axoplasm and invaginated or exvaginated, distorted or thickened myelin sheaths was greatly increased. In the portion distal to the first lesion degenerated remnants of large axon swellings with electron dense axoplasm filled with dark, shrunken organelles were found besides numerous non-enlarged fibers with condensed axoplasm and distorted myelin sheaths.

Discussion

It was the aim of these experiments to study some submicroscopic alterations in optic axons severed for a second time after they were separated from the eyeball. For the electron microscopic investigation, the stumps distal to the two lesions were chosen for two reasons. First, the events taking place in the axoplasm of distal fiber segments are not influenced by the cell body, such as by proximo-distal plasma flow. Secondly, the proximal stump of the first lesion in this experiment corresponded to the zone just next to the lamina cribrosa, i.e. the area praelaminaris, which has a special submicroscopic architecture and contains special types of organelles (Wendell-Smith *et al.*, 1966). Therefore, the proximal stumps of the two lesions were disregarded in this study.

It is evident from our findings that axons in the central nervous system remain capable of producing organelle accumulations distal to a second traumatic lesion for up to 6 h after separation from the perikarya of the cells. These changes do not differ from those developing in previously undamaged fibers, i.e. in the distal axon stumps at the site of primary fiber interruption. Accumulation of the same types of organelles was described by many authors for distal axon stumps of nerve fibers in peripheral nerves (de Webster, 1962; Lee, 1963) and in the central nervous system (Lampert and Cressmann, 1966; Schlote, 1966). The concentration of mitochondria and dense bodies 6 h after the crush lesion, and that of vesicles and tubules 12 h after the lesion is indicative of a biphasic process: the accumulation of mitochondria is probably caused by a segmentation and by displacement of preexisting organelles towards the stump, while the later appearing endoplasmic reticulum may result from a transformation and/or proliferation of preexisting axonal constituents *in loco*. The behaviour of separated fiber segments during these hours may be compared to that of anucleated protozoal organisms and anucleated algae in which plasma movements and formative processes persist for a limited time, depending mainly on their content of mitochondria and of messenger ribonucleic acid (Werz, 1969). It does not seem justified to attribute the accumulation of organelles in distal axon segments to the process of Wallerian degeneration which affects the axon for its entire length, and which is characterized by condensation of axoplasm, disappearance of neurofilaments and disintegration of mitochondria, accompanied by disruption of the myelin sheath. Alterations of this clearly degenerative type are not seen before 40 h (28 and 12 h, see Fig.1c), as also reported by other authors for other fiber systems (Alksne *et al.*, 1966). The accumulation of intact organelles in peritraumatic axons would be more appropriately interpreted as a *reactive* change in the axoplasm, according to the classification by Lampert (1967, 1968). The same phenomenon has been observed in pathologic conditions *without* fiber interruption (Schröder and Wechsler, 1965; Bubis and Luse, 1964; Hayano, 1967).

The appearance of unusual large mitochondria of incomplete or vacuolated type in distal fiber stumps of nerves recrushed after being severed 12 h earlier is tentatively interpreted as an abortive posttraumatic *reaction in the axoplasm of degenerating nerve fibers* not yet displaying submicroscopic alterations of degenerative type at the time of investigation. It may be of pathogenic significance that similar enlarged, vacuolated mitochondria in swollen axon segments were observed by Toga *et al.* (1970) in a brain biopsy of a 6 year old child suffering from neuroaxonal dystrophy.

In optic nerve fibers severed 28 h earlier only a redistribution of axoplasm could be evoked, as indicated by whorls of neurofilaments in the distal fiber stumps. No accumulation of other organelles than neurofilaments were observed lending further support to the idea, that the displacement of organelles and their accumulation in the stumps at earlier stages may be based on an active mechanism.

The focal clear axonal swellings along the fibers found frequently in the segments distal to the second lesion—observed more rarely also in the corresponding distal stumps of the first lesion—bear close resemblance to the swellings recently described by Mire *et al.* (1970) in distal segments of unmyelinated axons in cultures of rodent sensory ganglia 12 h or 24 h after transsection *in vitro*, or 5 to 7 days after nutritional deprivation. In the opinion of these authors, clear axon swellings of this type probably result from intraaxonal accumulation of ions and water caused by failing active extrusion of Na^+. This interpretation seems applicable also to the clear swellings in the degenerating optic nerve fibers where the energy supply for the sodium pump decreases during the slowly progressing degenerative process. As such swellings are more frequently seen in axons distal to the second lesion, an additional factor evidently favours the development of these swellings in the already degenerating, anew traumatized optic nerve.

Literature

Bubis, J. H., Luse, S. A.: An electron microscopic study of experimental allergic encephalomyelitis in the rat. Amer. J. Path. **44**, 299—327 (1964).

Alksne, J. F., Blackstadt, T. W., Walberg, F., White, L. E.: Electron microscopy of axonal degeneration: a valuable tool in experimental neuroanatomy. Berlin-Heidelberg-New York: Springer 1966.

Hayano, M.: Unusual axons found in experimental brain edema of cats. Arch. histol. jap. **28**, 483—501 (1967).

Kreutzberg, G. W.: Neuronal dynamics and axonal flow. IV. Blockage of intraaxonal enzyme transport by colchicine. Proc. nat. Acad. Sci. (Wash.) **62**, 722—738 (1969).

Lampert, P. W.: A comparative electron microscopic study of reactive, degenerating, regenerating and dystrophic axons. J. Neuropath. exp. Neurol. **26**, 345—368 (1967).

— Fine structural changes of myelin sheaths in the central nervous system. In: The structure and function of nervous tissue, Vol. I, pp. 187—204. Ed. G. H. Bourne. New York-London: Academic Press 1968.

— Cressmann, M. R.: Fine structural changes of myelin sheaths after axon degeneration in the spinal cord of rats. Amer. J. Path. **49**, 1139—1155 (1966).

Lee, C. J.: Electron microscopy of Wallerian degeneration. J. comp. Neurol. **120**, 65—80 (1963).

Martinez, A. J. Friede, R. L.: Accumulation of axoplasmic organelles in swollen nerve fibers. Brain Res. **19**, 183—198 (1970).

Mire, J. J., Hendelman, W. J., Bunge, R. P.: Observations on a transient phase of focal swelling in degenerating unmyelinated nerve fibers. J. Cell Biol. **45**, 9—22 (1970).

Schlote, W.: Der Aufbau von Schichtenkörpern im Axoplasma durchtrennter Opticusfasern distal der Läsion. J. Ultrastruct. Res. **16**, 548—568 (1966).

— Nervus opticus und experimentelles Trauma. Monographien aus dem Gesamtgebiete der Neurologie und Psychiatrie, Heft 131. Berlin-Heidelberg-New York: Springer 1970.

Schröder, J. M., Wechsler, W.: Ödem und Nekrose in der grauen und weißen Substanz beim experimentellen Hirntrauma. Acta neuropath. (Berl.) **5**, 82—111 (1965).

Toga, M., Berard-Badier, M., Gambarelli-Dubois, D.: La dystrophie neuroaxonale infantile ou maladie de Seitelberger. Etude clinique, histologique et ultrastructurale de deux observations. Acta neuropath. (Berl.) **15**, 327—350 (1970).

Webster, H. de F.: Transient, focal accumulation of axonal mitochondria during the early stages of Wallerian degeneration. J. Cell Biol. **12**, 361—384 (1962).

Wendell-Smith, C. P., Blunt, M. J., Baldwin, F.: The fine structural caracterization of macroglial cell types. J. comp. Neurol. **127**, 219—239 (1966).

Werz, G.: Morphogenetic processes in acetabularia. In: Inhibitors, Tools in Cell Res., pp. 167 to 186. Ed.: Th. Bücher and H. Sies. Berlin-Heidelberg-New York: Springer 1969.

Prof. Dr. W. Schlote
Institut für Hirnforschung der Universität
D-7400 Tübingen, Calwer Straße 3

Acta neuropath. (Berl.) Suppl. V, 49—53 (1971)

Fine Structural Changes of Neurites in Alzheimer's Disease *

Peter Lampert

Department of Pathology, University of California at San Diego,
La Jolla, California

Summary. Neurites in senile plaques of Alzheimer's disease show a variety of changes which in order of frequency consist of 1. accumulation of membrane-bounded, floccular dense bodies; 2. interlacing bundles of twisted tubules; 3. aggregates of mitochondria usually associated with membranous dense bodies; 4. arrays of irregular vesicular profiles, and 5. granular and vacuolar disintegration. A relationship between amyloid deposits and abnormal neurites in senile plaques could not be established. Except for the accumulation of twisted tubules similar axonal changes are observed in animals in peritraumatic regions and in dying back neuropathies. The theory (Terry and Wisniewski, 1970) that neurofibrillar tangles in nerve cell bodies produce axoplasmic stasis and subsequent accumulation of organelles in the terminal arborization of neurites is discussed.

Key-Words: Alzheimer's Disease — Senile Plaques — Amyloid — Neurofibrillary Tangles — Axoplasm.

Introduction

Neurofibrillar tangles and senile plaques are characteristic features of Alzheimer's disease. The tangles are composed of intraneuronal aggregates of twisted tubules (Terry, 1963). The plaques, according to Terry and Wisniewski (1970) are of four types, consisting of 1. small aggregates of abnormal neurites; 2. abnormal neurites with sparse extracellular amyloid and proliferated glial cells; 3. central core of amyloid surrounded by abnormal neurites and glial cells (classical type); 4. amyloid and gliosis with few or no abnormal neurites.

The structure of the abnormal neurites (dendrites and axons) of senile plaques varies considerably in regard to type and quantity of accumulated organelles. The purpose of this presentation is to demonstrate the varying morphology of the abnormal neurites and to compare these findings to those observed in experimental animals in which axons underwent reactive, degenerative, regenerative and dystrophic changes.

Materials and Methods

This study was done on a cortical biopsy from a 36-year old woman who developed behavioral changes at 32 years of age. Her mental status became progressively worse. Mannerisms, memory impairment, confusion and autism were prominent clinical features. Her mother had died of a similar disease and her sister, age 40, has the same symptoms. The biopsy was placed in phosphate-buffered glutaraldehyde, post fixed in osmium and embedded in Araldite. The material from the experimental conditions was obtained from the thoracic spinal cord of rats, 4 to 52 days after cordotomy, for the study of reactive, degenerating and regenerating axons and from the gracile and cuneate nuclei of rats kept on a vitamin E deficient diet for

* This study was supported by United States Public Health Research Grant NS-09053 from the National Institute of Neurological Diseases and Stroke, National Institutes of Health, Bethesda, Maryland.

5 to 10 months for the study of dystrophic axons. For details of these experiments see previous publications (Lampert, 1967). The electron micrographs were made with a Siemens Elmiskop 101 and a Zeiss 9S.

Results

The cortical biopsy was riddled with senile plaques. Many nerve cells were filled with neurofibrillar tangles and pigment granules. The tangles within nerve cells were composed of interlacing bundles of twisted tubules that were oriented parallel to each other. The tubules measured about 200 Å at their widest diameter. Twisting of these tubules occurred at regular periods spaced about 800 Å apart. Except for a few plaques that showed only extracellular amyloid between proliferated astrocytic processes, the vast majority of the plaques were composed of varying numbers of abnormal neurites. Unless synaptic junctions were identified unmyelinated neutries were considered to represent either axons or dendrites. When identifiable, abnormal changes were found in both axons and dendrites. The following alterations were characteristic of the various types of abnormal neurites: 1. densely packed mitochondria with or without membranous dense bodies; 2. membrane-bounded, floccular dense bodies (most frequent finding, Fig. 1); 3. irregular vesicular profiles (Fig. 2); 4. abundant twisted tubules usually associated with a few floccular dense bodies (Figs. 3, 4); 5. vacuolation (seen occasionally in dendrites); 6. granular disintegration of axoplasm (predominently found in myelinated axons in the white matter). The twisted tubules in the abnormal neurites were identical to those seen in the cell bodies of neurons. Amyloid filaments were found in extracellular spaces and within membrane-bounded compartments of glial cells. A clear relationship between amyloid and abnormal neurites could not be established. Amyloid was found between glycogen-filled glial processes and normal neurites and as massive deposits in the core of plaques surrounded by abnormal neurites. Clusters of abnormal neurites without detectable amyloid were, however, much more frequently encountered.

Discussion

Experimental studies on axonal injury have repeatedly confirmed the following facts. After transection the proximal and distal stumps of the severed axons swell. Neurotubules, filaments but particularly mitochondria and membranous dense bodies collect in these swollen axonal enlargements (Webster, 1962). Similar axonal changes also develop focally in uninterrupted axons, e. g., at sites of demyelination (Lampert, 1967). The accumulation of these organelles in the swollen stumps or at sites of focal damage has been interpreted as a reactive phenomenon. Since this phenomenon is most likely caused by axoplasmic stasis followed by settling of organelles at sites of arrested axonal flow, the term "stagnant" axoplasmic change rather than "reactive" might be more appropriate.

Fig. 1. Abnormal neurite in Alzheimer's disease showing membrane-bounded floccular dense bodies. × 30,000

Fig. 2. Irregular vesicular profiles. × 25,000

Fig. 3. Aggregates of interlacing bundles of twisted tubules. × 25,000

Fig. 4. Twisted tubules in abnormal neurite. × 60,000

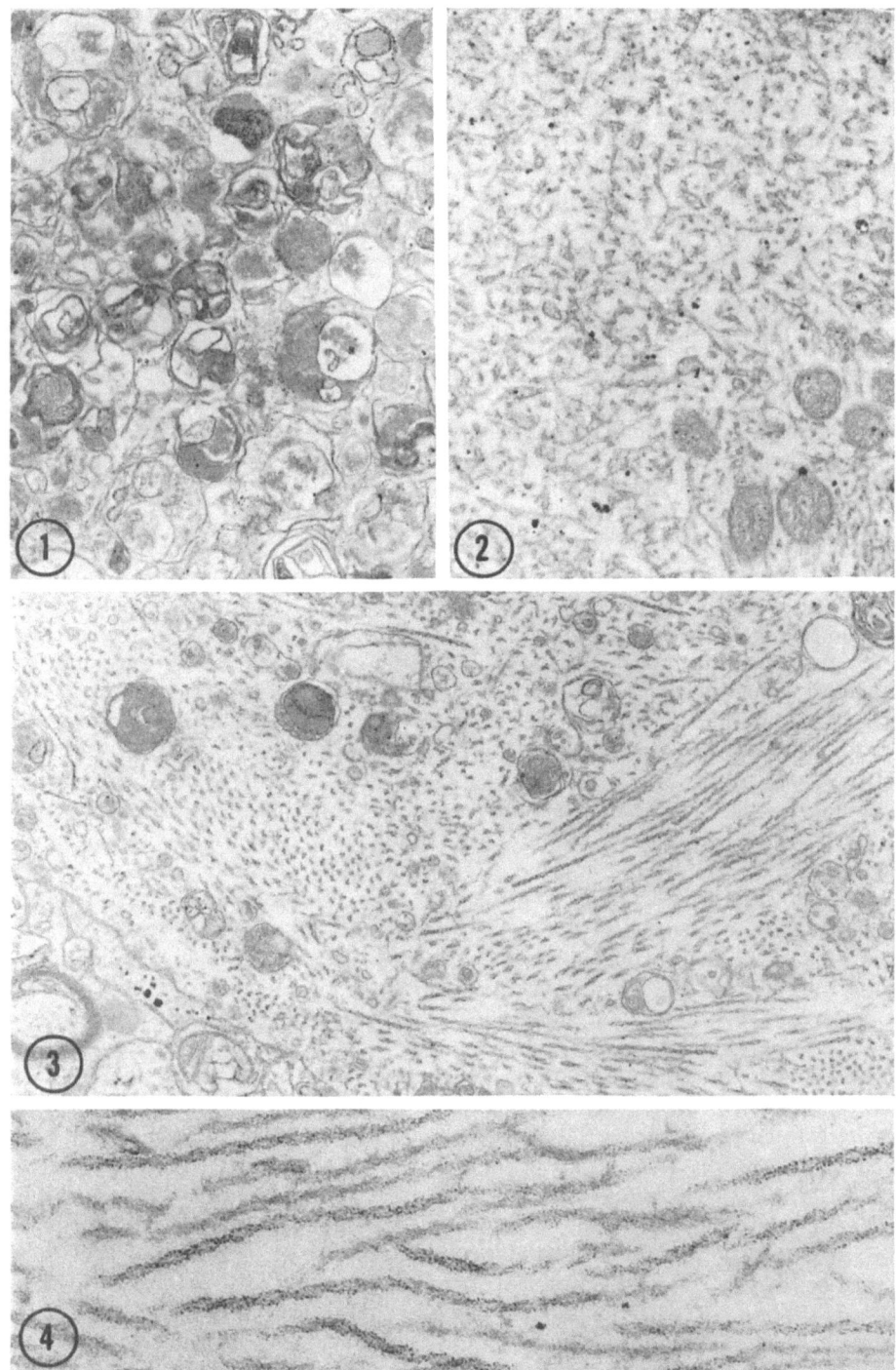

Figs. 1—4

In the enlarged, degenerating stumps of transected axons the accumulated mitochondria change into membrane-bounded floccular dense bodies (Lampert, 1967). Granular disintegration of neurofilaments is characteristic of degenerating axons at a distance from the peritraumatic region.

Regenerating axons show an axoplasm filled with neurofilaments and vesicular structures as well as mitochondria and a few membranous dense bodies. These latter organelles do not usually aggregate to the same degree as observed in "stagnant" axoplasm. Of particular interest is the observation that regenerated axonal sprouts undergo vacuolar degeneration after an abortive attempt at establishing functional connections (Lampert and Cressman, 1964).

Dystrophic axons as observed in Vitamin-E-deficient rats contain conglomerates of organelles that, in places, mimick the appearance of stagnant, degenerating or regenerating axoplasm. In addition other characteristic features are encountered which are not seen in the other experimental conditions, namely, granular dense material that is not bounded by membranes, glycogen granules within mitochondria, concentric arrays of membranes and aggregates of tubular rings (Lampert and Pentschew, 1965).

A comparison of the abnormal neurites in Alzheimer's disease with the axonal changes as seen in the above reviewed experimental conditions indicates the following. 1. Conglomerates of twisted tubules were not seen in the experimental animals. Such tubules are characteristic of altered nerve cells and neurites in man though not limited to Alzheimer's disease (Terry and Wisniewski, 1970; Schochet et al., 1968). 2. Collections of mitochondria and membranous dense bodies were identical to what is observed in stagnant axoplasm of distal degenerating stumps of transected axons. Abundant, membrane-bounded floccular dense bodies in abnormal neurities have been found consistently in senile plaques (Terry et al., 1964; Luse and Smith, 1964; Krigman et al., 1965). 3. Occasional neurites filled with irregular vesicular profiles and neurofilaments resembled regenerating axoplasm. Very similar axonal changes develop in axons following tri-ortho-cresyl phosphate intoxication (Bischoff, 1967; Prineas, 1969). 4. None of the features peculiar to dystrophic axons in Vitamin E deficiency were encountered in the abnormal neurites in Alzheimer's disease.

In regard to the pathogenesis of the abnormal neurites that form the bulk of senile plaques, several ideas must be mentioned. Since many of the abnormal neurites mimick the axonal changes as seen in the peritraumatic regions of the experimental animals, focal injury to neurites appears plausible. It is not known, however, what agent could produce such a change in so many points of the cortex. There is evidence suggesting that the deposition of amyloid is not the primary event. Amyloid is found in association with normal neurites (Wisniewsky et al., 1970); and abnormal neurites are encountered in the absence of detectable amyloid. If focal injury is responsible for the formation of senile plaques one must consider an agent capable of producing both axonal changes and amyloid deposits. At present, the more readily understood explanation for the formation of the abnormal neurites takes into account the characteristic neurofibrillar degeneration of the nerve cells in Alzheimer's disease. Neurofibrillar tangles are believed to severely impede axonal flow which would result in axoplasmic stasis and subsequent accumulation of organelles in the terminal arborization of the neurites (Terry and

Wisniewski, 1970). Experimentally, Wisniewski and Terry (1970) have been able to produce abnormal neurites in the cortex of rabbits that were subjected to drugs known to induce neurofibrillar changes in nerve cells. The fact that some of the neurites showed changes (Fig. 2) similar to what is characteristic of experimentally induced dying back neuropathies (Bischoff, 1967; Prineas, 1969) also supports the idea that senile plaques develop secondary to changes in the nerve cell bodies.

References

Bischoff, A.: The ultrastructure of tri-ortho-cresyl phosphate poisoning. 1. Studies on myelin and axonal alteration in the sciatic nerve. Acta neuropath. (Berl.) **9**, 158—184 (1967).

Krigman, M. D., Feldman, R. G., Bensch, K.: Alzheimer's presenile dementia—a histochemical and electron microscopic study. Lab Invest. **14**, 381—396 (1965).

Lampert, P. W.: A comparative electron microscopic study of reactive, degenerating, regenerating and dystrophic axons. J. Neuropath. exp. Neurol. **26**, 345—367 (1967).

— Cressman, M.: Axonal regeneration in the dorsal column of the spinal cord of adult rats. An electron microscopy study. Lab. Invest. **13**, 825—839 (1964).

— Pentschew, A.: An electron microscopic study of spheroid and convoluted bodies in dystrophic terminal axons. Acta neuropath. (Berl.) **4**, 158—168 (1964).

Luse, S. A., Smith, K. R.: The ultrastructure of senile plaques. Amer. J. Path. **44**, 553—563 (1964).

Prineas, J.: The pathogenesis of dying-back polyneuropathies. I. An ultrastructural study of experimental tri-ortho-cresyl phosphate intoxication in the cat. J. Neuropath. exp. Neurol. **28**, 571—597 (1969).

Schochet, S. S., Lampert, P. W., Lindenberg, R.: Fine structure of the Pick and Hirano bodies in a case of Pick's disease. Acta neuropath. (Berl.) **11**, 330—337 (1968).

Terry, R. D.: The fine structure of neurofibrillary tangles in Alzheimer's disease. J. Neuropath. exp. Neurol. **22**, 629—642 (1963).

— Gonatas, N. K., Weiss, M.: Ultrastructural studies in Alzheimer's presenile dementia. Amer. J. Path. **44**, 269—297 (1964).

— Wisniewski, H.: The ultrastructure of the neurofibrillary tangle and the senile plaque. In: CIBA Foundation Symposium on Alzheimer's disease and related conditions, pp. 143—165. London: Churchill 1970.

Webster, H. de F.: Transient, focal accumulations of axonal mitochondria during the early stages of Wallerian degeneration. J. Cell Biol. **12**, 361—384 (1961).

Wisniewski, H., Johnson, A. B., Raine, C. S., Kay, W. J., Terry, R. D.: Senile plaques and cerebral amyloidosis in aged dogs: A histochemical and ultrastructural study. Lab. Invest. **23**, 281—296 (1970).

— Terry, R. D.: An experimental approach to the morphogenesis of neurofibrillary degeneration and the argyrophilic plaque. In: CIBA Foundation Symposium on Alzheimer's disease and related conditions, pp. 223—240. London: Churchill 1970.

Peter Lampert M.D.
Department of Pathology
University of California at San Diego
La Jolla, Cal. 92037/U.S.A.

Acta neuropath. (Berl.) Suppl. V, 54—60 (1971)

Mitochondrial Changes in Axonal
Dystrophy Produced by Vitamin E Deficiency

Sydney S. Schochet, Jr.

Division of Neuropathology, Department of Pathology,
University of Iowa, Iowa City, Iowa

Summary. Diverse mitochondrial abnormalities constitute one of the conspicuous ultra-structural features of the dystrophic axons that develop in rats maintained on a vitamin E deficient diet. The alterations include enlargement accompanied by pleomorphism, swelling, derangement in the structure of cristae and two types of intramitochondrial deposits. Many of these changes are also observed in other types of cell injury and therefore cannot be considered a specific manifestation of vitamin E deficiency or axonal dystrophy. However, the non-autophagic dissolution of mitochondria leading to the accumulation of unbounded masses of granular dense material appears characteristic of the conditions of chronic neuronal injury that result in dystrophic axon formation.

Key-Words: Axonal Dystrophy — Vitamin E Deficiency — Mitochondria.

Chronic vitamin E deficiency in the rat is regularly accompanied by the development of discontinuous swellings along the course and at the distal termination of certain axons. This process, termed axonal dystrophy (Pentschew and Schwarz, 1962) is especially pronounced in the dorsal funiculi of the spinal cord and in the gracile and cuneate nuclei of the medulla. Ultrastructurally, the resulting fusiform or spheroidal enlargements are characterized by a complex admixture of normal and abnormal cytoplasmic organelles and are distinguishable from reactive, regenerative or degenerating axons (Lampert and Pentschew, 1963; Lampert *et al.*, 1964; and Lampert, 1967). The dramatic alterations in the mitochondria and resulting dense bodies constitute the subject of this report.

Material and Methods

Material from two groups of animals was used in this study. The first group[1] consisted of 14 inbred Fischer 344 rats of both sexes. These animals were maintained on a vitamin E deficient diet containing Torula yeast as a source of protein and supplemented with selenium as a source of factor 3 activity. The animals, sacrificed at intervals between 5 and 10 months of age, were perfused with $1^0/_0$ osmium tetroxide solution.

The second group consisted of 15 female Sprague-Dawley rats. These animals were maintained on a commercial vitamin E deficient diet (Nutritional Biochemicals Corp., Cleveland, Ohio) containing casein and no added selenium. These animals, sacrificed at intervals between 4 and 8 months of age were perfused with a picric acid—formaldehyde solution (Stefanini *et al.*, 1967).

After perfusion, tissue was obtained from the gracile and cuneate nuclei. The blocks from the aldehyde perfused animals were postfixed in $1^0/_0$ osmium tetroxide solution. Subsequently,

---

1 This group of animals had been prepared for previous studies (Lampert and Pentschew, 1963; Lampert *et al.*, 1964; and Lampert, 1967). Epon embedded tissue was made available through the courtesy of Dr. Peter W. Lampert.

the blocks were dehydrated in a graded series of alcohols and embedded in an epoxy resin. Sections 2 μ thick were stained with paraphenylenendiamine for screening. From selected blocks, thin sections were cut and stained with uranyl acetate and lead citrate prior to examination in a Philips 300 electron microscope.

Results

Almost identical mitochondrial changes were observed within the dystrophic axons from both groups of animals despite the differences in strain and type of vitamin E deficient diet. However, primary aldehyde fixation resulted in darker mitochondria with less contrast between the matrix and membranes. Within the axonal enlargements, there were usually large numbers of mitochondria clustered about irregular masses of finely granular osmophilic material (Fig. 1 a). The mitochondria were generally larger and more pleomorphic than in normal axons. Some of the mitochondria were markedly enlongated and folded but most were enlarged with irregular contours (i.e., bulbous). Although the surfaces of adjacent mitochondria were occasionally in contact, none were observed to protrude into one another.

The cristae displayed many alterations (Fig. 1 b, c). Often they were increased in number and apparently unattached to the inner membrane of the envelope. Particularly in the bulbous forms the arrangement of the cristae was frequently disorderly or even concentric. The individual cristae were variously laminar, angular or tubular. Often a single outer membrane surrounded several closed chambers derived from the inner membrane of the envelope. In the mitochondria altered in this manner, multiple groups of cristae were present, each group arising from the infolding of a separate inner membrane chamber. Intramitochondrial vesicles apparently derived from fragmentation and dilatation of portions of individual cristae were present. Still other cristae were in contact with and appeared to give rise to small myelin figures.

Many of the mitochondria appeared abnormally electron dense due to a very finely granular material that was dispersed uniformly throughout the matrix. Often this material condensed into irregular granular masses within the matrix (Fig. 1 b). These masses were more common in severely disarranged mitochondria. Accumulations of glycogen granules were present in some of the mitochondria, and were found in either the intracristal space or between the inner and outer membranes of the envelope. Some of the glycogen deposits were sufficiently large to compress and displace the other mitochondrial components.

Occasionally, severely altered mitochondria displayed focal to extensive dissolution of the outer membrane of the envelope (Fig. 1 c). Where exposed, the inner membrane was irregularly serrated. Further degeneration resulted in dissolution of the inner membrane and the mitochondrial contents, including the dense granular material and the altered cristae, spilled into the surrounding cytoplasm. During this process of lysis of the membranes of the envelope, no membranes corresponding to the periphery of autophagic vacuoles or cytolysosomes were recognized. The absence of isolating membranes distinguished this process of mitochondrial dissolution from the occasionally observed autophagic vacuoles in which small portions of cytoplasm and mitochondria were being degraded.

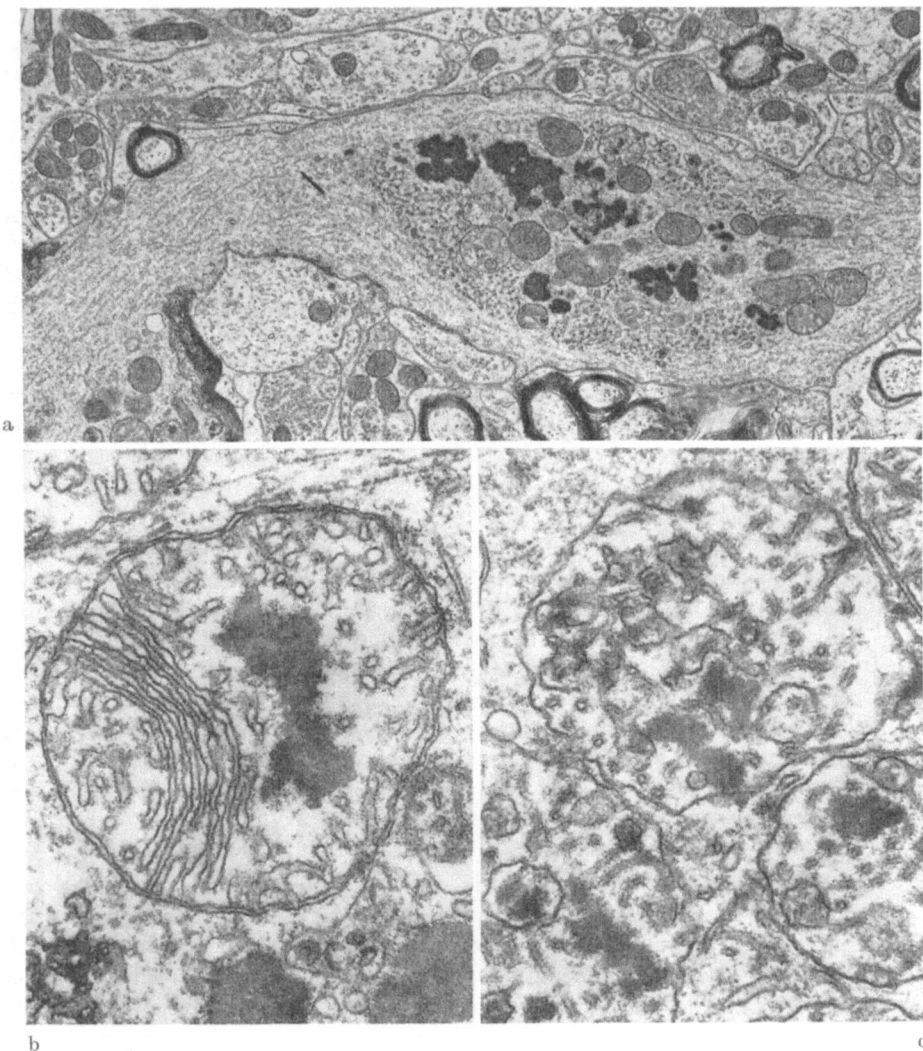

Fig. 1 a—c. Electron microscopic appearance of mitochondria in dystrophic axons produced by vitamin E deficiency.   a Note the dense granular material associated with altered mitochondria. ×14,000;   b Note the abnormal arrangement of cristae and the finely granular osmophilic material within the matrix compartment. ×42,000;   c Mitochondria undergoing dissolution of the membranes of the envelope. ×42,000

Discussion

Diverse mitochondrial alterations constitute one of the most conspicuous ultrastructure features of the dystrophic axons. The role of vitamin E deficiency in producing these changes is not clear for they have also been observed in the dystrophic axons of aged rats (Schochet, 1971). Many may be non-specific mitochondrial reactions to cellular injury. One of the common findings, mitochondrial enlargement accompanied by pleomorphism has also been observed in liver cells of rats maintained on a vitamin E deficient diet (Sulkin and Sulkin, 1962) or on a necrogenic diet deficient in both tocopherol and factor 3-selenium (Svoboda and Higginson, 1963). However, these same mitochondrial alterations have been prominent in various other situations such as in neurons of Gunn rats affected by bilirubin encephalopathy (Schutta et al., 1970) and in hepatocytes from mice on a diet deficient in essential fatty acids (Wilson and Leduc, 1963).

Many of the abnormal mitochondria were also swollen. Unlike mitochondrial enlargement in which there is an increase in structural components, swelling is due to an altered membrane permeability and imbibition of water. This is a ubiquetous change, perhaps reflecting a decrease P:0 ratio, that can accompany almost any type of cell injury (Trump and Ericsson, 1965). The various alterations in the structure of the cristae, such as disorderly arrangement, fragmentation and vesiculation are also found in many types of cellular injury and must be considered a non-specific reaction (Trump and Ericsson, 1965). The myelin figures occasionally present in mitochondria are considered to be derived from the phospholipids of the membranes in response to various stimuli (Le Beux et al., 1969).

Deposits of two types of granular osmophilic material were present in the abnormal mitochondria. Coarse granular material, apparently glycogen, was found in the envelope and the intracristal spaces. The larger deposits of this material displaced and compressed other mitochondrial components. Similar deposits of glycogen have been reported in various normal (Ishikawa and Pei, 1965; Berthold, 1966; Lin, 1965; and Yamamoto et al., 1969) and abnormal tissues (Schutta et al., 1970; Tandler and Shipkey, 1964; Hug and Schubert, 1970). The origin of these deposits in obscure since glycogen synthesis is not considered to occur in mitochondria.

The second type of deposit, consisting of finely granular osmophilic material occurred as irregular masses within the matrix. In the dystrophic axons, these deposits were more common in the severely altered mitochondria. Accumulations of this material have been seen following several types of cell injury (Svoboda and Higginson, 1963; Minick et al., 1965; Trump et al., 1965; Gritzka and Trump, 1968). The proximity to degenerating mitochondrial membranes led to the suggestion that they are composed of phospholipids (Trump et al., 1965); later work suggested that they may be denatured proteins from the matrix. This concept was supported by the rapid appearance of similar material in mitochondria denatured by boiling water, laser radiation or heavy metals (Gritzka and Trump, 1968). Less drastic conditions can also lead to the appearance of similar intramitochondrial masses of granular material, for they have been observed in the kidney of starved summer and early winter frogs (Karnovsky, 1963) and in various cells of a snake during and following hibernation (Yamamoto et al., 1969). These deposits are unlike the calcific deposits that have been observed in mitochondria inasmuch as they are not microcrystalline and are not closely embraced by cristae (Gritzka and Trump, 1968).

In the dystrophic axons, clusters of abnormal mitochondria commonly accompany or even surround unbounded intracytoplasmic masses of finely granular osmophilic material. Lampert (1967) suggested that these aggregates may be

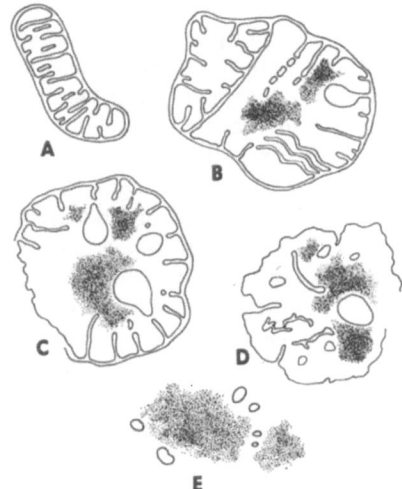

Fig. 2. Diagram of the successive steps during the non-autophagic mitochondrial dissolution leading to unbounded granular dense material and vesicles

derived from the confluence of similar appearing electron-dense material in the matrix of disintegrating mitochondria. The demonstration of abnormal mitochondria undergoing dissolution of the membranes of the envelope supports this hypothesis. Furthermore, it seems possible that some of the small vesicles associated with the intracytoplasmic dense material may be derived from degenerated cristae. Similar focal to extensive dissolution of the membranes of the mitochondrial envelope have been observed during *in vitro* necrosis of liver (Trump *et al.*, 1965) and renal tubular necrosis (Gritzka and Trump, 1968), and Cuprizone intoxication (Suzuki and Kikkawa, 1969).

Dissolution of the membranes is not the only process by which mitochondria are degraded in the dystrophic axons. Occasionally, single or double smooth membranes isolated small portions of cytoplasm, some of which contained mitochondria. The resulting structures appeared identical to autophagic vacuoles digesting mitochondria, a process that has been repeatedly demonstrated (Ashford and Porter, 1962; Elliott and Bak, 1964; Howes *et al.*, 1964; Swift and Hruban, 1964; Locke and Collins, 1965; Arstilla and Trump, 1968; Winborn and Bockman, 1968; and many others). This process of autophagic degradation clearly gives rise to some of the membrane bound dense bodies observed in the dystrophic axons.

Thus, many of the mitochondrial changes observed in this study are also encountered in other forms of cellular injury and cannot be regarded as unique to either vitamin E deficiency or axonal dystrophy. However, the process of non-autophagic dissolution of mitochondria leading to the accumulation of unbounded masses of granular dense material (Fig. 2) appears to be characteristic of the conditions of very chronic neuronal injury that result in dystrophic axon formation.

References

Arstila, A. U., Trump, B. F.: Studies on cellular autophagocytosis. Amer. J. Path. **53**, 687—733 (1968).

Ashford, T. P., Porter, K. R.: Cytoplasmic components in hepatic cell lysosomes. J. Cell Biol. **12**, 198—202 (1962).

Le Beux, Y., Hetenyi, G., Jr., Phillips, M. J.: Mitochondrial myelin-like figures: A non-specific reactive process of mitochondrial phospholipid membranes to several stimuli. Z. Zellforsch. **99**, 491—506 (1969).

Berthold, C.-H.: Ultrastructural appearance of glycogen in the B-neurons of lumbar spinal ganglia of the frog. J. Ultrastruct. Res. **14**, 254—267 (1966).

Elliott, A. M., Bak, I. J.: The fate of mitochondria during aging in *Tetrahymena pyriformis*. J. Cell Biol. **20**, 113—129 (1964).

Gritzka, T. L., Trump, B. F.: Renal tubular lesions caused by mercuric chloride. Electron microscopic observations: Degeneration of the pars recta. Amer. J. Path. **52**, 1225—1277 (1968).

Howes, E. L., Price, H. M., Blumberg, J. M.: The effects of a diet producing lipochrome pigment (ceroid) on the ultrastructure of skeletal muscle in the rat. Amer. J. Path. **45**, 599—631 (1964).

Hug, G., Schubert, W. K.: Idiopathic cardiomyopathy: Mitochondrial and cytoplasmic alterations in heart and liver. Lab. Invest. **22**, 541—552 (1970).

Ishikawa, T., Pei, Y. F.: Intramitochondrial glycogen particles in rat retinal receptor cells. J. Cell Biol. **25**, 402—407 (1965).

Karnovsky, M. J.: The fine structure of mitochondria in the frog nephron correlated with cytochrome oxidase. Exp. molec. Path. **2**, 347—366 (1963).

Lampert, P.: A comparative electron microscopic study of reactive, degenerating, regenerating, and dystrophic axons. J. Neuropath. exp. Neurol. **26**, 345—368 (1967).

— Blumberg, J. M., Pentschew, A.: An electron microscopic study of dystrophic axons in the gracile and cuneate nuclei of vitamin E deficient rats. J. Neuropath. exp. Neurol. **23**, 60—77 (1964).

— Pentschew, A.: An electron microscopic study of spheroidal and convoluted bodies in dystrophic terminal axons. Acta neuropath. (Berl.) **4**, 158—168 (1964).

Lin, H. S.: Microcylinders within mitochondrial cristae in the rat pinealocyte. J. Cell Biol. **25**, 435—442 (1965).

Locke, M., Collins, J. V.: The structure and formation of protein granules in the fat body of an insect. J. Cell Biol. **26**, 857—884 (1965).

Minick, O. T., Kent, G., Orfei, E., Volini, F. I.: Non-membrane enclosed intramitochondrial dense bodies. Exp. molec. Path. **4**, 311—319 (1965).

Pentschew, A., Schwarz, K.: Systemic axonal dystrophy in vitamin E deficient adult rats. Acta neuropath. (Berl.) **1**, 313—334 (1962).

Schochet, S. S., Jr.,: Comparison of axonal dystrophy resulting from vitamin E deficiency and aging. (In preparation) 1971.

Schutta, H. S., Johnson, L., Neville, H. E.: Mitochondrial abnormalities in bilirubin encephalopathy. J. Neuropath. exp. Neurol. **24**, 296—305 (1970).

Stefanini, M., De Martino, C., Zamboni, L.: Fixation of ejaculated spermatozoa for electron microscopy. Nature (Lond.) **216**, 173—174 (1967).

Sulkin, N. M., Sulkin, D.: Mitochondrial alterations in liver cells following vitamin E deficiency In: Fifth International Congress for Electron Microscopy (S. S. Breese, ed.), V. 2, vv-8. New York: Academic Press 1962.

Suzuki, K., Kikkawa, Y.: Status spongiosus of CNS and hepatic changes induced by cuprizone (biscyclohexanone) oxalyldihydrozone. Amer. J. Path. **54**, 307—325 (1969).

Svoboda, D. J., Higginson, J.: Ultrastructural hepatic changes in rats on a necrogenic diet. Amer. J. Path. **43**, 477—495 (1963).

Swift, H., Hruban, Z.: Focal degradation as a biological process. Fed. Proc. **23**, 1026—1037 (1964).

Tandler, B., Shipkey, F. H.: Ultrastructure of Warthin's tumor. J. Ultrastruct. Res. **11**, 292—305 (1964).

Trump, B. F., Ericsson, J. L. E.: Some ultrastructural and biochemical consequences of cell injury. In: The Inflammatory Process (B. W. Zweifach, L. H. Grant and R. T. McCluskey, eds.). New York: Academic Press 1965.
— Goldblatt, P. J., Stowell, R. E.: Studies on necrosis of mouse liver *in vitro*. Ultrastructural alterations in the mitochondria of hepatic parenchymal cells. Lab. Invest. **14**, 343—371 (1965).
Wilson, J. W., Leduc, E. H.: Mitochondrial changes in the liver of essential fatty acid-deficient mice. J. Cell Biol. **16**, 281—296 (1963).
Winborn, W. B., Bockman, D. E.: Origin of lysosomes in parietal cells. Lab. Invest. **19**, 256—264 (1968).
Yamamoto, T., Ebe, T., Kobayashi, S.: Intramitochondrial inclusions in various cells of a snake (*Elaphae quadrivirgata*). Z. Zellforsch. **99**, 252—262 (1969).

Sydney S. Schochet, Jr., M.D.
Department of Pathology
University of Iowa
Iowa City, Iowa 52240 /U.S.A.

Acta neuropath. (Berl.) Suppl. V, 61—69 (1971)

Permeability of Blood Vessels and Connective Tissue Sheaths in the Peripheral Nervous System to Exogenous Proteins

Y. Olsson, K. Kristensson

Neuropathological Laboratory, Institute of Pathology,
University of Göteborg, Sweden

I. Klatzo

Laboratory of Neuropathology and Neuroanatomical Sciences,
National Institute of Neurological Diseases and Stroke,
National Institutes of Health, Bethesda

Summary. Some observations on the permeability of blood vessels and connective tissue sheaths in the peripheral nervous system to exogenous proteins are reviewed. The perineurium and the vessels play a crucial role in the regulation of the internal milieu of the endoneurium in peripheral nerve by acting as diffusion barriers. However, the root sheaths of adult animals and the perineurium of immature mice and rats lack this property which makes it possible for various substances to diffuse into the endoneurium of the nerve roots and into nerve fasciculi of immature animals. Blood vessels in dorsal root ganglia and in the epineurium of the nerve trunks differ from those in the central nervous system and those in the endoneurium of peripheral nerve in being permeable to exogenous proteins.

Exogenous proteins which are brought into the endoneurium can diffuse widely in the extracellular spaces. Ultrastructural studies with peroxidase as tracer have shown that this protein can pass the basement membrane surrounding Schwann cells and enter the mesaxon. Some new observations on uptake and retrograde transport of exogenous proteins in axons of immature animals are also presented.

Key-Words: Permeability — Vasa nervorum — Perineurium — Axonal Flow.

Introduction

Previous studies on axons in peripheral nerve have elucidated various aspects of a proximo-distal flow of organelles, neurotransmittors and endogenous proteins labelled with radioactive amino acids (cf. Grafstein, 1969). The possibility that certain toxins and viruses may reach the central nervous system (CNS) by a transport in axons in the opposite direction has previously been proposed (Goodpasture, 1925; Sabin, 1937; Bodian and Howe, 1941), but is now generally discarded (Wright, 1953; Johnson and Mims, 1968; Zachs and Saito, 1969a). However, recent experimental data strongly indicate that this actually is one route by which certain viruses can reach the CNS after peripheral inoculation (Kristensson, 1970).

It is obvious that one condition for uptake and transport of various substances in axons of peripheral nerve is that they after systemic or peripheral administration are brought into direct contact with the axons. It is therefore important to determine how various macromolecular substances can enter the interior of the nerve fasciculi from the blood and from the site of peripheral administration. This presentation concerns the permeability of blood vessels and connective tissue sheaths in the peripheral nervous system (PNS) to exogenous proteins. Some new observations on uptake and transport of protein tracers in axons of immature animals are also presented.

Structure and Permeability of Blood Vessels in the Peripheral Nervous Systems

Peripheral Nerve. To provide a background for the following discussion on the vascular permeability some structural features of the blood vessels must be considered. When a nutrient artery reaches a nerve it forms a plexus of thin winding vessels. The epineurial vessels are connected with vessels situated between the perineurial cell layers which in turn communicate with the endoneurial vascular plexus. At the entrance and exit of blood vessels to and from the endoneurium, the vessels acquire a single perineurial sleeve which invests and accompanies them for a short distance into the endoneurium. Most vessels inside the endoneurium are capillaries which run lengthwise between the nerve fibres (for ref. see Lundborg, 1970; Olsson, 1971a).

The endoneurial blood vessels in peripheral nerve are surrounded by connective tissue containing large extracellular spaces. This organization is quite different from that in most parts of the CNS where the extracellular space is small and the glial cells closely invest the walls of capillaries. Only a few ultrastructural studies on the vasa nervorum have been reported (Olsson and Reese, 1969, 1971). A major difference between epineurial and endoneurial vessels in mouse sciatic nerve is the presence of tight junctions between endothelial cells in endoneurial vessels whereas epineurial vessels are joined by junctions of the open variety (Olsson and Reese, 1969, 1971). The tight junctions are pentalaminar and the apposing leaflets of the plasma membrane are fused. The open junctions contain a fine intermediate slit through which protein tracers like horseradish peroxidase can penetrate. However, it is not known if the mouse shares these ultrastructural properties of the vasa nervorum with other species.

Previous investigations of the vascular permeability in the PNS have been carried out with the same methods that have been applied in studies on the blood-brain barrier (BBB) (Waksman, 1963; Olsson, 1966; Mellick and Cavanagh, 1968). Serum proteins have in these studies been labelled with dyes, fluorescent and radioactive markers, which after intravenous (i.v.) administration have been visualized microscopically. Horseradish peroxidase has recently been used as protein tracer (Olsson and Reese, 1969, 1971), since a sensitive localization of this marker can be obtained by enzymatic action on an appropriate substrate (Graham and Karnovsky, 1966).

Following i.v. injection of fluorescent labelled albumin or gamma globulin, these proteins can almost immediately be traced to the lumen of epineurial vessels, and appear later in the connective tissue around the vessels (Olsson, 1966). The epineurial vessels therefore share with many other vessels in the body the ability to allow the passage of serum proteins across their walls (cf. Mancini, 1963). In such tissues there is normally a slow flow of serum proteins from the blood to the extracellular space. The proteins are then resorbed and conveyed back to the blood in lymphatics.

The permeability of the endoneurial blood vessels varies between different species (Waksman, 1963; Olsson, 1966, 1967, 1971b). Following their i.v. injection

in the rat and the mouse, fluorescent proteins are confined to the lumina of endoneurial blood vessels, and the tracers do not pass into the extracellular space of
the endoneurium (Olsson, 1966, 1968). However, in other species, such as guinea-
pig and hen, small amounts of proteins can be detected also outside endoneurial
blood vessels (Olsson, 1967, 1971 b).

The permeability of the endoneurial blood vessels in mouse sciatic nerve has
recently been studied with the peroxidase technique (Olsson and Reese, 1969,
1971). This tracer was stopped by the tight junctions between the endothelial
cells and was not transported across the endothelial cell cytoplasm by pinocytosis.
The endothelium of the endoneurial blood vessels in mouse sciatic nerve therefore
acts as a barrier to this tracer. The reason why proteins leak out from endoneurial
vessels in some other species is not known. Presumably, species differences in the
type of endothelial cell junctions are responsible.

Dorsal Root Ganglia and Spinal Nerve Roots. When albumin labelled with
Evans blue (EBA) is injected i.v. into mammals the CNS including the spinal
cord remains unstained but the dorsal root ganglia stain intensely blue by extra-
vasated tracer. Under a fluorescence microscope EBA can be seen in and outside
the lumen of blood vessels. The tracer rapidly penetrates the connective tissue
septa and occupies the spaces around neurons (Fig. 1). This phenomenon occurs
in all species thus far examined (Olsson, 1967, 1971 b). The vascular permeability
in dorsal root ganglia is therefore different from that in the CNS. The dorsal root
ganglia are richly vascularized and like other vessels in the PNS surrounded by
connective tissue containing large extracellular spaces. We have recently observed
that blood vessels in dorsal root ganglia of the rhesus monkey are fenestrated and
that some junctions are of the open variety. It is possible that the protein tracers
leak out from ganglionic vessels through either one of these regions but conclusive
evidence would require demonstration of an ultrastructural tracer passing these
areas of the vascular wall. Such information has not yet been obtained.

Few reliable data are available about the vascular permeability in spinal nerve
roots. However, some observations indicate that these vessels like those in the
ganglia are permeable to various protein tracers (Waksman, 1963; Olsson, 1968).

Structure and Permeability of Connective Tissue Sheaths Surrounding the Peripheral Nervous System

Peripheral Nerve. The epineurium, the perineurium and the endoneurium are
the terms introduced by Key and Retzius (1876) and still commonly used for the
various connective tissue compartments in peripheral nerve trunks. The different
fascicles of a nerve are embedded in loose connective tissue, i.e. the epineurium.
Each fascicle is surrounded by a perineurium, which is distinctly delineated from
the endoneurium (see review by Shantha and Bourne, 1969). The inner part of the
perineurium is formed by multiple layers of polygonal flattened cells surrounded
by basement membranes. The number of lamellae varies considerably from nerve
to nerve. Intramuscular nerve branches also loose their perineurial investment
immediately before the endorgan, where the nerve fibres are surrounded only by
the Schwann cells (Burkel, 1967; Saito and Zachs, 1969). In this area horseradish
peroxidase can diffuse into the endoneurium after intramuscular injection (Zachs
and Saito, 1969).

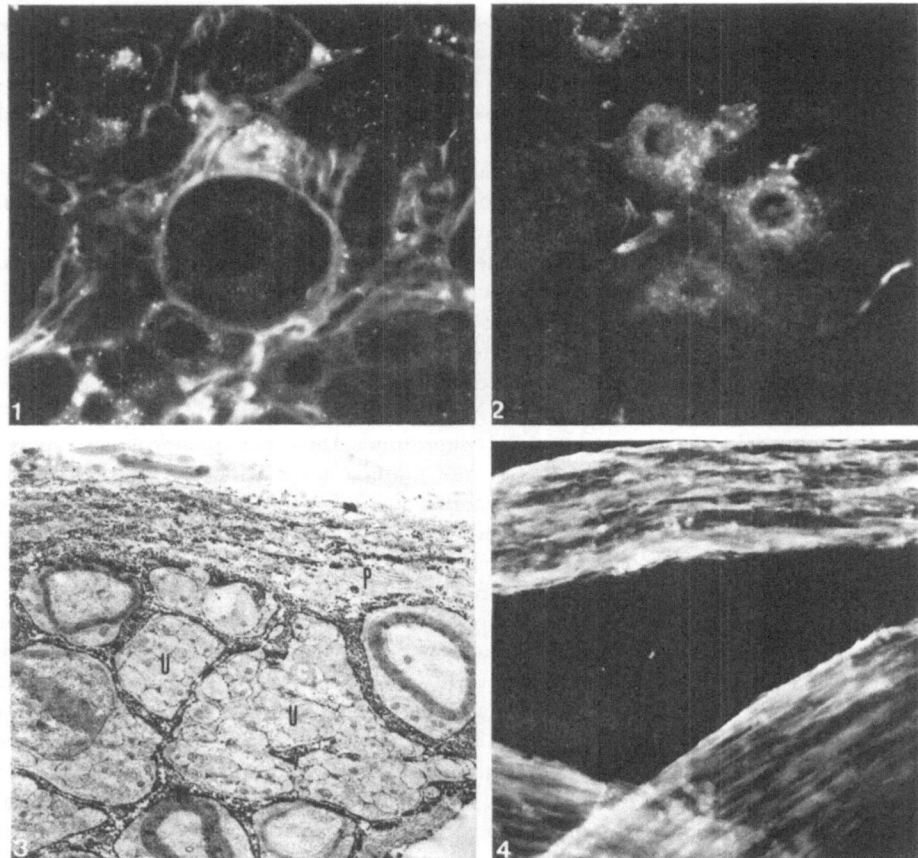

Fig. 1. Dorsal root ganglion after intravenous injection of albumin labelled with Evans blue (*EBA*). The fluorescent tracer has leaked out of the vessels and occupies spaces between neurons

Fig. 2. Ventral motoneurons in the spinal cord of a newborn mouse. EBA was injected in the gastrocnemius muscle and the fluorescent tracer has been transported to the neuronal cytoplasm. Autofluorescent products are not present in this age group

Fig. 3. Peroxidase injected around a sciatic nerve from an immature mouse has penetrated the perineurium (*P*) and spread in the extracellular space of the endoneurium. Note the presence of reaction product (tracer) in mesaxons of unmyelinated nerve fibres (*U*)

Fig. 4. Multiple fascicles of a newborn mouse sciatic nerve after injection of EBA around the nerve. The fluorescent tracer has penetrated the perineurium and spread in the endoneurium

Junctions between cells and basement membranes are particularly important for barrier functions in other parts of the organism (Karnovsky, 1967) and therefore deserve particular attention. Adjacent perineurial cells are joined by tight junctions (Olsson and Reese, 1969, 1971; Klemm, 1970). Since the perineurial cells at the site of the junctions sometimes loose their basement membrane the only complete investment around the nerve fasciculi is the cytoplasmic processes of the perineurial cells. From the morphological point of view the closely apposed perineurial cells connected with tight junctions are therefore well equipped to act as a diffusion barrier to various substances.

Physiological studies have shown that the connective tissue sheaths of peripheral nerves may act as a diffusion barrier to a broad range of substances including proteins (see Martin, 1964; Olsson, 1966). Recent ultrastructural observations with ferrithin (Waggener et al., 1965) and horseradish peroxidase (Olsson and Reese, 1969, 1971; Klemm, 1970) have provided conclusive evidence that the perineurium is the site of the diffusion barrier to proteins in the nerve sheaths. After injection around the sciatic nerve ferritin is stopped at the outer part of the perineurium presumably by basement membranes but peroxidase can penetrate the outer perineurial layers. In mouse sciatic nerve the diffusion of peroxidase is prevented by intermediate perineurial lamellae, which form complete circumferential belts around the nerve fasciculi. Here intercellular diffusion is prevented by the tight junctions and transport across the perineurial cell cytoplasm by pinocytosis is insignificant.

Studies on the structure and function of the perineurium have previously almost entirely been confined to various nerves in adult animals. However, we have recently obtained some interesting data in immature animals (Kristensson and Olsson, 1971). Following local injection of various proteins around the sciatic nerve of suckling rats and mice the tracers rapidly penetrated the perineurium and spread extensively in the endoneurium (Figs. 3, 4). The barrier function of the perineurium was not fully developed until about 3 weeks post partum. Newborn guinea-pigs, on the other hand, showed a normal barrier function.

Using horseradish peroxidase as tracer we have also studied electronmicroscopically the difference in permeability of the perineurium between mature and immature mice (Kristensson and Olsson, 1971). Wide gaps were present between some perineurial cells of newborn mice through which peroxidase diffused into the endoneurium. The difference in permeability of the nerve sheaths between mature and immature animals must therefore be due to differences in the apposition of the perineurial cells providing open pathways in the young but not in the adult mice.

Dorsal Root Ganglia and Spinal Nerve Roots. The dorsal root ganglia are covered with extensions of the perineurium and the epineurium. The ultrastructural features are similar to those in peripheral nerve (Lieberman, 1968).

Light microscopy did not provide much new information on the connective tissue covering of spinal nerve roots since Key and Retzius (1876) published their detailed observations on the anatomy of peripheral nerves. McGabe and Low (1969) recently described the ultrastructural appearance of the root sheaths in the rat subarachnoid space. The sheaths covering the roots was composed of loosely arranged cells only bound together by punctate junctions. The loose arrangement of the root sheath therefore provides an open pathway from the subarachnoid space to the endoneurium of the roots. This has presumably important implications regarding the transmission of various substances from the subarachnoid space to the roots but few experimental data are available with regard to this possibility. However, Klatzo and coworkers (1964) have observed a rapid penetration of protein tracers from the cerebrospinal fluid into the endoneurium of the roots.

Interestingly, the tracer spread extensively in the endoneurial connective tissue but stopped abruptly at the boundary with the spinal cord paranchyma.

Spread of Exogenous Proteins in the Endoneurium and in Axons of Immature Animals

Since various macromolecular substances under certain conditions may diffuse into the endoneurium of the PNS, it is particularly important to elucidate their further spread. Weiss and coworkers (1945) made a detailed study on the spread of various substances in the endoneurium of peripheral nerve and concluded that there is normally an endoneurial flow which is directed towards the periphery and not towards the spinal cord. It is also known that horseradish peroxidase which experimentally has been introduced into the endoneurium can diffuse extensively in the extracellular spaces between the nerve fibres (Olsson and Reese, 1969, 1971; Kristensson and Olsson, 1970). These studies also showed that the tracer can pass the basement membrane surrounding Schwann cells and penetrate the outer mesaxon of both myelinated and unmyelinated nerve fibres. Protein uptake into axons of adult animals has not yet been reported but a few vesicles in the endplate may contain peroxidase after intramuscular injection (Zachs and Saito, 1969). In dorsal root ganglia neurons may also contain protein tracer in cytoplasmic vesicles but their absolute numbers are few (Holtzman and Peterson, 1969).

Recent experimental observations also strongly indicate that uptake of EBA actually may occur in axons of immature animals under certain conditions (Kristensson, 1970). When this tracer was injected into the gastrocnemius muscle of suckling mice it diffused into the endoneurium of the sciatic nerve. Furthermore, red fluorescent granules were seen in the cytoplasm of motoneurons in the spinal cord (Fig. 2). Neurons containing tracer were restricted to the ipsilateral side and to a level of the cord that corresponded to the entrance of the nerve roots from the sciatic nerve. There was no abnormal permeability of blood vessels in the spinal cord and in adult mice the same phenomenon did not occur (Kristensson, 1970).

The remarkable and previously unrecognized phenomenon that a fluorescent protein tracer injected intramuscularly into suckling mice can be transferred to the originating motoneurons in the spinal cord seems to provide evidence for the presence of a mechanism for a rapid transport in axons of peripheral nerve directed opposite to the previously well known proximo-distal axonal flow (Kristensson, 1970). This finding supports the hypothesis advanced in some recent studies, that certain viruses can be transported inside axons to the CNS (Baringer and Griffith, 1970; Kristensson, 1970a; Kristensson et al., 1970). The similarity between the migration of the injected EBA and of such viruses was close: in both cases ipsilateral motoneurons were directly involved (Kristensson, 1970a, b).

Concluding Remarks

The entire peripheral somatic nervous system is surrounded by connective tissue sheaths with specialized structural and functional properties (see review by Shantha and Bourne, 1969). These sheaths are involved in the regulation of the internal milieu of the endoneurium, which in most areas can be kept different from that in surrounding tissues. The perineurium enclosing peripheral nerve fasciculi appears to play a crucial role for this regulation by acting as a diffusion barrier to a broad range of substances including proteins (see Martin, 1964; Olsson, 1966; Shantha and Bourne, 1969). This is presumably of utmost importance in various pathological processes. For instance, peripheral nerve trunks may pass through septic foci with no or only minor alterations of endoneurial structures probably since various toxins and infectious agents are prevented from diffusing into the endoneurium by the perineurium.

The connective tissue sheaths covering the spinal nerve roots in their passage through the subarachnoid space have a different structural organization (McGabe and Low, 1969) and different permeability properties (Klatzo *et al.*, 1964). In this area, the loose arrangement of the connective tissue cells provides an open pathway from the subarachnoid space to the endoneurium of the roots. This has presumably important implications for the development of some lesions mediated by infectious agents in the cerebrospinal fluid.

The regulation of the internal milieu of the endoneurium in PNS is carried out not only by the connective tissue sheaths but also by the endoneurial blood vessels (cf. Olsson, 1966). These vessels are impermeable or show a low permeability to protein tracers in most parts of the PNS except for dorsal root ganglia and spinal nerve roots (Olsson, 1968, 1971 b). Variations in permeability between such areas and between different species are presumably important for the distribution of lesions caused by some blood-born agents, for instance diphtheric and allergic polyneuritis (Waksman, 1963). In such diseases the pathological alterations are most severe in areas with permeable vessels whereas areas with impermeable vessels usually are unaffected by the disease.

Once inside the endoneurium, various agents including protein tracers can diffuse extensively (cf. Weiss *et al.*, 1945) and penetrate the basement membrane surrounding Schwann cells and then into mesaxons (Olsson and Reese, 1969, 1971; Klemm, 1970). Such tracers have extensive access to axonal membrane in unmyelinated fibres and the nodes of Ranvier is another area where exogenous proteins come in immediate contact to myelinated axons.

In adult animals the neurons and axons of the PNS show a low uptake of exogenous proteins under normal conditions. However, observations by one of us in immature animals show that exogenous agents including proteins actually can be taken up into axons and then be transported to the originating cell bodies in the spinal cord (Kristensson, 1970). The mechanism and detailed ways by which this uptake and disto-proximal transport occur have not yet been fully analyzed but such studies utilizing electron microscopic tracer techniques are now in progress. This phenomenon deserves particular attention since our data indicate that this presumably is one route by which certain neurovirulent viruses may reach the CNS.

Acknowledgement. We are indebted to Prof. Patrick Sourander for a most valuable support of our work in the Neuropathological Laboratory, Göteborg. Financial support was there obtained from the Swedish Medical Research Council, Projects no. B70-12X-82-05., K70-12X-3020-01A and B71-12X-3020-02A. Other data were obtained when one of us (Y. O.) worked as Visiting Scientist in the Laboratory of Neuropathology and Neuroanatomical Sciences, NINDS, NIH, Bethesda, Md.

References

Baringer, J. R., Griffith, J. F.: Experimental herpes simplex encephalitis: early neuropathological changes. J. Neuropath. exp. Neurol. **29**, 89—104 (1970).

Bodian, D., Howe, H. A.: Experimental studies on intraneural spread of poliomyelitis virus Bull. Johns Hopk. Hosp. **68**, 248—268 (1941).

Burkel, W. E.: The histological fine structure of perineurium. Anat. Rec. **158**, 177—190 (1967).

Goodpasture, E. W.: The axis-cylinders of peripheral nerves as portals of entry to the central nervous system for the virus of herpes simplex in experimentally infected rabbits. Amer. J. Path. **1**, 11—28 (1925).

Grafstein, B.: Axonal transport: Communication between soma and synapse. Advanc. Biochem. Psychopharm. **1**, 11—25 (1969).

Graham, R. C., Karnovsky, M. J.: The early stages of absorption of injected horseradish peroxidase in the proximal tubules of mouse kidney: Ultrastructural correlates with a new technique. J. Histochem. Cytochem. **14**, 291—299 (1966).

Holtzmann, E., Peterson, E.: Uptake of protein by mammalian neurons. J. Cell Biol. **40**, 863—869 (1969).

Johnson, R. T., Mims, C. A.: Pathogenesis of viral infections of the nervous system. New Engl. J. Med. **278**, 23—30 (1968).

Key, A., Retzius, A.: Studien in der Anatomie des Nervensystems und des Bindegewebes. Stockholm: Samson & Wallin 1876.

Klatzo, I., Miquel, J., Ferris, P. J., Prokop, J. D., Smith, D. E.: Observations on the passage of the fluorescein labeled serum proteins (FLSP) from the cerebrospinal fluid. J. Neuropath. exp. Neurol. **23**, 18—35 (1964).

Klemm, H.: Das Perineurium als Diffusionsbarriere gegenüber Peroxydase bei epi- und endoneuraler Applikation. Z. Zellforsch. **108**, 431—445 (1970).

Kristensson, K.: Morphological studies of the neuronal spread of herpes simplex virus to the central nervous system. Acta neuropath. (Berl.) **16**, 54—63 (1970).

— Transport of fluorescent protein tracer in peripheral nerves. Acta neuropath. (Berl.) **16**, 293—300 (1970).

— Lycke, E., Sjöstrand, J.: Spread of herpes simplex virus in peripheral nerves. Acta neuropath. (Berl.) **17**, 44—53 (1971).

— Olsson, Y.: The perineurium as a diffusion barrier to protein tracers. Differences between mature and immature animals. Acta neuropath. (Berl.) **17**, 127—138 (1971).

Liebermann, A. R.: The connective tissue elements of the mammalian nodose ganglion. A electron microscopic study. Z. Zellforsch. **89**, 95—111 (1968).

McGabe, J. S., Low, F. N.: The subarachnoid angle: An area of transition in peripheral nerve. Anat. Rec. **164**, 15—34 (1969).

Mancini, R. E.: Connective tissue and serum proteins. Int. Rev. Cytol. **14**, 193—222 (1963).

Martin, K. H.: Untersuchungen über die perineurale Diffusionsbarriere an gefriergetrockneten Nerven. Z. Zellforsch. **64**, 404—428 (1964).

Mellick, R. S., Cavanagh, J. B.: Changes in blood vessel permeability during degeneration and regenerating in peripheral nerves. Brain **41**, 141—160 (1968).

Olsson, Y.: Studies on vascular permeability in peripheral nerves. 1. Distribution of circulating fluorescent serum albumin in normal, crushed and sectioned rat sciatic nerve. Acta neuropath. (Berl.) **7**, 1—15 (1966).

— Phylogenetic variations in the vascular permeability of peripheral nerves to serum albumin Acta path. microbiol. scand. **69**, 621—623 (1967).

— Topographical differences in the vascular permeability of the peripheral nervous system. Acta neuropath. (Berl.) **10**, 26—33 (1968).

— The involvement of vasa nervorum in disease of peripheral nerves. In: Handbook of clinical neurology, vol. 15. Edit. by P. J. Vinken and G. W. Bruyn. North Holland Publishing Co. 1971 a.

— Studies on vascular permeability in peripheral nerve. IV. Distribution of intravenously injected protein tracers in the peripheral nervous system of various species. Acta neuropath. (Berl.) **17**, 114—126 (1971 b).

— Reese, T. S.: Inaccessibility of the endoneurium of mouse sciatic nerve to exogenous proteins. Anat. Rec. **163**, 22 (1969).

Olsson, Y., Reese, T. S.: Permeability of vasa nervorum and perineurium in mouse sciatic nerve to proteins studied by fluorescence and electron microscopy. J. Neuropath. exp. Neurol. (1971). In press.

Reese, T. S., Karnovsky, M. J.: Fine structural localization of a blood-brain barrier to exogenous peroxidase. J. Cell Biol. **34**, 244—256 (1967).

Sabin, A. B.: The nature and route of centripetal progression of certain neurotropic viruses along peripheral nerves. Amer. J. Path. **13**, 615—617 (1937).

Saito, A., Zachs, S. J.: Ultrastructure of Schwann and perineurial sheeths at the mouse neuromuscular junction. Anat. Rec. **164**, 379—390 (1969).

Shantha, T. R., Bourne, G. H.: The perineural epithelium—a new concept. In: The structure and function of nervous tissue, vol. I, pp. 379—459. New York-London: Academic Press 1968.

Waggener, J. D., Bunn, S. M., Beggs, J.: The diffusion of ferritin within the peripheral nerve sheath: an electron microscopy study. J. Neuropath. exp. Neurol. 24, 430—443 (1965).

Waksman, B. H.: Experimental study of diphthetic polyneuritis in the rabbit and the guinea-pig. III. The blood-nerve barrier in the rabbit. J. Neuropath. exp. Neurol. 20, 35—77 (1963).

Weiss, P., Wang, H., Taylor, A. C., Edds, Mac V., Jr.: Proximodistal connection in the endoneurial spaces of peripheral nerves demonstrated by colored and radioactive (isotope) tracers. Amer. J. Physiol. **143**, 521—540 (1945).

Wright, G. P.: Nerve trunks as pathways in infection. Proc. roy. Soc. Med. **46**, 319—330 (1953).

Zachs, S. J., Saito, A.: Uptake of exogenous horseradish peroxidase by coated vesicles in mouse neuromuscular junctions. J. Histochem. Cytochem. **17**, 161—170 (1969).

Dr. Y. Olsson
Institute of Pathology
Sahlgrenska sjukhuset
S-413 45 Göteborg, Sweden

Acta neuropath. (Berl.) Suppl. V 70—75 (1971)

Changes in Axonal Flow during Regeneration of Mammalian Motor Nerves

G. W. Kreutzberg and P. Schubert

Max-Planck-Institut für Psychiatrie, München

Summary. Measurements of axonal diameters in regenerating facial nerves of rats indicated a loss of axonal volume of approximately 60% in 14 days. These measurements were made in the intramedullary genu of the facial nerve thus indicating that transection of the distal portion of the nerve produces marked changes throughout the length of the injured axons.

Experimental studies on the transport of radioactive proteins in hypoglossal nerves of guinea pigs showed a significant increase of the radioactive material transported into the regenerating nerves, assumed to be mainly the fast component.

The slowly moving component of axonal flow appeared to be affected as well. Preliminary data suggest a redistribution rather than a change in the rate of transport in regenerating axons.

Key-Words: Axonal Flow — Regeneration — Motor Nerve — Axonal Diameter.

There can be no doubt that the concept of axonal flow by P. Weiss is of outstanding importance for the understanding of regeneration in peripheral nerves. In the classical study by Weiss and Hiscoe (1948) the role of axonal flow for the maintenance of the axon, and the consequences of interrupting the stream of axoplasm, have been discussed in the context of regeneration and Wallerian degeneration. Since then many of the changes occuring in axons proximal or distal to the site of transection have been thought to be dependent on axonal flow (Lubińska, 1964).

In a study of the regenerating facial nerve with conventional silver-impregnation technique we recently observed changes in fiber diameter in a part of the nerve previously neglected (Kreutzberg and Schubert, 1971). These changes probably indicate disturbances of axonal transport due to interrupting the continuity of the axon.

In this study, facial nerves in rats were transected unilaterally at the stylomastoid foramen and the axons were measured in the intramedullary genu of the facial nerve, i.e. ca. 13 mm proximal to the cut level. Statistically significant reduction of axonal diameters was found in this location as early as 48 h after the operation. The caliber of the axons decreased during the first postoperative week and then stabilized at about 40% of the normal mean diameter during the second and third week (s. Table). This equals volume loss of 60% in the axon which raises the question as to the fate of this material.

If the missing material was transported by axonal flow towards the periphery, one should be able to account for it at the cut end of the axon, probably in the axon swellings proximal to the site of transection. The amount of structures and

Table

Days after operation	Change in mean diameter on op. side %	Days after operation	Change in mean diameter on op. side %
1	− 5	14	− 40
2	− 11	21	− 37
3	− 9	35	− 28
4	− 19	120	− 17
6	− 31	135	− 13
8	− 29	240	− 13
10	− 38	365	− 15

organelles in these endbulbs and their size has surprised investigators. A local synthesis of this material has been postulated but was ruled out by experimental evidence (Kreutzberg, 1967).

Rough calculations showed that the reduction in axoplasm along the central part of the axon was in the same order of magnitude as the amount of material piled up in the endbulb: A facial nerve axon of 16 mm length and 4μ diameter looses 11% of its diameter in 48 h. If the lost volume (ca. $42.000 \mu^3$) is added to a 4μ thick axon, we end up with an axon swelling of 800μ length and 8.9μ diameter. This is the size of endbulbs frequently seen in the proximal stump of transected nerves.

On the basis of this rough calculation it seems reasonable to assume that the axonal enlargements in the proximal stump are filled with axoplasm displaced from central portion of the fibers. This assumption suggests marked changes in axonal flow during regeneration. Among the many factors that may be involved, changes in the speed of transport have been postulated by Grafstein and Murray (1969) for the regenerating optic nerve of gold fish.

To bring more light on this problem we studied axoplasmic transport in regenerating axons, using radioactive tracers. Similar to Miani (1963) we applied a radiochemical (^{3}H-lysine) to the calamus scriptorius of the 4th ventricle. To avoid tissue destruction the radiochemical was dropped on the surface rather than injected into the tissue (Fig. 1). The tritiated amino acid was taken up by the motoneurons of the hypoglossal and vagal nuclei and was incorporated into peptides and proteins which were transported down the axons towards the periphery. The amount of radioactivity in the nerves may either be measured by liquid scintillation counting or it can be demonstrated by autoradiography. Such methods have been used widely for studying axonal transport (Taylor and Weiss, 1965; Droz and Leblond, 1963; Ochs et al., 1967; McEwen and Grafstein, 1968; Karlsson and Sjöstrand, 1968; Lasek, 1968). There is evidence from these investigations of at least two different types of intraaxonal transport of proteins. According to the speed, they are refered to as slow component (ca. 1—3 mm per day) and fast component (ca. 40—400 mm per day).

In a first series of experiments we studied changes occuring in the so-called fast component at different stages of regeneration. In adult guinea pigs the hypoglossal nerve was transected unilaterally at the tendon of the digastric muscle. The animals were allowed to survive for 3, 5, 10, 17, 28, 42 and 60 days. Two days

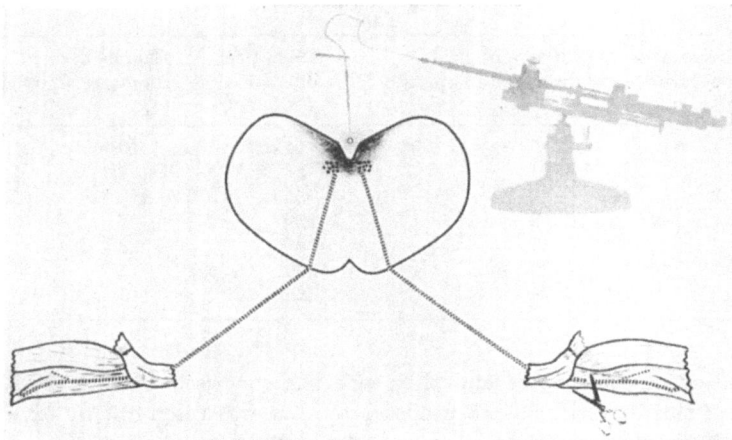

Fig. 1. Diagram illustrating the experimental procedure. By means of a microsyringe 8 µC of ^{3}H-lysine (spec. act. 5.3 C/mM) was dropped on the floor of the fourth ventricle (1 µC/µl) at intervalls of 10 min. This provided a uniform and concentrated supply of radiochemical to both vagal and hypoglossal nuclei, confirmed by autoradiography (blackened area). The radioactivity within the extramedullary part of the operated (right) and control (left) hypoglossal nerve was measured by means of scintillation counting

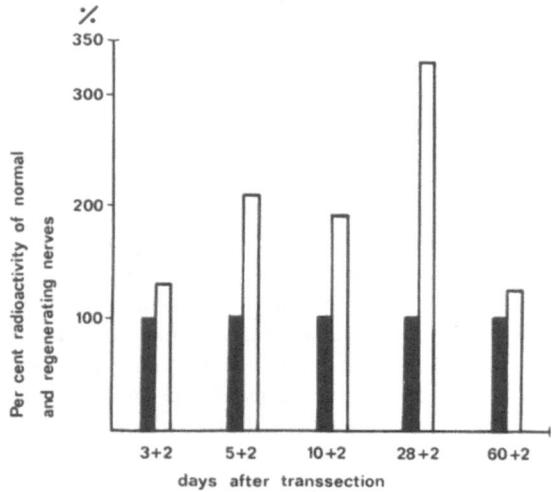

Fig. 2. Increasing of the total amount of radioactivity in regenerating hypoglossal nerves (white columns) at different times after transection expressed per 100% activity of the corresponding control nerves (black columns). Each pair of columns gives the mean value for 2 animals. ^{3}H-lysine was applied after transection, 2 days before sacrifice

before sacrifice radioactive lysine was applied to the hypoglossal nuclei as described above.

Results: 1. Total amount of radioactivity was significantly higher in the regenerating nerves (Fig. 2). 2. If the distribution of the radioactivity along the nerves was studied it was found that the increase in activity started just proximal to the

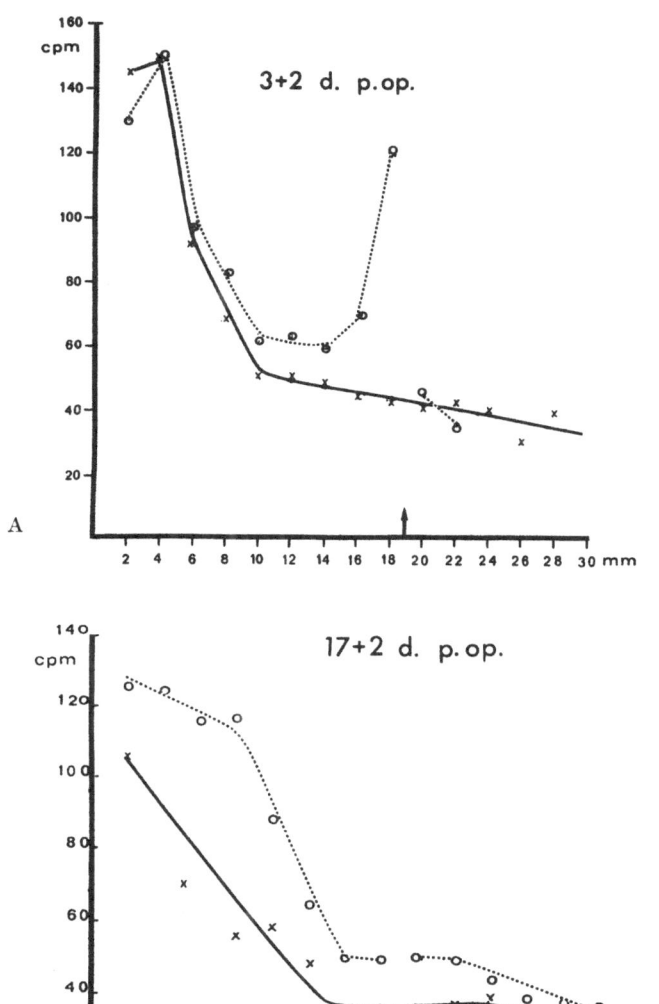

Fig. 3 A and B. Distribution of radioactivity within regenerating (----) and control (— —) hypoglossal nerves, 2 days after application of ^{3}H-lysine, indicating changes in "fast transport". The ordinate gives cpm/2 mm nerve, the abscissa gives the distance from the medulla. A 5 days after transection radioactivity is increased in the proximity of the transection (arrow), whereas the distribution of activity in the more proximal parts resembles that in the control nerve; B 19 days after transection radioactivity is increased over the whole length of the nerve as compared to control, even beyond the point of transection

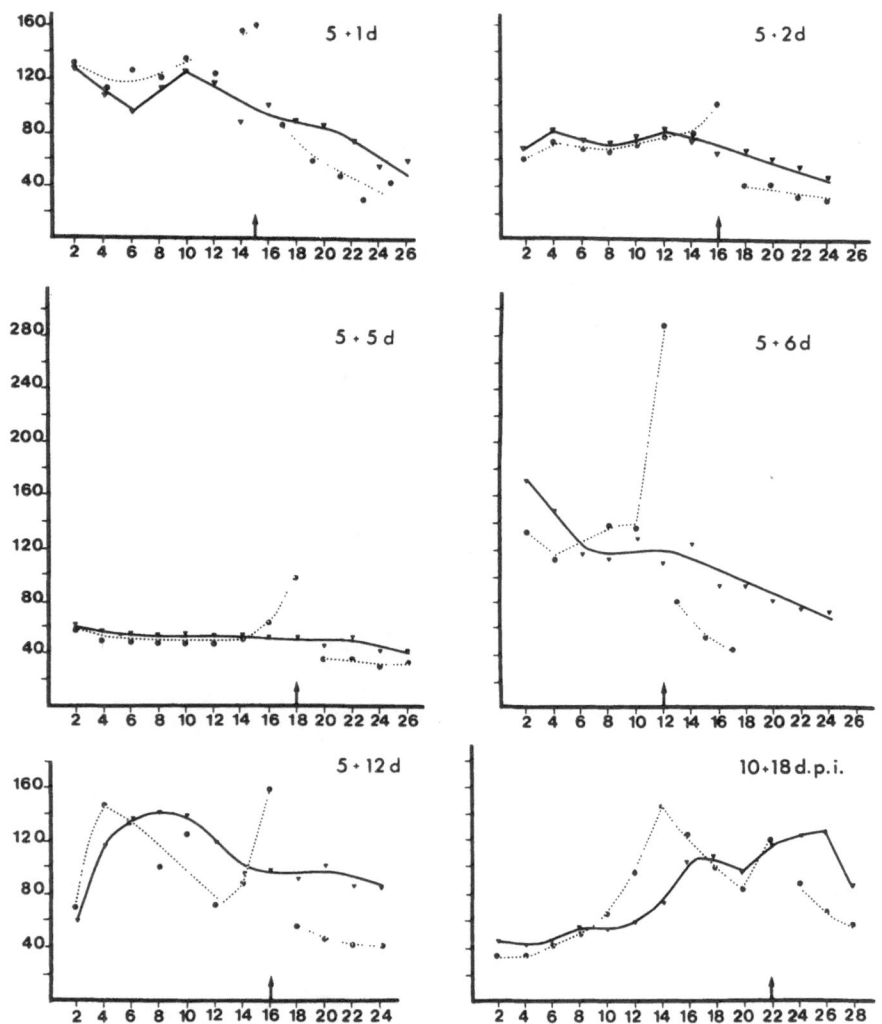

Fig. 4. Distribution of radioactivity in regenerating (----) and control (———) hypoglossal nerves suggesting changes in "slow transport". ³H-lysine was applied 5 days resp. 10 days (1 animal) before transection and the animals were allowed to survive the transection 1 to 17 days. At later stages (17 and 28 days p.i.) a wave of radioactivity is apparent with differing in shape for regenerating and control nerves

lesion (Fig. 3 A). At later stages there was more labelled material throughout the regenerating nerve when compared with the control side (Fig. 3 B). The distances this material had travelled during the 48 h between application of the ³H-lysine and sacrifice of the animal were compatible with the assumption that most of it belonged to the fast component.

Analysing the results not in absolute figures but in percentages, we could not convince ourselves of a change in the velocity of the transport during regeneration.

In the next series of experiments we reversed the sequence of transection and application of the radiochemical. First, ^{3}H-lysine was applied to the calamus scriptorius and 5 days later the right hypoglossal nerve was transected; the animals were killed after 1, 2, 5, 6 and 12 days. In one animal the nerve was cut 10 days after the application of ^{3}H-lysine and the animal was killed 18 days there after. Radioactivity was measured along the nerves in 2 mm segments by means of liquid scintillation counting.

The results (Fig. 4) showed surprisingly little differences for the regenerating and control nerves in the animals sacrificed 1 to 6 days after nerve transection. A significant increase in radioactivity was found only in the cut ends of the nerves, probably due to a piling up of the fast component. In these experiments not enough time was allowed to elapse to show a change in the slow component.

In the animals with long survival periods (5 + 12 days and 10 + 18 days) the slow component had reached the peripheral portion of the nerve as demonstrated by increasing activity. Differences in the distribution of the radioactivity were especially apparent in the 10 + 18 days experiment. The regenerating nerves showed a peak of radioactivity at the 14 mm point while no such peak was seen on the control side. The total radioactivity in the two nerves over the length of 28 mm was equal (10 879 c p m vs. 11 296 c p m). The significance of this peak is not fully understood at present; it does not seem to indicate an increasing velocity in axonal flow which has been demonstrated clearly in poikilothermic animals (Grafstein, 1970).

References

Droz, B., Leblond, C. P.: Axonal migration of proteins in the central nervous system and peripheral nerves as shown by autoradiography. J. comp. Neurol. **121**, 325—345 (1963).

Grafstein, B.: Role of axonal transport in nerve regeneration. Acta Neuropath. (Berl.) Suppl. V, 144—152 (1971).

— Murray, M.: Transport of protein in gold fish optic nerve during regeneration. Exp. Neurol. **25**, 494—508 (1969).

Karlsson, J. O., Sjöstrand, J.: Transport of labelled proteins in the optic nerve and tract of the rabbit. Brain Res. **11**, 431—439 (1968).

Kreutzberg, G. W.: Autoradiographic study on incorporation of leucine-H³ in peripheral nerves during regeneration. Experientia (Basel) **23**, 33 (1967).

— Schubert, P.: Volume changes in the axon during regeneration. Acta neuropath. (Berl.) **17**, 220—226 (1971).

Lasek, R. J.: Axoplasmic transport in cat dorsal root ganglion cells as studied with ^{3}H-leucine. Brain Res. **7**, 360—377 (1968).

Lubińska, L.: Axoplamic streaming in regenerating and in normal nerve fibers. Progr. Brain Res. **13**, 1—66 (1964).

McEwen, B. S., Grafstein, B.: Fast and slow components in axonal transport of protein. J. Cell Biol. **38**, 494—509 (1968).

Miani, N.: Analysis of the somato-axonal movement of phospholipids in the vagus and hypoglossal nerves. J. Neurochem. **10**, 859—874 (1963).

Ochs, S., Johnson, J., Ng, M. H.: Protein incorporation and axoplasmic flow in motoneuron fibres following intracord injection of labelled leucine. J. Neurochem. **14**, 317—331 (1967).

Taylor, A. C., Weiss, P.: Demonstration of axonal flow by the movement of tritium-labelled protein in mature optic nerve fibers. Proc. nat. Acad. Sci. (Wash.) **54**, 1521—1527 (1965).

Weiss, P., Hiscoe, H. B.: Experiments on the mechanism of nerve growth. J. exp. Zool. **107**, 315—395 (1948).

Dr. G. W. Kreutzberg, Dr. P. Schubert
Max-Planck-Institut für Psychiatrie
D-8000 München 23, Kraepelinstr. 2
Deutschland

Acta neuropath. (Berl.) Suppl. V, 76—85 (1971)

Nuclear, Cytoplasmic and Axoplasmic RNA in Experimental Neuroaxonal Dystrophy

Henrik A. Hartmann

University of Wisconsin Medical School, Madison, Wis. U.S.A.

Summary. While RNA has been measured in the axoplasm of marine animals ($0.04\ \mu\mu g/\mu^3$) and mammals ($0.006\ \mu\mu g/\mu^3$), a higher concentration of $0.23\ \mu\mu g/\mu^3$ was measured in experimentally produced dystrophic axons from rats. The increased amount of RNA may be derived by flow from the neuronal cell body, by *de novo* synthesis in the axoplasm itself or by migration from the surrounding sheath cells.

An origin of axonal RNA from the neuronal cell body is favored since an increased turnover of RNA was measured in the nucleus and cytoplasm of the dystrophic neurons while the amount of RNA in the cell body remained constant.

It cannot be excluded however that some RNA had been synthesized within the axon. Likewise the different base ratio of RNA from the axonal balloons could speak for a migration of RNA to the axon from the surrounding sheath cells.

Key-Words: Axoplasmic RNA — Nuclear RNA — Cytoplasmic RNA — Axonal flow — Neuroaxonal Dystrophy.

Introduction

The abundant basophilic material in the nerve cell body, known as Nissl substance to the light microscopist, to-day has its ultrastructural correlate in the ribosomes and its biochemical correlate in the ribonucleic acids, RNA. The earlier concept of RNA originating in the nucleolus (Casperson, 1936), and migrating to the cytoplasm, has now been recognized as one of the many importance events in the function of the cells. The validity of the genetic code (Watson, 1965), is being tested for a number of different cell types.

In case of the nerve cell a special concept was developed (Hydén, 1943, 1960), namely that increased neuronal activity was accompanied by production of RNA, proteins and lipids in the nerve cell. Also the validity of that concept has been tested under a number of different conditions. The highly specialized portions of a nerve cell, such as the axons, lacking basophilia as well as ribosomes, escaped scrutiny for RNA, until microchemical methods (Edstrøm, J. E., 1953) made measurements reliable, first in marine animals (Edstrøm, J. E., *et al.*, 1962) and later in mammals (Koenig, E., 1965). With the presence of axonal RNA beeing proven, the questions arise: "What roles do axonal and cell body (nuclear and cytoplasmic) RNA play in the normal axonal flow of proteins (Weiss, 1944, 1948)?" Finally: "Are the same factors altered during the condition known as axonal dystrophy?" (Seitelberger, 1957).

Axonal RNA

The *concentration* of axonal RNA has now been measured in several species, and we have added data from our experiments (Hartmann *et al.*, 1968a) to those given in a recent review (Lasek, 1970) completing the Table 1. The Mauth-

Table 1. *Concentration of axonal RNA in various animals*

Animal	Nerve	$\mu\mu g/100\ \mu^3$	Reference
Goldfish	Mauthner	0.03—0.07	Edstrøm, A., (1964a)
Crayfish	Stretch receptor	0.06	Grampp and Edstrøm, J. (1963)
Squid	Giant axon	0.018—0.025	Lasek, (1970)
Cat	XI	0.006	Koenig, E. (1965b)
Rat	Anterior intraspinal axonal balloon[a]	0.23	Hartmann *et al.* (1968)

[a] From rats given β-β iminodipropionitrile.

ner axon of goldfish (Edstrøm, A., 1964a) was 0.03—0.07 $\mu\mu g$ RNA/100 μ^3. Although this is only 1/40 of the concentration in the Mauthner cell body, when the volume of the entire axon was calculated, it contained about 4 times more RNA than the cell body. Crayfish stretch receptor (Grampp and Edstrøm, J. E., 1963) had a similar concentration, 0.06 $\mu\mu g$ RNA/100 μ^3. The giant axon of the squid (Lasek, 1970) had only a slightly lower concentration, 0.018—0.025 $\mu\mu g$ RNA/100 μ^3. Thus there are quite similar values for axonal RNA from marine animals, the average being about 0.04 $\mu\mu g$ RNA/μ^3.

The mammalian axons are difficult to obtain in large quantity. The XI nerve of the cat (Koenig, E., 1965) was utilized to obtain pure axoplasm which was found to contain only 0.005 $\mu\mu g$ RNA/μ^3, a value which is only 15% of that in marine axons. At the same time it should not be forgotten that other investigators (Rahmann, 1965, 1966), found no uptake of H^3-Cytidine and H^3-Uridine in the nerve fibers of mouse and fish. It is questionable, however, if autoradiographic technique on the light microscopic level is sensitive enough to decide this important point. After depositing P^{32} orthophosphate on the calamus scriptorius of the rabbit (Miani, 1963, 1966) labelled RNA with sedimentation characteristics of ribosomal RNA was recovered from the hypoglossal and vagus nerves. Rat brain has also been found to have RNA in the synaptosomes (Balázs and Cooks, 1967). After injection of orotic acid into the spinal cord (Austin *et al.*, 1966; Austin and Morgan, 1967), labelled RNA was recovered from the sciatic nerve. The last two experiment are mainly cited to emphasise the overwhelming evidence for the presence of RNA in normal axoplasm, realizing the limitations which exist with respect to the purity of the fractions.

The distribution of RNA throughout the axon was also investigated in the Mauthner axon (Edstrøm, A., 1964a). There was a proximodistal concentration decrease in the cranial two thirds of the axon from 0.05 to 0,03 $\mu\mu g$ RNA/100 μ^3. Along the distal one third of the axon the concentration again increases until it reached 0.07 $\mu\mu g$ RNA/100 μ^3 near the end. Presumably the concentration of RNA undergoes changes with functional activity. Thus it was found (Jakoubek and Edstrøm, J. E., 1965) that after the goldfish had been rotated for 30 min, there was a significant reduction of axonal RNA concentration which lasted until 3 hours later when the concentration again was found to be normal in the Mauthner axon. On the other hand a severe trauma, transection of the spinal cord of

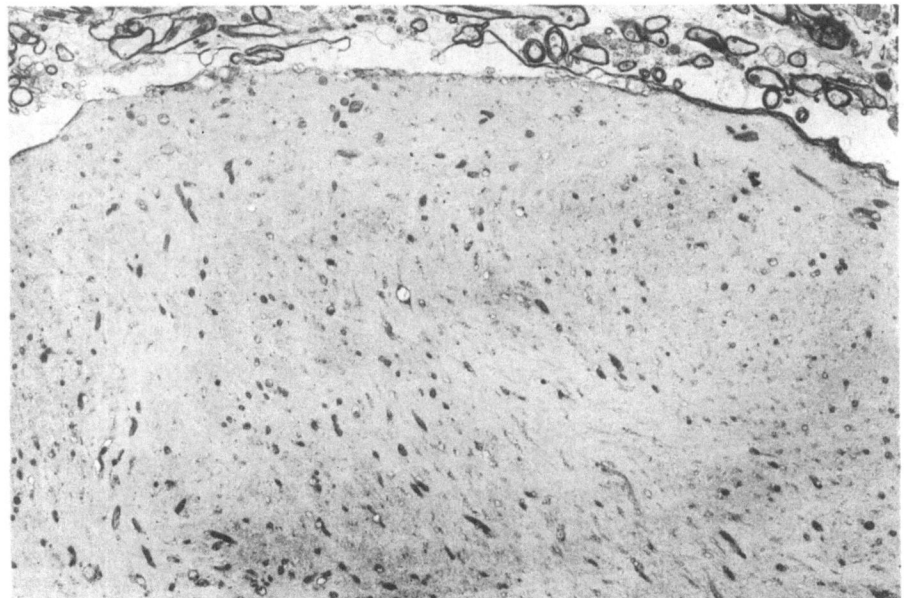

Fig. 1. Segment of axonal balloon from anterior motoneuron of rat, fed β-β iminodipropionitrile for 6 weeks. Dense tangles of neurofibrils intermingled with mitochondria, often cystically degenerated. $\times 7,5000$

gold fish (Edstrøm, A., 1964b), caused no change in the RNA content of the Mauthner axon when measured 2 and 30 days after the operation.

Under pathological conditions, such as swelling of the axons, (Hartmann *et al.*,
1968a), the large axonal balloons were high in RNA, 0.23[1] $\mu\mu g/100\,\mu^3$. This corresponds to 30 times the concentration found in normal cat axoplasm (Koenig,
1965) (Table 1). It is not possible however to say whether this high RNA concentration involves the axons uniformly, or whether it only occurs in these localized
swellings which are produced experimentally by feeding of β-β iminodipropionitrile to rats (Chou and Hartmann, 1964). Ultrastructurally, these balloons are
packed with neurofibrils, lysosomes and mitochondria which are increased in
number and cystically degenerated (Fig. 1 and 2) (Chou and Hartmann, 1965).

The *axonal RNA base composition* was first reported to be different from that
in the cell body RNA (Edstrøm, J. E., *et al.*, 1962). Later work, also on the
Mauthner axon, showed that an important nucleotide fraction other than RNA
was responsible for this difference, and it was concluded that the base composition
of RNA in the axon is similar to that of the cell body, namely ribosomal in type
(Edstrøm, A., 1964a). When axonal balloons (Hartmann *et al.*, 1968a) were examined the base ratio of RNA was different in that A/U = 0.61 (Table 2) compared
to 0.90 in the cell bodies from control rats. Unfortunately normal axoplasm from

---

[1] High RNA conc. might be due to shrinkage of axons during histological processing
(Anderson et al., 1970). Corrected for a shrinkage of 4.8 times would thus give a conc.
of 0.048.

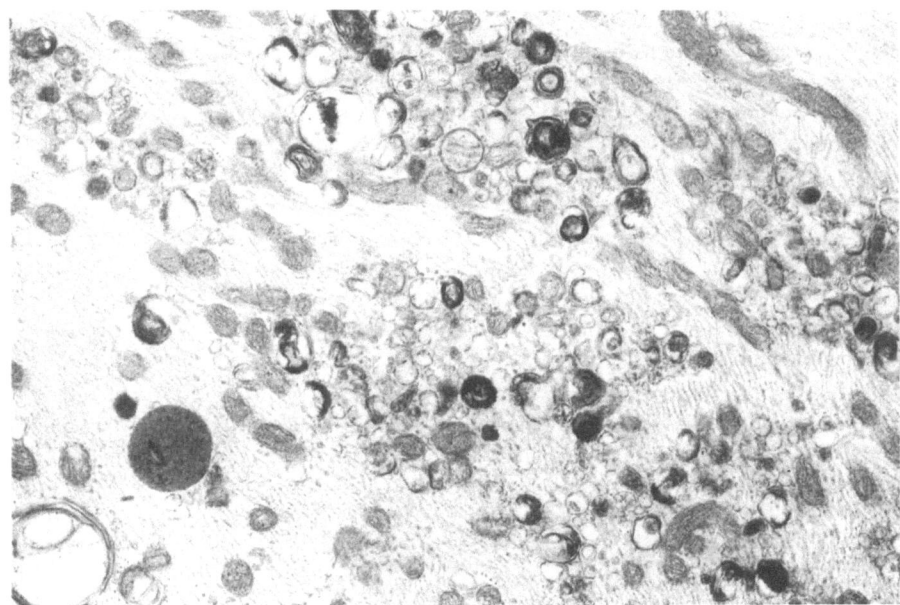

Fig. 2. Area of an axon with accumulation of mitochondria, lysosome-like bodies and vesicles between bundles of neurofilaments. ×24,000

mammals is difficult to isolate in pure condition, which explains why so few data are available. Cat accessory nerve (Koenig, 1965), free of myelin was found to have A/G = 0.57, and in the same type of material (Koenig, 1967) 85—96°/₀ of a radioactive precursor was found in a RNAase undigestible fraction. There have also been reports that spinal cord transection (Edstrøm, A., 1964b) and that functional activity (Jakoubek and Edström, J., 1965) will change the base composition of axonal RNA.

Sedimentation analysis of axonal RNA has been reported only recently (Edström, A., *et al.*, 1969). When Mauthner fibers alone were used, exclusively low molecular RNA with sedimentation rate of 4 S was found to incorporate H³-Uridine and H³-Cytidine. When the entire spinal cord was incubated in vitro with precursors, in addition to 4S higher molecular RNA, 16S and 28—30 S, were found in the same fiber. In other words, the fiber itself seems capable of synthesizing only 4S RNA, while the higher molecular RNA must have migrated from elsewhere. *Sensitivity of RNA synthesis to Actinomycin* (Edstrøm, A., *et al.*, 1969) has also been reported, indicating that the synthesis is dependent on a so-called messenger RNA.

The kinetics of axonal RNA could perhaps simplest be narrowed down to three possibilities. The RNA could be 1. produced in the cell body and transported down the axon, it could be 2. transported into the axon from the surroundings, or it could be 3. synthesized within the axon itself. The conclusion that some investigators (Miani *et al.*, 1966) arrived to after injection of P³² orthophosphate into the IVth ventricle and recovering the label from the axon, was that the axon itself was the only way of RNA migration from the cell body. Others (Austin *et al.*, 1966) injecting labelled orotic acid into fowl spinal cord, could find no exchange between axoplasm and adjacent tissue in the hypoglossal neurons. Perhaps the strongest argument in favor of a movement of RNA from the cell body and down the axon is the gradient of RNA (Edstrøm, A., 1964a, 40:1) (Hartmann *et al.*, 1968a, 23:1) (Koenig, 1965, 1000:1).

The study of incorporation of H^3-uridine in the newt, *Triturus* (Singer and Green, 1968), supposedly supports the second possibility, namely that RNA is synthesized in the Schwann cell and transport inward to the myelin sheath and axon. Although the resolution obtained in this autoradiographic study raises some questions, the experiment did show that transected nerves incorporated the precursor speaking against exclusive RNA synthesis in the neuronal cell body.

The third possibility, namely that RNA might be synthesized in the axoplasm itself was suggested when H^3-orotic acid and H^3-adenine were incorporated into axonal RNA (Koenig, 1967). In the absence of ribosomes in the axoplasm, mitochondria were suggested as a possible site for such synthesis. Sedimentation studies (Edstrøm, A., *et al.*, 1969) showed that Mauthner axon could synthesize 4S RNA in absence of the cell body.

Conclusions Regarding Axonal RNA

In normal axons there is RNA, apparently differing somewhat in concentration in different animals. The base ratios and the sedimentation characteristics seem to be similar to that of RNA in the cell body. Only 4S RNA has been found to be synthesized in the axon, so presumably 28S and 18S must have migrated from elsewhere.

In dystrophic axons there is higher concentration of RNA, at least in the axonal balloons. Its base ratio is abnormal with a low A/U, while the sedimentation characteristics presently are unknown.

Nuclear and Cytoplasmic RNA

It has been postulated (Hydén, 1960) that adequate stimulation might increase the concentration of RNA and protein in the nerve cell, whereas prolonged, intense stimulation might decrease them. The experimental evidence was originally based on rotation of rabbits (Hamberger and Hydén, 1949) which increased the concentration of RNA in the vestibular ganglion cells, and running of rabbits until exhaustion which caused a decreased concentration of RNA in the motor cells (Gomirato, 1954). In the last decade many investigators have conducted experiments testing Hydén's postulate. Supporting evidence came from the work on sympathetic ganglion in cat (Pevzner, 1965) showing that both electric stimulation and daily injections of adrenalin increased the nucleic acid content. Likewise the Purkinje cells from the cerebellum of rabbits which had been rotated (Jarlstedt, 1966, 1968) showed a moderate increase of RNA. It was also shown that chemicals, such as Tricyano-amino-propene, when injected into rabbits would increase the RNA by $25^0/_0$ in the Deiter cells, and at the same time change the base ratio of RNA (Egyhazi and Hydén, 1961).

Table 2. *Base ratios of RNA from anterior motoneurons*

	Control cells	Dystrophic cells	Axonal balloons[a]
Adenine	19.1	18.1	16.7
Guanine	29.5	29.5	30.8
Cytosine	20.2	29.1	25.4
Uracil	21.2	23.4	27.1
A/U	0.90	0.77	0.61

[a] Hartmann *et al.* (1968a) (from rats given β-β iminodipropionitrile).

Table 3. *Nuclear and cytoplasmic RNA from anterior horn cells and Deiter cells. A comparison*

	Anterior horn cells[a]		Deiter cells[b]	
	Nuclear	Cytoplasmic	Nuclear	Cytoplasmic
	Control			
Adenine	18.7	19.0	21.3	19.7
Guanine	28.7	29.4	26.6	33.5
Cytosine	29.4	28.4	30.8	28.8
Uracil	23.3	23.2	21.3	18.0
	Stimulated			
	IDPN[c]		TRIAP[d]	
Adenine	19.3	19.4	21.5	20.5
Guanine	28.7	27.7	30.0	34.6
Cytosine	28.2	28.9	30.4	26.7
Uracil	23.7	23.9	18.1	18.2

[a] Hartmann and Lin (1970);   [b] Hydén and Egyhazi (1962);   [c] β-β iminodipropionitrile; [d] Tricyano-amino-propene.

Other investigators were unable to demonstrate any changes that would support the postulate. Crustacean stretch receptors showed no difference in RNA level after electrical stimulation (Grampp and Edstrøm, J. E., 1963), and also showed no differences in base composition (Edstrøm, J. E., and Grampp, 1965). Even nerve cells which had undergone severe neurofibrillary degeneration due to aluminum phosphate injections (Embree *et al.*, 1957), showed no increase or decrease of RNA. Nerve cell bodies, belonging to axons which were severely dystrophic after administration of β-β iminodipropionitrile (INPN), also showed no increase in RNA. (Slagel *et al.*, 1966), but a transitory shift in base ratio, A/U from 0.90 to 0.77 (Hartmann *et al.*, 1968a) could be demonstrated (Table 2). Furthermore the view was advocated that the base composition of nuclear RNA can vary depending on the functional situation (Hydén and Egyhazi, 1962). It was found that even in normal Deiter cells significant differences existed between the base ratios of nuclear and cytoplasmic RNA, and after stimulation with Tricyano-amino-propene these differences became more pronounced (Table 3). When the same technique was applied to the anterior motor horn cell, from rat spinal cord (Hartmann and Lin, 1970), there were no significant changes in RNA base

Table 4. *H³ uridine incorporation into neurons after iminodipropionitrile (IDPN)*

Hours		Control	IDPN
1	Nucleus	2.84	4.94*
	Cytoplasm	0.09	0.41*
24	Nucleus	2.50	1.84
	Cytoplasm	1.18	0.05*

* $p < 0.05$.

Units: tracks/10 μ^2; material: autoradiography of spinal ganglion neurons from: Hartmann *et al.* (1968 b).

ratios between nuclear and cytoplasmic RNA from normal nerve cells. Also when cells were taken from rats with neuroaxonal dystrophy, after application of β-β iminodipropionitrile, no significant differences were found between the nuclear RNA bases (Table 3). There was however a significant drop in Guanine from the cytoplasm when compared both to nuclear RNA from the same experimental cells and from the control cells. On the basis of these and many other experiments it seems reasonable to conclude that *many nerve cells do not respond to stimulation with any change in content or composition of* RNA. More specifically in the case of experimental neuroaxonal dystrophy, the RNA content of cell bodies from the anterior motor horn remains at $670-700$ $\mu\mu$g during 12 weeks. (Hartmann *et al.*, 1968a).

If on the other hand incorporation of RNA precursor is studied, a more kinetic picture develops. In brain material, as in other tissue, incorporation is first seen in the nuclear RNA and much later in the cytoplasm (Bondy, 1966). In autoradiographic material of mice spinal ganglion (Hartmann *et al.*, 1968b), considerable number of grains were observed over the nuclei as early as 15 min after the injection of precursors and maximum incorporation was achieved after 30 min. Even after one hour, the cytoplasm showed only a few grain (Table 4). After 24 hours the cytoplasm shows maximal labeling. These data are in keeping with many others which show that the RNA is synthesized in the nucleus and later moves out into the cytoplasm. In the autoradiographs of spinal ganglia of mice which had been given IDPN, the grain counts gave the following results (Hartmann *et al.*, 1968b): 1. one hour after the injection of H³-Uridine both nuclear and cytoplasmic RNA showed significantly higher counts than in the controls. 2. At 24 hours both nuclear and cytoplasmic labelling was lower in the experimental rats. On the basis of those findings it was concluded that it is *highly probable that there is much more rapid turnover of RNA in the nerve cells from the experimental animals*, which had been stimulated by β-β iminodipropionitrile.

The effect of electrical stimulation on the RNA of a single nerve cell from a mollusc showed similar results (Peterson and Kernell, 1970). When the ganglionic nerves of a certain giant neuron (R2) were stimulated, marked increases in the amounts of labelled RNA in the nucleus as well as in the cytoplasm occured. On the basis of such experiments one might rephrase Hydén's postulate and say that *many types of stimuli may increase newly synthesized RNA which in turn may influence production of proteins in the nerve cell.*

Our knowledge of nuclear and cytoplasmic RNA has been expanded by such techn ques as succrose gradient centrifugation and agarose gel electrophoresis. While the ribosomal type of RNA has been characterized as 28S and 18S, transfer RNA is 4S. In addition to nucleolar ribosomal precursor RNA, many other nuclear RNA types have been described (Weinberg and Penman, 1968). In the brain the same main types of RNA have been found (Samli and Roberts, 1969; Saborio and Aleman, 1970), but it is still an open question if there are any RNA types specific to the brain.

Conclusions Regarding Nuclear and Cytoplasmic RNA

In normal anterior horn cells the base ratio of nuclear is the same as that of cytoplasmic RNA, and the same types of RNA (28S, 18S and 4S) are present in both.

In dystrophic neurons there is no change in the content (amount) of RNA and only transitory changes in the base ratio of cytoplasmic RNA, however the turnover of both nuclear and cytoplasmic RNA is increased.

Conclusions Regarding RNA in Normal and Dystrophic Neurons

RNA in the cell body of the neuron, like in other cells, is synthesized in the nucleus and migrates from the nucleolus to the cytoplasm where most of it gets bound in ribosomes to the membranes of the endoplasmic reticulum. Some of the RNA migrates down the axon where it is present in low concentration but in considerable amounts because of the large volume of the axon. However, some of the axonal RNA might be synthesized in the axon, and some of it might migrate in from the surrounding Schwann cells.

In neuroaxonal dystrophy there is an increased turnover of RNA in the cell body, which does not lead to an increased level in the cell body, but an increased concentration in the axon. However this increase might also be partly due to increased axonal synthesis, or migration from the surrounding Schwann cells.

References

Andersson, E., Edstrøm, A., Jarlstedt, J.: Properties of RNA from giant axons of crayfish. Acta physiol. scand. 78, 491—502 (1970).

Austin, L., Bray, J., Young, R.: Transport of proteins and ribonucleic acid along nerve axons. J. Neurochem. 13, 1267—1269 (1966).

— Morgan, I. G.: Incorporation of radioactively labelled leucine into synaptosomes from rat cerebral cortex in vitro. J. Neurochem. 14, 377—387 (1967).

Balázs, R., Cooks, W. A.: RNA metabolism in subcellular fractions of brain tissue. J. Neurochem. 14, 1035—1055 (1967).

Bondy, S. C.: The ribonucleic acid metabolism of the brain. J. Neurochem. 13, 955—959 (1966).

Casperson, T. O.: Über den Aufbau der Strukturen des Zellkernes. Skand. Arch. Physiol. 73, Suppl. 8 (1936).

Chou, S. M., Hartmann, H. A.: Axonal lesions and waltzing syndrome after IDPN adminis-tration in rats. Acta neuropath. (Berl.) 3, 428—450 (1964).

— — Electronmicroscopy of focal neuroaxonal lesions produced by β-β iminodipropionitrile (IDPN) in rats. Acta neuropath. (Berl.) 4, 590—603 (1965).

Edstrøm, A.: The ribonucleic acid in the Mauthner neuron of the goldfish. J. Neurochem. **11**, 309—314 (1964a).
— — The effect of spinal cord transection on the base composition and content of RNA in the Mauthner nerve fiber components. J. Neurochem **11**, 557—559 (1964b).
— Edstrøm, J. E., Hökfeldt, T.: Sedimentation analysis of ribonucleic acid extracted from isolated Mauthner nerve fiber components. J. Neurochem. **16**, 53—66 (1969).
Edstrøm, J. E.: Ribonucleic acid concentration in individual nerve cells. Biochim. biophys. Acta. (Amst.) **12**, 361—386 (1953).
— Eichner, D., Edstrøm, A.: The ribonucleic acid of axons and myelin sheaths from Mauthner axons. Biochim. biophys. Acta (Amst.) **61**, 178—184 (1962).
— Grampp, W.: Nervous activity and metabolism of ribonucleic acids in the crustacean stretch receptor neuron. J. Neurochem **12**, 735—741 (1965).
Egyhazi, E., Hydén, H.: Experimentally induced changes in the base composition of the ribonucleic acids of isolated nerve cells and their oligodendroglial cells. J. biophys. biochem. Cytol. **10**, 403—410 (1961).
Embree, L. J., Hamberger, A., Sjøstrand, J.: Quantitative cytochemical studies and histochemistry in experimental neurofibrillary degeneration. J. Neuropath. exp. Neurol. **26**, 427—436 (1967).
Grampp, W., Edstrøm, J. E.: The effect of nervous activity on ribonucleic acid of the crustacean stretch receptor neuron. J. Neurochem. **10**, 725—732 (1963).
Gomirato, G.: Quantitative evaluation of the metabolic variations in the spinal motor root cells studied by biophysical methods and following adequate stimulation. J. Neuropath. exp. Neurol. **13**, 359—368 (1954).
Hamberger, C. A., Hydén, H.: Production of nucleoproteins in the vestibular ganglion. Acta oto-laryng. (Stockh.) Suppl. **75**, 53—82 (1949).
Hartmann, H. A., Lin, J.: Nuclear and cytoplasmic RNA in experimental neuroaxonal dystrophy. J. Neuropath. exp. Neurol. **29**, 135 (1970).
— — Shively, M. C.: RNA of nerve cell bodies and axons after β-β iminodipropionitrile. Acta neuropath. (Berl.) **11**, 275—281 (1968a).
— Shively, M. C., Kitiyakara, A.: H³-uridine incorporation into RNA of nerve cells from mice stimulated by iminodipropionitrile. Fed. Proc. **27**, 2230 (1968b).
Hydén, H.: Protein metabolism in the nerve cell during growth and function. Acta physiol. scand. 6, Suppl. **17**, 5—132 (1943).
— In: The cell, Vol. IV, p. 274. J. Brachet and A. Mirsky, ed. New York-London: Academic Press 1960.
— Egyhazi, E.: Changes in the base composition of nuclear ribonucleic acid of neurons during a short period of enhanced protein production. J. Cell Biol. **15**, 37—44 (1962).
Jarlstedt, J.: Functional localization in the cerebellar cortex studied by quantitative determinations of Purkinje cell RNA. Acta physiol. scand. **67**, 243—252 (1966).
— In: Macromolecules and the function of the neuron, pp. 324—333. Z. Lodin, S. P. R. Rose ed. Amsterdam: Excerpta Medica Foundation 1968.
Jakoubek, B., Edstrøm, J. E.: RNA changes in the Mauthner axon and myelin sheath after increased functional activity. J. Neurochem. **12**, 845—849 (1965).
Koenig, E.: Synthetic mechanisms in the axon II. RNA in myelin free axons of the cat. J. Neurochem. **12**, 357—361 (1965).
— Synthetic mechanisms in the axon IV. *In vitro* incorporation of H³-precursosrs into axonal protein and RNA. J. Neurochem. **14**, 437—446 (1967).
Lasek, R. J.: The distribution of nucleic acids in the giant axon of the squid. J. Neurochem. **17**, 103—109 (1970).
Miani, N.: Analysis of the somatoaxonal movements of phospholipids in the vagus and hypoglossal nerves. J. Neurochem. **10**, 859—874 (1963).
— di Girolamo, A., di Girolamo, M.: Sedimentation characteristics of axonal RNA in rabbit. J. Neurochem. **13**, 755—759 (1966).
Peterson, R., Price, Kernell, D.: Effects of nerve stimulation on the metabolism of ribonucleic acid in a molluscan giant neuron. J. Neurochem. **17**, 1075—1085 (1970).
Pevzner, L. Z.: Topochemical aspects of nucleic acid and protein metabolism within the neuron-neuroglia unit of the superior cervical ganglion. J. Neurochem. **12**, 993—1002 (1965).

Rahmann, H.: Zum Stofftransport im Zentralnervensystem der Vertebraten. Autoradiographische Untersuchungen mit P^{32}-orthophosphate, H^3-Histidin, H^3-Cytidin und H^3-Uridin an Mäusen und Fischen. Z. Zellforsch. **66**, 878—890 (1965).

— Zum Vorkommen von RNS im Nervenfaserbereich. Experientia (Basel) **22**, 762—764 (1966).

Saborio, J. L., Alemán, V.: Study of RNA in subcellular fractions from rat brain. Simultaneous incorporation of C^{14}-Uridine and H^3-Methyl-Methionine. J. Neurochem. **17**, 91—101 (1970).

Samli, M. H., Roberts, S.: Properties of RNA fractions from nuclei of brain cells which stimulate incorporation of amino acids by brain ribosomes. J. Neurochem. **16**, 1565—1580 (1969).

Seitelberger, F.: Zur Morphologie und Histochemie der degenerativen Axonveränderungen im Zentralnervensystem, III. Congr. Intern. Neuropath., Brussel: Acta méd. belg. (Brüssel) 128—147 (1957).

Singer, M., Green, M. R.: Autoradiographic studies of uridine incorporation in peripheral nerve of the newt. J. Morph. **124**, 321—344 (1968).

Slagel, D. E., Hartmann, H. A., Edström, J. E.: The effect of iminodipropionitrile on the ribonucleic acid content and composition of mesencephalic V cells, anterior horn cells, glial cells and axonal balloons. J. Neuropath. exp. Neurol. **25**, 244—253 (1966).

Watson, J. D.: Molecular biology of the gene. New York: W. A. Benjamin 1965.

Weinberg, R. A., Penman, S.: Small molecular monodisperse nuclear RNA. J. molec. Biol. **38**, 289—304 (1968).

Weiss, P.: Damming of axoplasm in constricted nerve, a sign of perpetual growth in nerve fibers. Anat. Rec. **88**, 464—465 (1944).

— Hiscoe, H. B.: Experiments on the mechanism of nerve growth. J. exp. Zool. **107**, 315 to 395 (1948).

Henrik A. Hartmann
University of Wisconsin Medical School
Madison, Wisconsin/U.S.A.

Acta neuropath. (Berl.) Suppl. V, 86—96 (1971)

The Dependence of Fast Transport in Mammalian
Nerve Fibers on Metabolism

SIDNEY OCHS

Department of Physiology, Indiana University Medical Center, Indianapolis, Indiana

Summary. A fast transport of labelled components in the myelinated fibers of cat sciatic nerve was found after injection of the L7 dorsal root ganglion with ^{3}H-leucine. Fast transport was shown by a crest of activity which moved outward in the nerve at a regular rate of close to 400 ± 35 mm/day without change in its shape. The transport inside the axons is independent of a propulsive force exerted from the soma. After incorporated materials are supplied by the soma to the fiber, the somas can be destroyed without effect on the subsequent movement of material in the fibers. The mechanism of transport was shown thereby to be present all along the length of the fiber. It was also found to be closely dependent on oxidative phosphorylation in studies made in an *in vitro* system where fast transport is maintained by O_2. Fast transport was rapidly blocked with N_2 or oxidative blocking agents such as CN or DNP present in the Ringer solution. The energy derived from oxidative phosphorylation is most likely transferred through ATP to a sliding transport filament mechanism involving microtubules and/or neurofilaments which is believed to underly fast axoplasmic transport.

Key-Words: Fast Transport — Axoplasmic Transport — Oxidative Metabolism — Nerve — Sliding Transport Filament.

Introduction

The fast axoplasmic transport system which moves material down the mammalian nerve fibers at a rate close to 400 mm/day (Ochs, Sabri and Johnson, 1969; Ochs and Ranish, 1969) has been differentiated from the more well-known slow axoplasmic flow with a rate of several mm/day (Dahlström and Häggendal, 1966; Sjöstrand and Karlsson, 1969; Barondes, 1967; Lubińska, 1964; McEwen and Grafstein, 1968; Grafstein, 1969; Ochs and Johnson, 1969; Lasek, 1970; Ochs, 1970a). Fast transport is of special interest because it appears to be more closely related to the maintenance of normal nerve function and in the case of motor nerve fibers to continued neuromuscular transmission than the slow transport system (Ochs, 1970b). As will be described in this brief review, fast transport can be maintained *in vitro* when the excised nerve is supplied with oxygen (Ochs and Ranish, 1970; Ochs and Hollingsworth, 1970). The underlying mechanism of transport was shown to be locally present all along the axons and to be more closely dependent on oxidative metabolism than glycolysis.

Characteristics of Fast Transport *in vivo*

Transport was studied in the long lengths of nerve fibers of the cat sciatic nerve after injecting the lumbar seventh dorsal root (L7) ganglion with a small volume of ^{3}H-leucine (Ochs *et al.*, 1969). A sufficient time is allowed for incorporation of the precursor into proteins and a subsequent downflow of labelled materials in the fibers. After sectioning the nerve and sampling each segment, a plateau of

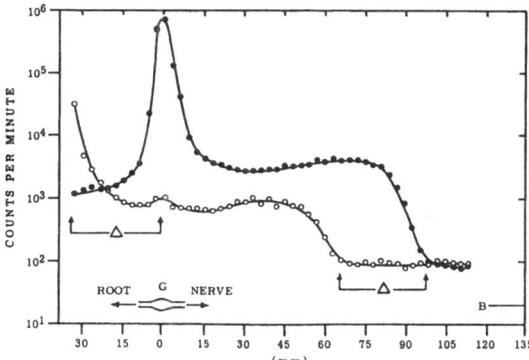

Fig. 1. Comparison of peaks and rate of fast transport in sensory and motor fibres. The L7 motoneuron region was injected with ^{3}H-leucine on the left side of the cord (o), the L7 ganglion on the right side (•). Six hours later the nerves were removed for sampling. The antero-posterior displacement (△) of the peaks is comparable to the antero-posterior displacement of the cord motoneurons and ganglion cell bodies (▲). (From Ochs and Ranish, 1969)

activity is found distal to the high level of activity remaining in the ganglion with still more distally a rise to a crest which then drops sharply to base-line levels of activity (Fig. 1). A similar crest of activity was found in the sciatic nerve after injecting the L7 motoneuron region in the ventral horn of the spinal cord except that its crest has a more proximal position. The displacement of the crests after injecting the L7 dorsal root ganglion and L7 spinal cord motoneuron region matches closely the anatomical antero-distal displacement of the L7 motoneuron and L7 dorsal root ganglion somas. This indicates that the rate of fast transport is similar in the sensory and motor nerve fibers (Ochs and Ranish, 1969).

Using the L7 spinal root ganglion, as more time elapses between ganglion injection and nerve removal, the crest of activity in the sciatic nerve takes a more distal position in the nerve. Taking the intersection of the front of the crest to the center of the ganglion distance and the time of removal after injection, a rate of 401 ± 35 mm/day was found for 35 animals (Ochs, Sabri and Ranish, 1970). This method supplants earlier measures of the rate where an exponentially declined outflow of activity from the CNS or distal root ganglion intersecting the base-line was used (cf. Ochs, Dalrymple and Richards, 1962; Miani, 1963; Ochs and Johnson, 1969; Lasek, 1968). The crest is a more satisfactory measure of movement especially as the shape of the crest does not show much alteration with distance along the nerve. This is the case not only for the cat but as well for the monkey sciatic nerve, and in goat sciatic nerve where even at a distance of 35 cm a typical crest indicative of fast axoplasmic transport was found with a rate of approximately 390 mm/day.

Fast transport in the axon is not dependent upon the soma acting as a force to move materials down the axons, i.e. the transport mechanism is present locally all along the nerve fiber. This was shown by first injecting the L7 ganglion with ^{3}H-leucine and then at some later time making a ligation just distal to the ganglion

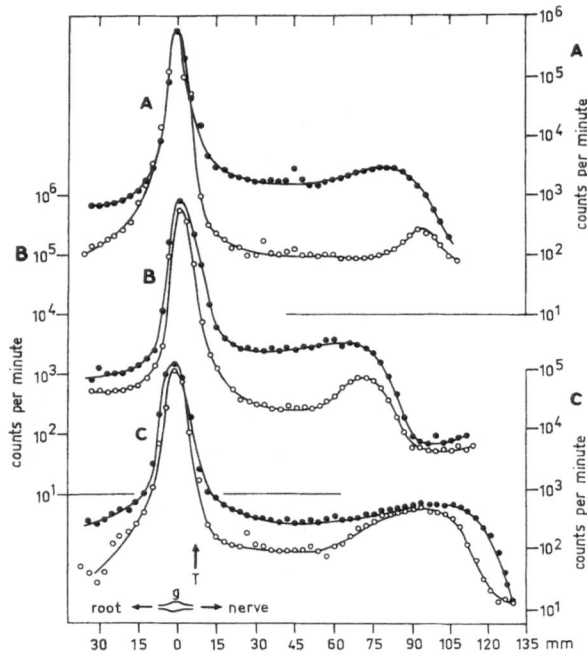

Fig. 2. A The L7 ganglia on the two sides were injected with ³H-leucine and 1 h later the nerve on one side (○) was ligated just distal to the ganglion (T). Six hours later control and ligated nerves were removed. The control side (●) shows a crest typical of 7 h of downflow, the ligated nerve shows a peak at this same position. B As in A, except that the S1 ganglion was injected and the nerve was ligated just below the S1 ganglion 2 h after ³H-leucine injection. Nerves were removed 6 h after injection. C Nerve ligation was made just distal to the L7 ganglion on one side 3 h after injection. (From Ochs and Ranish, 1970a)

or destroying the ganglion so that no further materials could exit from the cell body into the fibers. The labelled materials which had gained entry to the fibers continues to move at the usual rate (Ochs *et al.*, 1970). This is shown in Fig. 2 where ligations were made just distal to the ganglion at either 1, 2 or 3 h after injection of the ganglia and allowing an additional period of time for further downflow of the labelled materials which had entered the fibers.

On comparison of the position of the peaks in the ligated nerves it was found that the active materials which first gained entry to the nerve, i.e. the peak moved down in the 1 h ligation, takes up the most advanced position at the front of the crest of activity. The later additions shown by the 2 and 3 h ligation experiments, fill out the crest and the plateau behind the crest.

The transport mechanism in the axon is to be differentiated from the synthetic processes in the cell body which determine the kind and amount of materials manufactured by the soma and then transported down the axon. Subcellular fractionation of either ventral roots or nerves at different times after injection of ³H-leucine near the cell bodies showed that some higher molecular weight

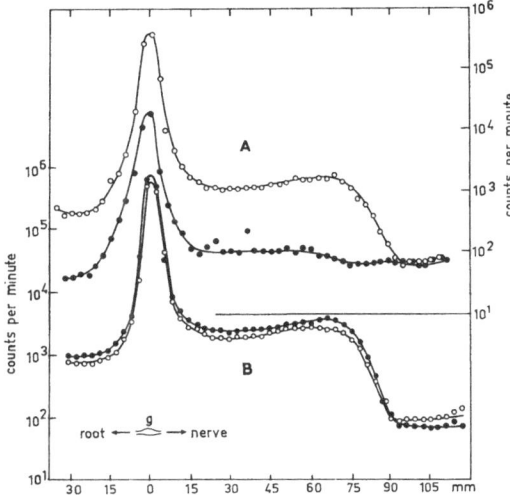

Fig.3. A Cycloheximide (17. 8 mM injected into the left L7 ganglion (•) and Ringer solution into the right (○) 20 min before injection of ³H-leucine into each ganglia. Nerves removed 4 h later. B Cycloheximide (17.8 mM) injected into the right L7 ganglion (○) and Ringer solution into the left (•) 30 min after ³H-leucine was injected into each ganglion. Nerves removed 5 h after ³H-leucine injection. (From Ochs et al., 1970)

protein, polypeptides and a highly labelled component of small particulates are moved down by the fast axoplasmic transport system while the slow transport system carries down a richer complement of higher molecular weight soluble protein (Kidwai and Ochs, 1969; Ochs et al., 1969; Ochs, 1970; James et al., 1970; James and Austin, 1970).

The rate of synthesis in the neuron cell bodies is relatively rapid. This was shown by injection of the protein synthesis blocking agents puromycin and cyclo-heximide in concentrations adequate to block protein synthesis either before or after the injection of the precursor ³H-leucine (Ochs et al., 1970). If either of these protein synthesis blocking agents were injected ¹/₂ to 1 h before the precursor there was a marked and almost complete block of downflow of labelled materials (Fig.3). On the other hand if either of these agents were injected 10—20 min afterwards, they were almost completely ineffective. These findings indicate that the time of synthesis in the cell bodies is relatively short, probably taking no longer than 10 min. These results are also in accord with the cell bodies being the major if not the sole site of synthesis.

However, the possibility still exists that some small amount of protein synthesis can take place locally in the axon and/or at the terminals where evidence for a local mechanism of synthesis has been reported by Austin and Morgan (1967) and by Autilio et al. (1968).

In vitro Transport and Oxidation Metabolism

If nerves are left in situ in killed animals, fast axoplasmic transport fails within 15 min indicating that fast transport is closely dependent on a supply of blood-

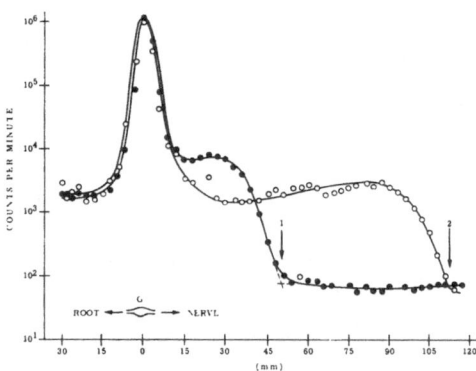

Fig. 4. The L7 ganglia were injected with [³H]-lysine and the animal was killed 3 h later. The control nerve, L7 ganglion and dorsal root, removed from the right side (○) shows a crest with the distal displacement shown by arrow 1 as expected of a fast transport lasting 3 h. The opposite nerve (●) was placed in a chamber containing oxygen and kept moist with Ringer solution at 38°C for an additional 4 h. The displacement of the crest in this preparation show by arrow 2 is in accord with a fast axoplasmic transport for a period of 7 h, consistent with a 401 ± 35 mm/day flow rate

transported oxygen for its maintenance (Ochs *et al.*, 1969). This was shown to be the case by using an *in vitro* technique where oxygen could be supplied to the nerve. The ganglia were first injected with ³H-leucine as usual and a downflow of materials into the nerve fibers allowed for several hours and the animal killed. The nerves were then removed as quickly as possible. One was taken for sampling and the other placed into a chamber with just enough Krebs-Ringer solution present to keep it moist. The chamber was flushed and filled with oxygen (or better a 95% oxygen + 5% CO_2 gas mixture) and kept at 38°C for several hours. The downflow pattern found in these nerves showed that fast transport occurs *in vitro* at approximately the same rate previously found for *in vivo* downflow (Fig. 4). The crest of activity had extended to a distance typical of a full 7 h of downflow, i.e. for the 3 h of downflow which had taken place in the animal plus the 4 h while in the chamber.

In experiments where the nerve had been subjected to the same conditions except that nitrogen was used to fill the chamber instead of oxygen, a rapid failure of transport was seen. Little more than an additional 15 min of downflow, was seen. This is apparent in the example of Fig. 5 where an additional 3 h was allowed with the nerve in the nitrogen filled chamber. The dependence on oxidative metabolism was similarly shown by the block of downflow when NaCN was added to the Ringer solution moistening nerves and with oxygen present (Fig. 6). The rapid failure of fast axoplasmic transport would be expected from the block of the terminal cytochrome oxidase in the electron transport chain (Lehninger, 1965).

Dinitrophenol was of particular interest because it is an uncoupler of oxidative phosphorylation (Webb, 1966). This agent effected as rapid a block of fast axoplasmic transport as nitrogen asphyxiation or NaCN (Fig. 7).

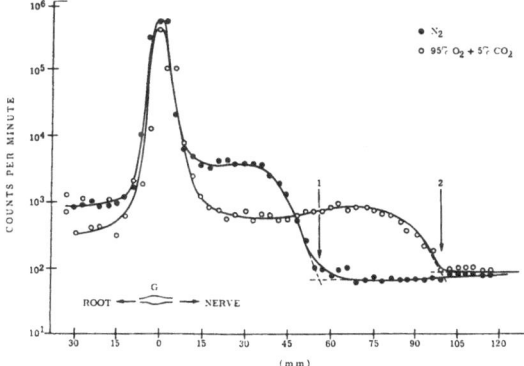

Fig. 5. *Nitrogen asphyxiation.* Nerves removed from an animal sacrificed 3 h after L7 ganglion injection with ³H-leucine. The nerve from one side (o) was placed in a chamber for 3 h while kept moist with Ringer-lactate solution at a temperature of 38°C and exposed to a 95% O_2 + 5% CO_2. *In vitro* transport to a distance expected of a continued fast transport (arrow 2) was found. The other nerve exposed to nitrogen (•) shows no further advance beyond that which had taken place during the 3 h in the animal

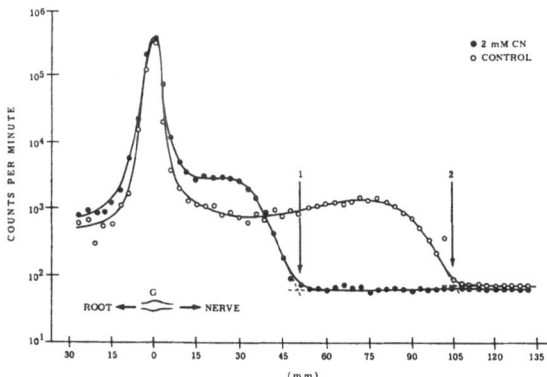

Fig. 6. *Block of fast transport by NaCN.* Control nerve (•) removed 3 h after L7 ganglion injection and placed in a chamber containing 95% O_2 + 5% CO_2 for 3 h of *in vitro* transport. Downflow occurred as expected for the total time of 6 h (arrow 2). The opposite nerve (o) was exposed to a 2 mM solution of NaCN. No movement beyond that occurring in the animal was apparent (arrow 1)

The estimated time of block of fast transport by all these metabolic blocking agents occurred within approximately 15 min, a time similar to the reported 10—33 min survival time found for nerve action potentials after initiation of N_2 asphyxiation (Gerard, 1932; Wright, 1964, 1947). In repeating these experiments a somewhat short survival time of approximately 10 min was found (Ochs, Hollingsworth and Helmer, 1970). In any case, the close similarity of the two times suggested that a common supply of ATP is used to supply the sodium pump to maintain the ion levels required for nerve excitability and action poten-

92   S. Ochs:

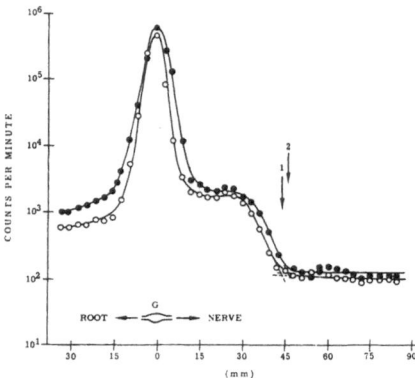

Fig.7. *Fast transport block by DNP*—Both L7 ganglia were injected and the control nerve (•) removed 3 h later shows the usual 3 h downflow (arrow 1). The other nerve was placed in a chamber for 3 more hours containing 95% O_2 + 5% CO_2 and exposed to 2 mM DNP. It shows little extra downflow (arrow 2)

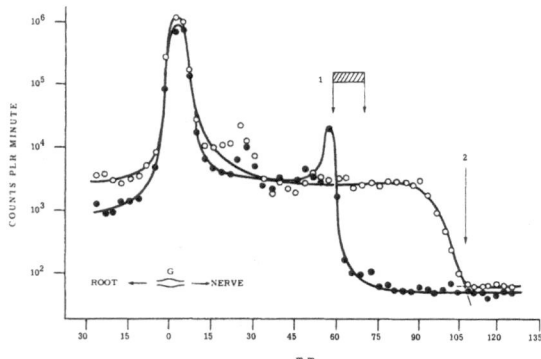

Fig.8. Nerves placed in chambers 3 h after L7 dorsal root injection with ³H-leucine. A short length of nerve on one side (•) was covered with 1 cm plastic strips and petrolatum to prevent entry of oxygen. This region is indicated by arrow 1 and the hatched r. Arrow 2 at the foot of the control (o) nerve shows the expected fast transport during the 3 h the nerves were in the chamber for *in vitro* downflow. Transport beyond the forward edge of the locally anoxic region was blocked with a damming of activity just behind it

tials (Hodgkin and Keynes, 1955; Baker, 1965) and as well the fast transport mechanism. In the relatively small diametered mammalian nerve fiber, K^+ is depleted rapidly and Na^+ gained after the sodium pump is stopped as compared to the giant axon. In accordance with this hypothesis experiments in our laboratory with M. I. Sabri have shown a fall in ATP and creatine phosphate and a rise in P in sciatic nerves asphyxiated by nitrogen at the time when fast transport fails.

The local nature of the energetic supply to the underlying transport mechanism was studied by asphyxiating a short length of nerve transporting labelled compounds *in vitro*. Failure of transport into the locally asphyxiated region is shown

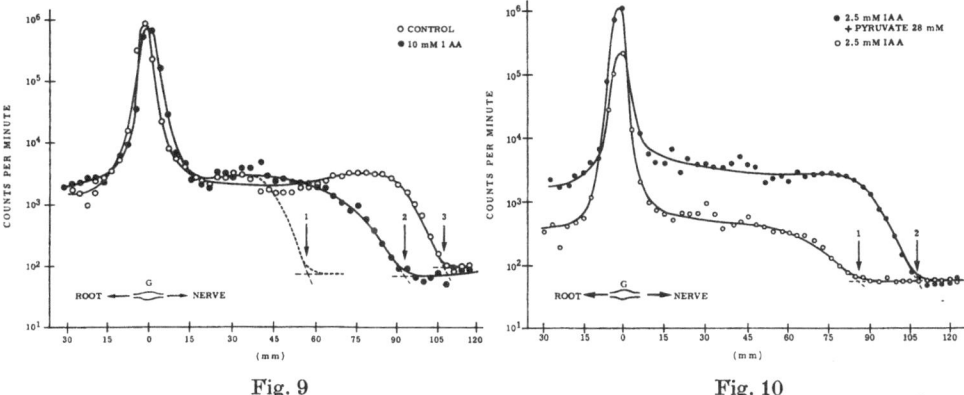

Fig. 9   Fig. 10

Fig.9. Effect of IAA on nerve. The nerves were removed 3 h after ganglion injection which would give the expected downflow indicated by the dashed line and its intersection with the baseline at arrow 1. One nerve (o) was placed in a chamber and oxyginated for 3 h and shows the usual fast transport expected of the total 6 h (arrow 3). The other nerve was similarly treated except that it was exposed to a 10 mm IAA solution (•). It shows a decrementing downflow and failure after about 2 h of *in vitro* downflow (arrow 2. Ochs and Smith, 1971)

Fig.10. Effect of a higher concentration of exogenous pyruvate producing a normal appearing curve of downflow. Both nerves were treated with 2.5 mM IAA in an experiment similar to that of Fig.9. With 28 mM pyruvate added (•) the pattern appears normal. The nerve (o) shows the usual declining pattern seen with IAA treatment. (Ochs and Smith, 1971)

by a damming of activity at the anterior part of the asphyxiated region (Fig.8). The oxidative enzymes required are present in the mitochondria which appear also to be transported down the nerve fibers (Friede, 1959; Barondes, 1966; Kapeller and Mayor, 1969).

Relation of *in vitro* Transport to Glycolysis

In contrast to the rapid block of fast transport found after interruption of oxidative metabolism, exposure of nerves *in vitro* to iodoacetic acid (IAA) causing a block of glycolysis fast transport to continue in decrementing fashion for about 2 h before a block of transport eventually occurred (Ochs and Smith, 1970). With IAA, a characteristic sloping diminution in the front of activity and a failure of a full extent of transport is apparent (Fig.9).

This is not due to a delay in the entry of IAA into the nerve fibers which enters within 10 min to block glyceraldehyde phosphate dehydrogenase (Sabri and Ochs, 1970) a sulfhydryl enzyme required for glycolysis to proceed (Webb, 1966).

When either pyruvate or L-lactate was supplied as an exogenous metabolite to IAA blocked nerves, a reversal of the pattern of decreased axoplasmic transport was seen (Fig.10). The isoenzyme composition of lactic dehydrogenase in nerve found by Sabri and Khan in this laboratory has a high heart muscle (H) isoenzyme content compared to the mainly muscle (M) isoenzyme content typical of skeletal muscle (Kaplan, 1963), thus allowing L-lactate to enter the tricarboxylic acid cycle.

Conclusion and a Note on Mechanism

A variety of cells showing streaming or pseudopodial movement and having actinomyosinoid properties which require ATP and Ca^{2+} (Jahn and Bovee, 1969) are of interest with respect to transport in the nerve. The microtubules and/or neurofilaments found in nerve fibers appear likely to act as a molecular substrate for transport (Ochs, 1966; Porter, 1966; Schmitt, 1968; Ochs, 1970b). It has previously been pointed out for the slow axoplasmic transport system that these linearly organized elements are not themselves being manufactured in the soma to be moved out into the axons as the labelled components (Ochs, 1967). This was indicated in studies using stretch to bead nerves followed by freeze substitution (Ochs, 1965). Constricted regions rich in microtubules and neurofilaments showed no greater amount of activity in radioautographs of labelled nerves (Ochs, 1967).

The inference from those studies was that the transported materials are moved down the axon along the neurotubules and/or neurofilaments rather than that these elements themselves are being transported. A new hypothesis advanced to account for fast transport is that a protein "transport" filament is being continuously produced in the cell body and it enters the axon (Ochs, 1970b). In analogy to muscle, the transport filament slides along the microtubules and/or neurotubules by means of cross-bridges activated by ATP.

Particulates, proteins and polypeptides, components associated with fast transport (Ochs et al., 1969) are bound to the postulated transport filament and thus carried down the nerve fiber.

The task remains to demonstrate this hypothesis. Further understanding of this mechanism promises to give new insights into neural function and its pathological alterations in both the peripheral and central nervous system.

Acknowledgements. Thanks are due to my associates in this work, Drs. Sabri and J. Johnson and Mr. N. Ranish and Mrs. Carolyn Smith and to the assistance of Mrs. Mary Ann Neel and Mrs. Carolynn Pankoke. Thanks are also due to Mr. James Glore and the Illustration Department. The work on which this review is based was supported by NIH NB-8706, NSF GB 7234X1 and the Hartford Foundation.

References

Austin, L., Morgan, I. G.: Incorporation of ^{14}C-leucine into synaptosomes isolated from rat cerebral cortex in vitro. J. Neurochem. **14**, 377—387 (1967).

Autilio, L. A., Appel, S. H., Pettis, B., Gambeth, P. L.: Biochemical studies of synapses in vitro. I. Protein Synthesis. Biochemistry **7**, 2615—2622 (1968).

Baker, P. F.: Phosphorus metabolism of intact crab nerve and its relation to the active transport of ions. J. Physiol. (Lond.) **180**, 383—423 (1965).

Barondes, S. H.: On the site of synthesis of the mitochondrial protein of nerve endings. J. Neurochem. **13**, 721—727 (1966).

— Axoplasmic transport. Neurosci. Res. Progr. Bull. **5**, 307—419 (1967).

Dahlström, A., Häggendal, J.: Studies on the transport and life-span of amine storage granules in a peripheral adrenergic neuron system. Acta physiol. scand. **67**, 278—288 (1966).

Friede, R. L.: Transport of oxidative enzymes in nerve fibers; a histochemical investigation of the regenerative cycle in neurons. Exp. Neurol. **1**, 441—466 (1959).

Gerard, R. W.: Nerve metabolism. Physiol. Rev. **12**, 469—592 (1932).

Grafstein, F.: Axonal transport: Communication between soma and synapse. Advanc. Biochem. Psychopharm. **1**, 11—25 (1969).

Hodgkin, A. L., Keynes, R. D.: Active transport of cations in giant axons from Sepia and Loligo. J. Physiol. (Lond.) **128**, 28—60 (1955).

Jahn, T. L., Bovee, E. C.: Protoplasmic movements within cells. Physiol. Rev. **49**, 793—862 (1969).

James, K. A. C., Austin, L.: The binding in vitro of colchicine to axoplasmic proteins from chicken sciatic nerve. Biochem. J. **117**, 773—777 (1970).

— Bray, J. J., Morgan, I. G., Austin, L.: The effect of colchicine on the transport of axonal protein in the chicken. Biochem. J. **117**, 767—771 (1970).

Kapeller, K., Mayor, D.: An electron microscopic study of the early changes proximal to a constriction in sympathetic nerves. Proc. roy. Soc. B **172**, 39—63 (1969).

Kaplan, N. O.: Symposium on multiple forms of enzymes and control mechanisms. Bact. Rev. **27**, 155—169 (1963).

Kidwai, A. M., Ochs, S.: Components of fast and slow phases of axoplasmic flow. J. Neurochem. **16**, 1105—1112 (1969).

Lasek, R. J.: Axoplasmic transport in cat dorsal root ganglion cells as studied with ^{3}H-l-leucine. Brain Res. **7**, 360—377 (1968).

— Protein transport in neurons. Int. Rev. Neurobiol. (in press) (1970).

Lehninger, A. L.: The Mitochondrion. New York: W. A. Benjamin 1965.

Lubińska, L.: Axoplasmic streaming in regenerating and in normal nerve fibers in mechanisms of neural regeneration. Progr. Brain Res. **13**, 55—66 (1964).

McEwen, B., Grafstein, B.: Fast and slow components in axonal transport of protein. J. Cell Biol. **38**, 494—508 (1968).

McIlwain, H.: Biochemistry and the central nervous system, 3rd ed. London: Churchill 1966.

Miani, N.: Analysis of the somato-axonal movement of phospholipids in the vagus and hypoglossal nerves. J. Neurochem. **10**, 859—874 (1963).

Ochs, S.: Beading of myelinated nerve fibers. Exp. Neurol. **12**, 84—95 (1965).

— Axoplasmic flow in neurons. Macromolecules and behavior. J. Gaito, (Ed.). New York: Appleton-Century-Crofts 1966.

— Axoplasmic transport of protein and the beading phenomenon in axoplasmic transport. S. Barondes (Ed.). Neurosci. Res. Progr. Bull. **5**, 337—340 (1967).

— Fast axoplasmic transport of proteins and polypeptides in mammalian nerve fibers. Protein metabolism of the nervous system. A. Lajtha (Ed.). New York: Plenum Press 1970 a.

— Axoplasmic flow-the fast transport system in mammalian nerve fibers. In Macromolecules and Behavior, 2nd Ed. J. Gaito (Ed.). New York: Appleton-Century-Crofts (in press) 1970 b.

— Hollingsworth, D.: Dependence of fast axoplasmic transport in nerve on oxidative metabolism. J. Neurochem. **18**. 107—114 (1971).

— Dalrymple, D., Richards, G.: Axoplasmic flow in ventral root nerve fiber of the cat. Exp. Neurol. **5**, 349—363 (1962).

— Hollingsworth, D., Helmer, E.: Dependence of fast axoplasmic transport in mammalian nerve on metabolism and relation to excitability. Biophys. Soc. Abst. **10**, 114 a (1970).

— Johnson, J.: Fast and slow phases of axoplasmic flow in ventral root nerve fibers. J. Neurochem. **16**, 845—853 (1969).

— Ranish, N.: Metabolic dependence of fast axoplasmic transport in nerve. Science **167**, 878—879 (1970).

— — Characteristics of the fast transport system in mammalian nerve fibers. J. Neurobiol. **1**, 247—261 (1969).

— Sabri, M. I., Johnson, J.: Fast transport system of materials in mammalian nerve fibers. Science **163**, 686—687 (1969).

— — Ranish, N.: Somal site of synthesis of fast transported materials in mammalian nerve fibers. J. Neurobiol. **1**, 329—344 (1970).

— Smith, C. B.: Fast axoplasmic transport in mammalian nerve in vitro after block of glycolysis with iodoacetic acid (in press) (1971).

Porter, K. R.: Cytoplasmic microtubules and their functions. In: Principles of biomolecular organization. Ciba Foundation Symposium. G. E. W. Wolstenholme, and M. O. O'Connor (Eds.). Boston: Little Brown & Co. 1966.

Sabri, M. I., Ochs, S.: The action of iodoacetic acid on glyceraldehyde 3-phosphate de-
    hodrogenase (GADP) in mammalian nerve. Physiologist **13**, 299 (1970).
Schmitt, F. O.: The molecular biology of neuronal fibrous proteins. Neurosci. Res. Progr.
    Bull. **6**, 114—119 (1968).
Sjöstrand, J., Karlsson, J. O.: Axoplasmic transport in the optic nerve and tract of the rabbit:
    A biochemical and radioautographic study. J. Neurochem. **16**, 833—844 (1969).
Webb, J. L.: Enzymes and metabolic inhibitors, Vol. 3. New York: Academic Press 1966.
Wright, E. B.: A comparative study of the effects of oxygen lack on peripheral nerve. Amer. J.
    Physiol. **147**, 78—89 (1946).
— The effects of asphyxiation and narcosis on peripheral nerve polarization and conduction.
    Amer. J. Physiol. **148**, 174—184 (1947).

                              Dr. Sidney Ochs
                              Department of Physiology
                              Indiana University Medical Center
                              1100 West Michigan Street
                              Indianapolis, Indiana 46202
                              U.S.A.

Acta neuropath. (Berl.) Suppl. V, 97—103 (1971)
© by Springer-Verlag 1971

Slow and Rapid Transport of Protein
to Nerve Endings in Mouse Brain *

Samuel H. Barondes

Department of Psychiatry, University of California, San Diego

Summary. The site of synthesis of a number of classes of proteins of nerve endings have been studied. Our results indicate that the general class of soluble proteins, which includes microtubular protein, are transported relatively slowly. In contrast, fucosyl glycoproteins are representative of a group of proteins which are transported to nerve endings at a more rapid, but measurable rate. Evidence is also presented for local incorporation of glucosamine into nerve ending macromolecules. These studies indicate the variable sites of synthesis and rates of transport of different protein components of nerve endings in mouse brain.

Key-Words: Axonal Transport — Protein Synthesis — Nerve Endings.

In the last few years, most research on axoplasmic transport has been concerned with documenting and characterizing the two widely differing rates of transport of protein in axons—"slow" flow and "fast" flow. Convincing evidence for these two classes of transport of proteins in the axon came from studies of transport of protein in defined axon populations, either leaving (sciatic nerve, Ochs *et al.*, 1970) or entering (optic nerve, McEwen and Grafstein, 1968) the central nervous system. This evidence is considered extensively by other participants in this symposium and will not be restated here. Our own studies of axoplasmic transport have not been done with peripheral or cranial nerves. Rather, they have been concerned with the brain, and with determining the rate with which proteins synthesized in the nerve cell body reach nerve endings, and presumably regulate their function.

Our studies show that some newly synthesized protein appears at nerve terminals within minutes after its synthesis (Droz and Barondes, 1969). Some of this protein appears to be mitochondrial protein which is locally synthetized at nerve terminals (Barondes, 1968). However, some of the newly synthesized protein which appears at nerve terminals is rapidly transported there through the axoplasm. The present brief report will describe some of the evidence for rapid transport of fucosyl glycoproteins to nerve endings in the mouse brain. It will also demonstrate the slower transport to nerve endings of soluble proteins, including a 60,000 molecular weight protein which has been identified as microtubular protein. The major purpose of this report is to indicate that the slow and fast forms of axoplasmic transport, shown so clearly in peripheral nerve, are also found in the brain and that different populations of proteins arrive at nerve terminals at these two major rates.

---

* Supported by Grant MH-18282 from the U.S.P.H.S.

Demonstrating "Fast" and "Slow" Transport in Brain

Studies of the transport of proteins to nerve endings in the mouse brain are conducted by a method which is described in detail in previous publications (Barondes, 1968). In essence, a radioactive precursor of protein or glycoprotein is injected intracerebrally into groups of mice, the animals are sacrificed by decapitation at various times from 15 min to several weeks after the injection, the cerebral hemispheres are homogenized and separated into fractions including a nerve ending fraction (synaptosome fraction), and the relative rate of incorporation of the radioactive precursor into proteins or glycoproteins of the nerve ending fraction is compared with that in the various other subcellular fractions. Incorporation into components of the nerve ending fraction is interpreted as being due to axoplasmic transport of proteins synthesized in the nerve cell body, if there is a *lag* between incorporation into whole brain components and appearance of the incorporated protein in nerve ending components. Incorporation into the various whole brain components is taken to reflect the rate of incorporation into nerve cell bodies, since this should not differ from the rate of incorporation into the glia.

The soluble component of the nerve ending fraction, which is obtained by water lysis and ultracentrifugation of the isolated nerve ending fraction has been a major subject of interest since it represents the purest component of the nerve ending fraction. This is because the major contaminants of this fraction are particulate and release little protein with water lysis. Major attention is therefore paid to the relative rate of appearance of labelled protein in the soluble component of the nerve ending fraction as compared with incorporation of label into the proteins of the soluble components of whole brain. In addition, incorporation into the particulate component of the nerve ending fraction is contrasted with incorporation into the various particulate components of whole brain.

In extensive studies with radioactive leucine it has been shown that the protein of the soluble component of the nerve ending fraction contains only five per cent as much label as the soluble protein of whole brain when measured one hour after intracerebral injection of radioactive leucine, and that this percentage rises in the ensuing days. Several days after injection of the precursor the specific activity of the soluble protein of nerve endings exceeds that of the specific activity of the soluble protein of whole brain (Barondes, 1968). These studies are believed to reflect slow transport of soluble protein from nerve cell bodies to nerve terminals by analogy with the slow transport of the major portion of soluble proteins, in optic nerve (McEwen and Grafstein, 1968). Therefore, this method is clearly suitable for studying slow transport of soluble protein to nerve endings in mouse brain because of the long lag before the specific activity of the soluble protein of nerve endings becomes maximal, and because the soluble protein of the nerve endings is quite free of contamination by the soluble proteins from other components of the brain.

Greater limitations exist when one studies transport of the protein of particulate components of the nerve ending because there is more contamination with particulate components from the rest of the brain; and when one attempts to study rapid flow, where the lag is relatively short because of the short axons of brain neurons. To be sure, it can be demonstrated that some protein associated with

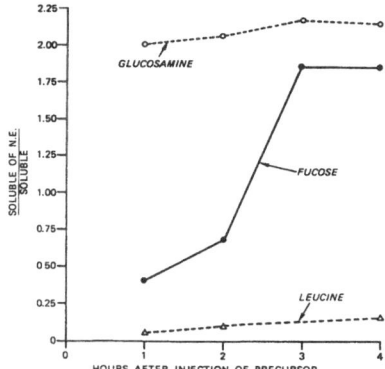

Fig. 1. Ratio of specific activity of soluble macromolecules of nerve endings to those of whole brain at relatively short times after injection. Young adult mice were injected intracerebrally with radioactive leucine or fucose or glucosamine, sacrificed one or more hours later, and their cerebral hemispheres were homogenized and fractionated to yield the soluble components of the whole homogenate and of the nerve ending of fraction (for details see Barondes, 1968). After determination of the radioactivity incorporated into the (non-lipid) acid precipitable component of these fractions, the ratio of their specific activities was plotted. (For details of the data with leucine see Barondes, 1968; for fucose and glucosamine see Zatz and Barondes, 1971)

some particulate components of the nerve endings are transported with the slow phase (Barondes, 1968). However, the site of synthesis of labeled proteins which are very rapidly associated with the nerve ending fraction, are difficult to determine, not only because of problems of contamination but because of an important property of our technique.

The technique which we have employed for studying axoplasmic transport in brain differs in one important respect from that used in studies in peripheral nerve. In the latter labeled precursor is introduced into the region of the nerve cell bodies (for example, the ventral horn of the spinal cord or the retina) and has relatively little access to the region of the nerve terminals which are far away. In our method labeled precursor is injected into the brain so that both nerve terminals and nerve cell bodies are exposed to the radioactive precursor. This raises the important problem that rapid appearance of labeled macromolecules at nerve endings could be due either to local synthesis in nerve endings or to rapid transport. The only hope for distinguishing between these two possibilities is to demonstrate a lag, no matter how brief, between incorporation of the labeled precursor into components of the nerve cell body and incorporation into the nerve endings. In recent studies using radioactive fucose (Zatz and Barondes, 1971) as precursor we have found clear evidence for transport of fucosyl glycoproteins to nerve endings at a rate which far exceeds the rate of transport of the bulk of soluble protein.

In the first hour after intracerebral injection of radioactive fucose the ratio of incorporation into the soluble fucosyl glycoproteins of nerve endings, as compared with the soluble fucosyl glycoproteins of whole brain, is extremely low. However, in the ensuing few hours there is a sudden rapid increase in the relative labeling of the soluble fucosyl glycoproteins of nerve endings (Fig. 1). The lag which precedes the rapid increase in specific activity of the soluble fucosyl glycoproteins of nerve endings is most probably due to the short delay between synthesis of these glycoproteins in the nerve cell body and their arrival at the nerve ending. It should be noted that the lag is not so great as it is for the transport of proteins labeled with leucine since the leucine labeled proteins have a low specific activity even three to four hours after injection of the precursor and do not attain a high specific activity for several days. It appears, therefore, that fucosyl glycoproteins are transported with the rapid component of axoplasmic flow whereas the bulk of soluble proteins are transported to nerve terminals at a slower rate. Therefore, under certain circumstances, the technique can clearly resolve a rapid component of axoplasmic transport in the brain.

The limitation of the technique, namely simultaneous exposure of nerve ending and the other parts of the neuron to labeled precursor is also, in some respects, as asset. Because of this, it is possible to attempt to determine if there is local macromolecular biosynthesis at the nerve endings themselves. This is shown in studies with glucosamine done simultaneously with the fucose studies (Fig. 1). At the earliest time studied (one hour) glucosamine is incorporated into the soluble macromolecules of nerve endings to the same extent as into the soluble macromolecules of whole brain. Furthermore, the ratio of glucosamine incorporated in the soluble macromolecules of nerve endings to that in the soluble macromolecules of whole brain remains fairly constant over the ensuing hours. Since incorporation of glucosamine into the soluble component of the nerve ending fraction is relatively insensitive to treatment with acetoxycycloheximide which blocks the biosynthesis of polypeptide acceptors for glycoproteins, it appears that a macromolecular acceptor exists at nerve endings into which glucosamine can be locally incorporated (Barondes and Dutton, 1969; Zatz and Barondes, 1971).

We conclude that, using injected leucine, fucose or glucosamine as precursors, we can demonstrate three different origins of soluble macromolecules of nerve endings. The studies with leucine indicate slow transport of soluble proteins to nerve endings because of the long lag which we find. The studies with fucose indicate the rapid transport of some fucosyl glycoproteins because the lag is much shorter. Studies with glucosamine indicate there is a potentiality for locally incorporating glucosamine into macromolecular acceptors at nerve endings, since no lag is found and because of the results with acetoxycycloheximide (Barondes and Dutton, 1969).

Transport of Microtubular Protein Nerve Endings

Microtubules are of great interest to students of axoplasmic transport since they are known to be an extremely abundant component of axons and could play some role in directing or mediating axoplasmic transport (Schmitt, 1969). In the past few years evidence has been presented that microtubular protein, the subunit of microtubules is composed of monomers with a molecular weight of 60,000 (Weisenberg *et al.*, 1968), and that this protein binds colchicine (Borisy and Taylor, 1967), is precipitable by vinblastine (Marantz *et al.*, 1969), and can be purified

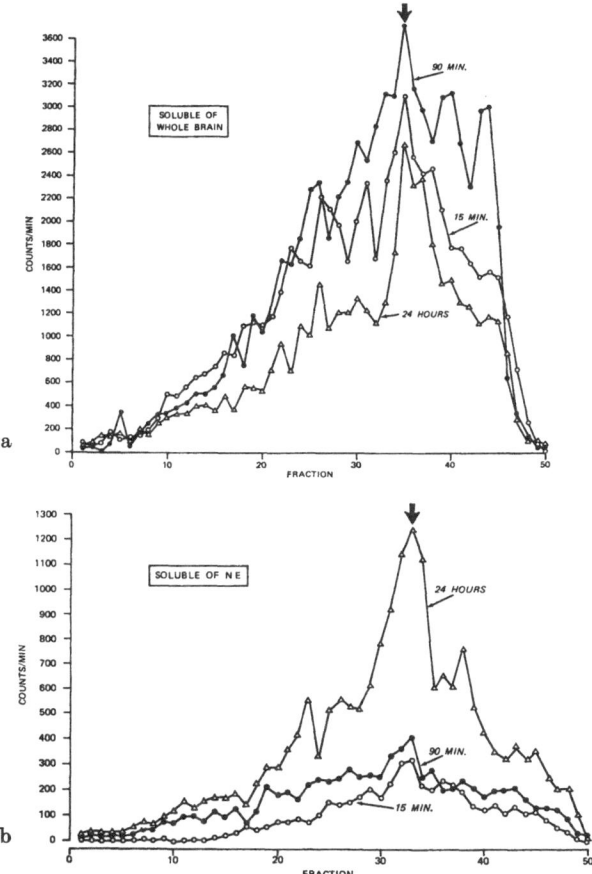

Fig. 2a and b. Polyacrylamide gel electrophoresis of labeled protein from the soluble fraction of whole brain and of nerve endings. Five day old mice were injected intracerebrally with ³H-leucine, sacrificed 15 min to 24 hours later and the soluble protein from whole brain homogenates and from nerve endings was obtained as in Fig. 1. The proteins were reduced, alkylated electrophoresed, and fractionated in a system which separates disaggregated proteins on the basis of molecular weights (Shapiro *et al.*, 1967). Internal standards of ¹⁴C-labelled microtubular protein with a molecular weight of approximately 60,000 migrated to the point indicated by the heavy arrow. (Unpublished data of G. Dutton and S. Barondes)

from vinblastine precipitates. This protein represents a major component of the total labeled soluble protein found in developing mouse brain after intracerebral injection of radioactive leucine (Dutton and Barondes, 1969). Extensive studies with Feit, Dutton and Shelanski, which will be published in detail elsewhere, have shown that more than 20% of the soluble protein obtained by lysis of an isolated nerve ending fraction is microtubular protein as determined by co-migration in polyacrylamide gel electrophoresis systems when run along with authentic

microtubular protein and also as demonstrated by peptide mapping and vinblastine precipitation. Based on these studies we have found the metabolism of
microtubular protein in mouse brain can be estimated from studies of the incorporation into and turnover of 60,000 molecular weight soluble protein subunits.
Polyacrylamide gel electrophoresis patterns of labeled soluble proteins of whole
five day old mouse brain at various times after intracerebral injection of radioactive leucine are shown in Fig. 2. A major peak of radioactive protein with a
molecular weight of 60,000 is observed 15 and 90 min after injection of the radioactive precursor. The specific activity of this protein and other soluble proteins
of whole brain has decreased by 24 hours due to turnover. In striking contrast
the specific activity of the 60,000 molecular weight protein in the soluble component of the nerve ending fraction increases markedly in the interval between
15 min and 24 hours after injection of the precursor. In other experiments we
have found that the protein from the soluble fraction of isolated nerve endings
which corresponds to this 60,000 molecular weight protein peak is precipitable
by vinblastine and, after suitable purification, has a peptide map which is similar
to authentic microtubular protein.

The prominence of the 60,000 molecular weight protein in the soluble component of nerve endings should be apparent from the figure. In earlier studies with
adult mice its relative prominence shortly after injection of labeled leucine led us
to emphasize that same soluble microtubular protein was transported to nerve
terminals at a rapid rate. The present experiments and many others confirm that
soluble microtubular protein is transported to nerve endings. They also clearly
show that its overall rate of transport is similar to that of transport of most
other soluble proteins. In essence then we conclude that most microtubular
protein moves to nerve endings with the "slow component" of axoplasmic
transport. This conclusion is consistent with studies of the rate of transport
of bound colchicine presumably moving with microtubules in axons of the optic
nerve (Grafstein et al., 1970).

References

Barondes, S. H.: Further studies of the transport of protein to nerve endings. J Neurochem.
15, 343—350 (1968).
— Dutton, G. R.: Acetoxycycloheximide effect on synthesis and metabolism of glucosamine
containing macromolecules in brain and nerve endings. J. Neurobiol. 1, 99—110 (1969).
Borisy, G. G., Taylor, E. W.: The mechanism of action of colchicine: binding of colchincine-
³H to cellular protein. J. Cell Biol. 34, 525—533 (1967).
Droz, B., Barondes, S. H.: Nerve endings: rapid appearance of labeled protein shown by
electron microscope radioautography. Science 165, 1131—1133 (1969).
Dutton, G. R., Barondes, S. H.: Microtubular protein: synthesis and metabolism in developing
brain. Science 166, 1637—1638 (1969).
Grafstein, B., McEwen, B. S., Shelanski, M. L.: Axonal transport of neurotubule protein.
Nature (Lond.) 227, 289—290 (1970).
Marantz, R., Ventilla, M., Shelanski, M.: Vinblastine induced precipitation of microtubule
protein. Science 165, 498—499 (1969).
McEwen, B. S., Grafstein, B.: Fast and slow components in axonal transport of protein. J.
Cell Biol. 38, 494—508 (1968).
Ochs, S., Sabri, M. I., Ranish, N.: Somal site of synthesis of fast transported materials in
mammalian nerve fibers. J. Neurobiol. 1, 329—344 (1970).

Schmitt, F. O.: Fibrous proteins and neuronal dynamics .In: Cellular dynamics of the neuron. pp. 95—111. ed. by S. H. Barondes. New York: Academic Press 1969.

Shapiro, A. L., Vinuela, E., Maizel, J., Jr.: Molecular weight estimation of polypeptide chains by electrophoresis in SDS-polyacrylamide. Biochem. biophys Res. Commun. 28, 815—844 (1967).

Weisenberg, R. C., Borisy, G. G., Taylor, E. W.: The colchicine-binding protein of mammalian brain and its relation to microtubules. Biochemistry 7, 4466—4478 (1968).

Zatz, M., Barondes, S. H.: Rapid transport of fucosyl glycoproteins to nerve endings in mouse brain. J. Neurochem. (in press) (1971).

Samuel H. Barondes, M.D.
University of California
San Diego
La Jolla, California 92037/U.S.A.

Acta neuropath. (Berl.) Suppl. V, 104—108 (1971)

Transport of S-100 Protein in Mammalian Nerve Fibers and Transneuronal Signals

Nicolò Miani

Department of Anatomy, Università Cattolica del S. Cuore Roma, Italy

Summary. The brain-specific acidic protein S-100 is a migratory protein from soma to terminals of the glossopharyngeal and vagus nerves of rabbit (axonal transport of S-100 protein).

Autoradiographic analyses indicate that certain proteins including probably the S-100 conveyed to the nerve endings of the otic ganglion migrate beyond them, towards the ancillary cells of the axo-dendritic synapses and eventually to the postsynaptic neurons (transynaptic transfer of S-100).

Key-Words: S-100 Protein — Transneuronal Signals — Radioactivity — Axonal Transport.

This report is concerned with the flow along the axon, and the behaviour at the synaptic terminal, of a protein called S-100 by Moore (1965).

It is well known that the S-100 protein is specific for the nervous system and conserves its immunological identity throughout phylogenesis (Levine and Moore, 1965; Moore *et al.*, 1968; Kessler *et al.*, 1968; Calissano *et al.*, 1969). Such attributes indicate that the biological function of the S-100 is highly specific.

Experimental studies designed to localize the protein have yielded somewhat equivocal results (Perez and Moore, 1968; Hydén and McEwen, 1966), although it is suggested that the S-100 is largely, if not exclusively, a glial protein (Perez *et al.*, 1970; Cicero *et al.*, 1970).

When tritiated leucine and lysine (100 μc, fifty/fifty per animal) is deposited on the floor of the fourth ventricle of adult rabbits under direct vision through a window in the atlanto-occipital membrane, the nuclei of the medulla oblongata just below the floor and the surrounding structures synthesize labelled substances that thereafter flow down the hypoglossal, vagus and glossopharyngeal nerves (Miani, 1963). In order to obtain a negligible background of radioactivity in the body, the calamus scriptorius and the surrounding structures must be carefully kept free of cerebrospinal fluid by continuous drainage of the cisterna magna throughout the labelling experiment.

Five days after labelling the vagus and hypoglossal nuclei, 30 per cent of the radioactivity of the homogenate of cervical vagus and hypoglossal nerves was in the supernatant (Table 1). When the soluble proteins were fractionated on DEAE-Sephadex A-50 column under an appropriate gradient of sodium chloride (Moore and McGregor, 1965), a typical pattern of protein and radioactivity was obtained (Fig. 1). It can be seen the neutral and basic proteins eluted in the first 20 fractions contain only 14 per cent of the radioactivity, whereas the acidic proteins, especially those bound most tightly to the DEAE-Sephadex, are highly radioactive.

Table 1. *Distribution of protein and radioactivity in fractions from cervical vagus and hypoglossal nerve of 5 rabbits at 5 days after labelling the related nuclei*

Fractions	Protein (mg)	Radioactivity % (DPM×10⁶)		Specific activity DPM×10³/mg protein
Homogenate	91.1	100.0	(4.98)	54.6
Insoluble	70.0	68.0	(3.40)	48.5
Supernatant (100,000 g$_{av}$)	20.8	30.1	(1.50)	71.8
Supernatant excluded from Sephadex G-25 column	20.6	30.0	(1.49)	72.3

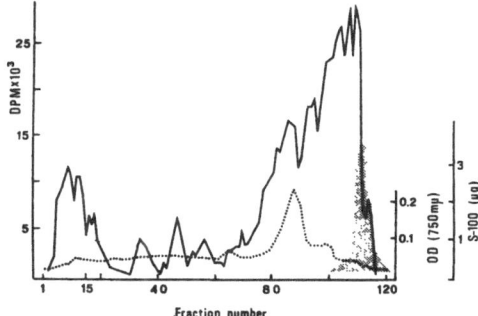

Fig. 1. Protein and radioactive chromatographic patterns of soluble proteins from cervical vagus and hypoglossal nerve of rabbits 5 days after labelling the vagus and hypoglossal nuclei

Further separation of the column chromatography fractions by polyacrylamide gel electrophoresis (Davis, 1964), showed that the actual number of different resolvable proteins containing radioactivity was 20 to 40 among a total of at least 100 protein bands. By micro complement-fixation assay (Moore and Perez, 1966), the S-100 protein has been localized at the right end of the chromatogram (Fig. 1). where the radioactivity falls from the maximum. Acrylamide gel electrophoresis of the corresponding fraction tubes confirms that the S-100 was localized in the band moving at the front and that the protein was radioactive. From this starting point, indicating that S-100 is a migratory protein, we searched for its rate of flow along the vagus nerve and arrival at the synaptic terminals of the salivatory component of the glossopharyngeal nerve, that is, to the otic ganglion. This could be accomplished by separating the soluble proteins of nerves or of ganglia directly by 7.5% polyacrylamide electrophoresis and measuring the S-100 content as well as the radioactivity in the 2 mm thick gel slice containing the front.

Fig. 2 shows the specific activity of the S-100 protein in 3 segments of the vagus nerve as a function of the time after labelling the corresponding nuclei in the medulla oblongata. The specific activity of S-100 in the bulbar structures reached a maximum 15 hours after the beginning of the experiment with tritiated leucine and lysine (not shown in Fig. 2); thereafter the group of labelled S-100

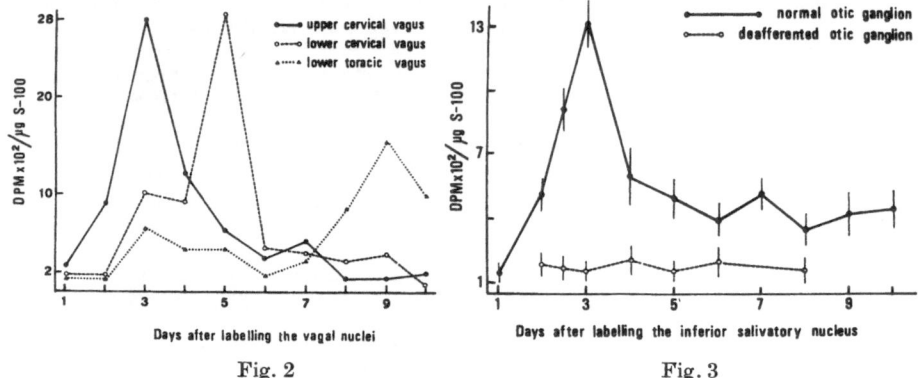

Fig. 2   Fig. 3

Fig. 2. Specific activity of the S-100 protein in 3 segments of the vagus nerve at different time
intervals after labelling the vagus nuclei

Fig. 3. Specific activity of the S-100 protein in otic ganglia at different time intervals after
labelling the inferior salivatory nucleus

molecules flowed down the vagus nerve. The lower thoraco-subdiaphragmatic
segment of the nerve was reached 9 days after labelling. The lower thoraco-subdiaphragmatic segments under analysis, as the cervical ones, were 40 mm long
and were 230 mm from the bulbar origin of the nerve.

We choose to express the displacement of the labelled S-100 molecules in
terms of group velocity (g_v). Under the present experimental conditions, the group
velocity of the S-100 protein was 25 mm per day in the vagus nerve; the motion
of the group was uniform from just below the nodose ganglion to the diaphragmatic
level of the vagus nerve, that is, within a traffic line of 180 mm. The specific
activity in the lower thoraco-subdiaphragmatic segment appeared reduced as
compared to that of the upper and lower cervical vagus, because of the loss of
efferent fibers proximally and perhaps also the half-life of the S-100 in the axonal
compartment.

The otic ganglion is a small structure, but excellent for exploring the arrival
of the S-100 conveyed by salivatory fibers. Sectioning of the preganglionic salivatory fibers interrupts the traffic of radioactive material, and the blank for the
ganglion may be determined. Each experiment of this series required collecting
at least 3 normal and as many deafferented ganglia.

In the deafferented ganglia the general background of radioactivity was very
low and did not change with time (Fig. 3). On the contrary, in the normal ganglia,
the S-100 protein reached the synaptic terminals soon and accumulated there up
to 3 days after labelling the salivatory nucleus in the bulb. We estimate the group
velocity of S-100 molecules in the preganglionic salivatory fibers about 20 mm
per day.

In summary, these experiments prove that S-100 molecules synthesized in the
vagus and glossopharyngeal nuclei flow downwards and reach the nerve endings.

The next question is concerned with the destination of the S-100 protein that
reachs the nerve ending. The immunological identity of the S-100 throughout the

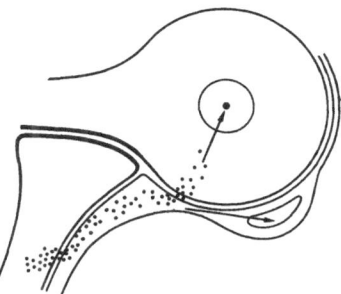

Fig. 4. Diagrammatic representation of migration of labelled substances from pre- to post-synaptic neuron in the otic ganglion of rabbit

phylogenesis and its chemico-physical characteristics could suggest that the protein is intended for the postsynaptic cell in particular for the nucleus of the postsynaptic neuron where it would interact with histones that also are known to conserve their immunological identity during evolution. It follows, therefrom, that histones would gain a specific imprint for their repressing genetic activity.

In order to test this hypothesis, the otic ganglion was choosen for two series of experiments: (1) To analyze autoradiographically the transfer of labelled substance from pre- to post-synaptic neurons; (2) To isolate the migrated S-100 from post-synaptic neurons.

In terms of autoradiographic reaction, the activity of the otic ganglion was low at any time interval after labelling the related salivatory nucleus in the bulb, but the signal-to-noise ratio was high, because the general background of radio-activity in the organ was very low. Moreover, there was the possibility to prevent the signals from arriving at the ganglion by interrupting its afferent salivatory fibers, as shown above.

Three days after labelling the salivatory nucleus with $100\mu c$ of tritiated leucine and lysine, fifty/fifty, silver grains can be seen inside the axons of nonmyelinated fibers (Miani *et al.*, 1970) as well as in the synaptic terminals. In addition, discrete foci of labelling appeared in the processes of the satellite cells and scattered silver grains in the perikarya of the ganglion cells or over the neuron-glial contacts. Dendritic processes also showed labelling. In both neurons and satellite cells the labelling was not related to cytoplasmic organelles. Finally, radioautographic studies showed labelled material in the nuclei of nerve cell bodies and satellite cells.

The deafferented ganglia displayed no activity inside the perikarya and dendritic processes. Although qualitative in nature, the results indicate that no more than 5 to 10 per cent of the total activity invaded the neuroplasma of ganglion cells within four days after labelling the salivatory nucleus.

Considered together, the autoradiographic data suggest the following successive events in the otic ganglion, as schematically indicated in Fig. 4: (i) radioactive material from salivatory nucleus is conveyed to synaptic terminals; (ii) some molecules migrate to postsynaptic neurons; (iii) the transfer of labelled molecules from pre- to postsynaptic neurons is mediated primarly by the satellite cells; (iiii) the nuclei of the postsynaptic neurons seem to be the destination of some of the transferred molecules. The satellite cells around the synaptic apparatus, therefore, would be involved in the transfer process of molecules from pre- to post-synaptic neurons, though a direct neuron-to-neuron migration could not be ruled out.

According to the hypothesis mentioned above, S-100 protein is a candidate for transneuronal signals. Since autoradiographic data indicate that some labelled substances reach the nuclei of the postsynaptic neurons, we attempted to isolate labelled S-100 from nuclei of the otic ganglion. Because of technical difficulties we have not yet obtained satisfactory results.

References

Calissano, P., Moore, B. W., Friesen, A.: Effect of calcium ion on S-100, a protein of the nervous system. Biochemistry 8, 4318—4326 (1969).

Cicero, T. J., Cowan, W. M., Moore, B. W., Suntzeff, V.: The cellular localization of the two brain specific proteins, S-100 and 14-3-2. Brain Res. 18, 25—34 (1970).

Davis, B. J.: Disc electrophoresis. Ann. N. Y. Acad. Sci. 121, 404—427 (1964).

Hydén, H., McEwen, B. S.: A glial protein specific for the nervous system. Proc. nat. Acad. Sci. (Wash.) 55, 354—358 (1966).

Kessler, D., Levine, L., Fasman, G.: Some conformational and immunological properties of a bovine brain acidic protein (S-100). Biochemistry 7, 758—764 (1968).

Levine, L., Moore, B. W.: Structural relatedness of a vertebrate brain acidic protein as measured immunochemically. Neurosci. Res. Progr. Bull. 3, 5—11 (1965).

Miani, N.: Analysis of the somato-axonal movement of phospholipids in the vagus and hypoglossal nerves. J. Neurochem. 10, 859—874 (1963).

— De Renzis, G., Olivieri Sangiacomo, C., Michetti, F., Correr, S., Caniglia, A.: Axonal transport and transynaptic transfer of S-100 protein. (In preparation.)

Moore, B. W.: A soluble protein characteristic of the nervous system. Biochem. biophys. Res. Commun. 19, 739—744 (1965).

— McGregor: Chromatographic and electrophoretic fractionation of soluble proteins of brain and liver. J. biol. Chem. 240, 1647—1653 (1965).

— Perez, V. J.: Complement fixation for antigens on a picogram level. J. Immunol. 96, 1000—1005 (1966).

— — Gehring, M.: Assay and regional distribution of a soluble protein characteristic of the nervous system. J. Neurochem. 15, 265—272 (1968).

Perez, V. J., Moore, B. W.: Wallerian degeneration in rabbit tibial nerve: changes in amounts of the S-100 protein. J. Neurochem. 15, 971—977 (1968).

— Olney, J. W., Cicero, T. J., Moore, B. W., Bahn, B. A.: Wallerian degeneration in rabbit optic nerve: cellular localization in the central nervous system of the S-100 and 14-3-2 proteins. J. Neurochem. 17, 511—519 (1970).

Dr. Nicolò Miami
Department of Anatomy
Università Cattolica del S. Cuore
Roma, Italy

Acta neuropath. (Berl.) Suppl. V, 109—118 (1971)
© by Springer-Verlag 1971

Dynamic Condition of Protein in Axons and Axon Terminals *

B. Droz

Département de Biologie, Commissariat à l'Énergie Atomique, Saclay

H. L. Koenig

Laboratoire de Cytologie, Faculté des Sciences, Paris

Summary. Radioautographic studies performed with labeled amino acids visualize the complexity of the dynamic state of protein in nerve endings. One protein fraction, at least, is replaced at a rate of 4% per day. On the one hand, the loss of used protein in presynaptic axon terminals seems to be balanced by the arrival of new migratory proteins, synthesized in the nerve cell bodies and conveyed along the axons at various velocities. On the other hand, the slight local incorporation of amino acids observed in nerve endings rises the question whether proteins are synthesized *in situ*; this is probably true for mitochondria. However, the configurational change of a protein by addition of an amino acid or by linkage with a peptide would be a possible mean to modulate the biological activity of presynaptic nerve endings.

Key-Words: Axonal Transport — Radioactivity — Protein Synthesis — Nerve Endings.

It is now well established that protein molecules present in axons and nerve endings turn over continuously (see review in Barondes, 1967, 1969; Droz, 1969; Grafstein, 1969). In our presentation, we will briefly discuss the mechanisms involved in the replacement or alteration of axonal proteins in presynaptic nerve terminals.

Possible Origins of Axoplasmic Proteins

Various sources have been proposed to account for the renewal of protein in axonal processes:

1. *The nerve cell body* was considered as a probable purveyor of axoplasmic protein eventually transported along the axon (Weiss and Hiscoe, 1948). Such an axonal migration of protein was shown to take place in various peripheral nerves and in the central nervous system (Droz and Leblond, 1963). Velocities of transport ranging from a few millimeters to several hundred millimeters per day were recorded (Grafstein, 1967; Lasek, 1968; Ochs and Johnson, 1969; Sjøstrand, 1970; Schonbach and Cuénod, 1970).

2. *The glial cells*, which closely encompass the axon, synthesize proteins which, according to Singer and Salpeter (1966), would be transferred to the axon through the myelin sheath.

3. *The axon and its terminals* would be able to manufacture a part of their own proteins by local synthesis (Edström, 1969; Koenig, 1970; Austin et al., 1970).

---

* A la mémoire de Nicole Granboulan.

Radioautographic Study of Protein Renewal in Nerve Endings

To investigate the possible mechanisms by which proteins are renewed in nerve endings, we have used radioautography. The limits of confidence of this technique for the detection of labeled proteins were tested on nerve ending fractions of mouse brain: the biochemical analysis showed that 87 to 94 per cent of the total radioactivity contained in "synaptosomes" was firmly bound to protein (Droz and Barondes, 1969).

Our radioautographic study of the renewal of protein in nerve endings was performed on the giant calices present in the ciliary ganglion of the chicken (Koenig and Droz, 1970). This material was selected mainly because: 1. the volume occupied by the presynaptic axon terminals is large enough to yield a reliable estimation of the label content; 2. the axonal length, that is the distance between the nerve cell bodies in the Edinger-Westphal nucleus and their axon terminals in the ciliary ganglion, is known to average 6 millimeters.

After a stereotaxic injection of a labeled amino acid into the third cerebral ventricle of 2-week-old chickens, the ciliary ganglia were removed at various time intervals and radioautographs were prepared for light (Kopriwa and Leblond, 1962) and electron microscopy (Granboulan and Granboulan, 1965). Under these conditions, it was hoped that the tracer, first incorporated into protein synthesized by the nerve cell bodies of the Edinger-Westphal nucleus, then transported along the preganglionic axons, would finally reach the giant calices.

Arrival and Fate of Migratory Proteins in Nerve Endings

One hour after the intraventricular injection of leucine-^{3}H, only a few silver grains overlaid the preganglionic nerve endings. Three hours after the administration of tritium labeled glutamic acid, leucine, phenylalanine or lysine, a clear-cut radioautographic reaction was located over the presynaptic calices; in contrast, the preganglionic axons were poorly labelled as compared to their terminals (Fig. 1). Thus, in the absence of axonal flow of free amino acids (Di Giamberardino, 1970), the early appearance of the label in nerve endings corresponds probably to the arrival of protein moving at a velocity faster than 50 mm per day.

With time, the radioautographic reaction was progressively enhanced over the nerve endings and reached a maximal value by 18 hours; at later time intervals, the preganglionic axons were heavily labeled (Fig. 2). It is concluded that the late appearance of radioactivity in preterminal axons and in their terminals is due to a massive transport of protein migrating at a rate of 1—3 mm per day.

Electron microscope radioautographs showed that silver grains were distributed over mitochondrial profiles, areas containing membranes or synaptic vesicles at 3 hours as well as 48 hours after the intraventricular injection of lysine-^{3}H (Figs. 3 and 4). Cell fractions of ciliary ganglia indicated that 3 or 6 days after the intraventricular injection of leucine-^{3}H, 50 or 73 per cent of the radioactivity was recovered in soluble proteins and only 7 or 8 per cent in synaptic vesicles (Israel and Koenig, unpublished).

Assuming that the disappearance of the label corresponds to a first order reaction, the decay curve of the radioactivity concentration in nerve endings indicates a turnover rate of 4 per cent per day. Thus, the mean time of sojourn of protein in presynaptic calices is about 25 days. Similar turnover times have been reported by von Hungen et al., (1968) in the synaptosomal fraction of brain cortex in rats.

The axonal delivery of neuroplasmic protein to postsynaptic structures (Korr et al., 1967) remains a controversial subject. It was thought that the postsynaptic ganglion cell would be a suitable material to look for a possible transsynaptic migration of protein. Sparse silver grains indeed were constantly found over the ganglion cell bodies (Figs. 1 and 2). To decide whether the dim reaction observed over the postsynaptic ganglion cells was due to labelled protein discharged from the presynaptic calyx or to a local incorporation of labelled amino acid having leaked into the bloodstream, ciliary ganglia were wrapped in a piece of "spongel" soaked with a concentrated puromycin solution, prior to the intraventricular injection. Under these conditions, 3 and 48 hours later, the label had accumulated in presynaptic calices, whereas no reaction occured over the postsynaptic nerve cell bodies. These data indicate that the slight reaction observed in postsynaptic nerve cell bodies is due to a leakage of the labelled amino acid in the course of the intraventricular injection rather than to a transsynaptic transfer of labelled protein. A similar conclusion was reached by Hendrickson (1969) in the optic nerve terminals.

Local Incorporation of Amino Acids into Nerve Endings

A local synthesis of protein has been reported to take place in nerve ending fractions of the brain (Morgan and Austin, 1968; Autilio et al., 1968; Gordon and Deanin, 1968) but, as noted by Barondes (1969), brain fractionation makes it difficult to separate synaptosomes from any contaminant capable of synthesizing protein. To answer the question whether preganglionic nerve endings were able or not to incorporate labelled amino acids into protein, ciliary ganglia of young chickens were excised and incubated in vitro with leucine-^{3}H for 1 hour. To impede a nonspecific binding of labelled leucine on preformed proteins, large amounts of non-radioactive leucine were added to the chase medium and to the formaldehyde solution used as fixative[1]. Radioautographs of the peripheral region of ciliary ganglia incubated under various conditions were compared (Figs. 5—10).

After an incubation with leucine-^{3}H, a strong radioautographic reaction spread over the nerve cell bodies and the initial segments of the thin axons of the ganglion cells (Fig. 5); the thick axons of the preganglionic nerves, which were associated with labelled Schwann cells, displayed no reaction or, at most, stray silver grains. Thus, when an artifactual retention of the label is prevented, our radioautographic data indicate that the delivery of protein from Schwann cells to axons would be, if it occurs at all, a very restricted process.

Electron microscope radioautographs showed the presence of the tracer in presynaptic calices (Fig. 8). The concentration of the label in these nerve endings was less than one third of that measured in the perikaryon of ganglion cells

---

1 When unlabelled leucine, at a concentration 1000 times higher than that of the radioactive leucine, is added to the formaldehyde solution, the unlabelled leucine passes massively through the cell membrane which is permeated by the fixative. Thus, the labelled leucine bound on protein by weak linkages such as ionic bonds may be efficiently washed out. On the contrary, the labelled leucine incorporated into proteins by means of strong peptide bond is not exchanged and may produce a radioautographic reaction.

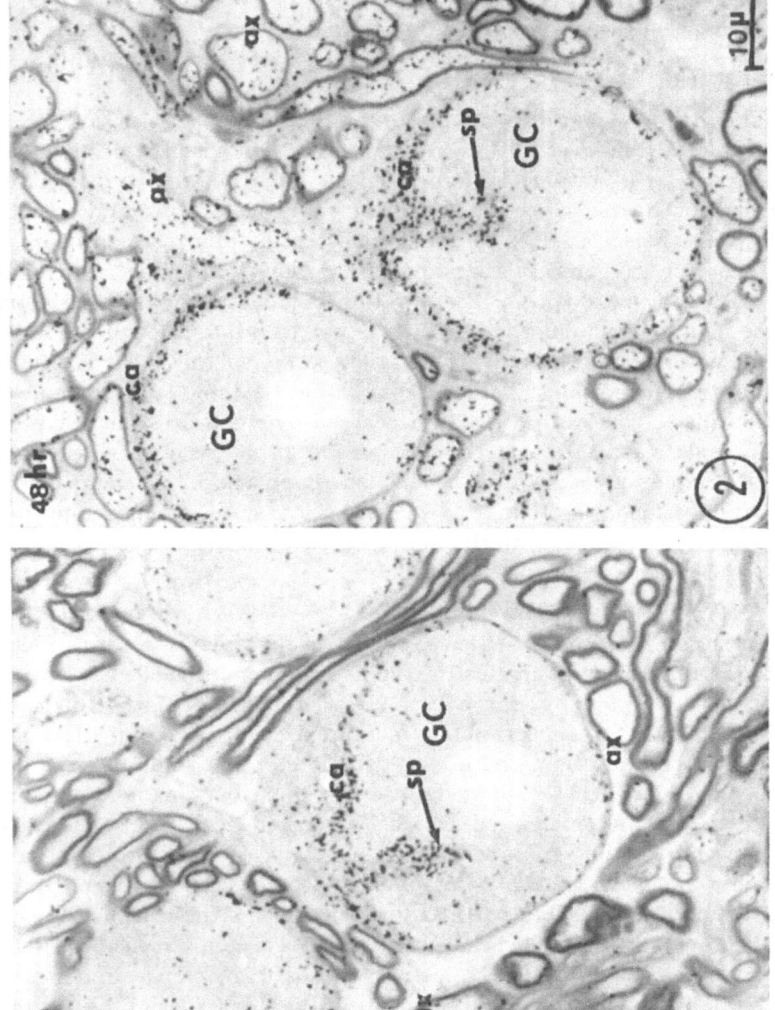

Plates I and II. Accumulation of radioactivity in giant nerve endings of the ciliary ganglion of chicken 3 and 48 hours after an injection of lysine-^{3}H into the third cerebral ventricle.

Fig. 1. At 3 hours, the radio-autographic reaction is promi-nent over the presynaptic calyx (*ca*) and its spur (*sp*). Very few silver grains are seen over the preganglionic axons (*ax*)

Fig. 2. By 48 hours, an inten-sified reaction persists over the calyx (*ca*) and its spur (*sp*). Numerous silver grains ac-cumulate over the pregang-lionic axons (*ax*). At both times, a small number of silver grains are scattered over the postganglionic nerve cell body (*GC*)

Figs. 3 and 4. At 3 and 48 hours, silver grains are located over areas rich in synaptic vesicles (*sv*) and over mitochondrial profiles (*mi*) present in pre-synaptic calices (*ca*). The post-synaptic perikaryon of the ganglion cell (*GC*) is free of label

Plate I

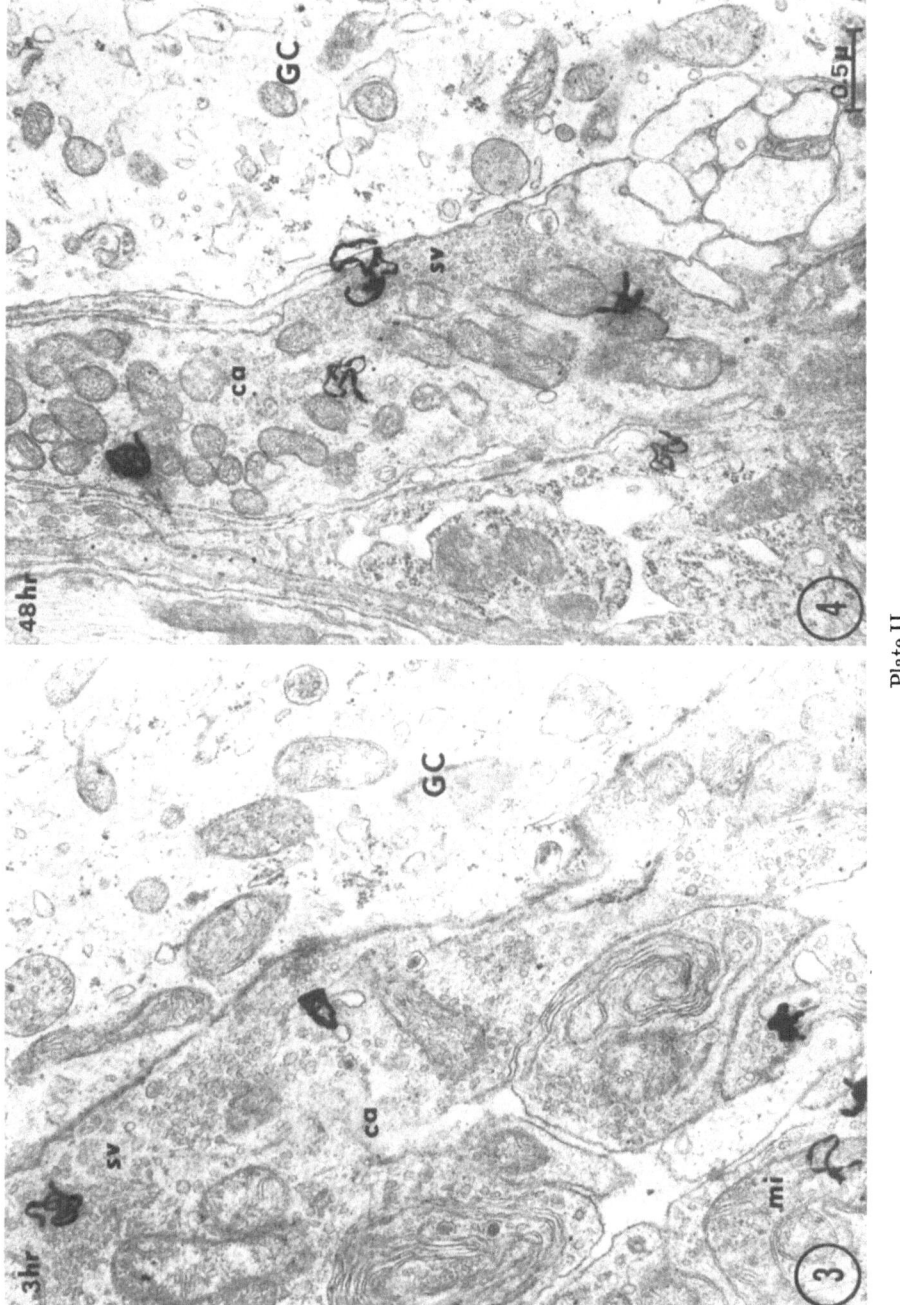

Plate II

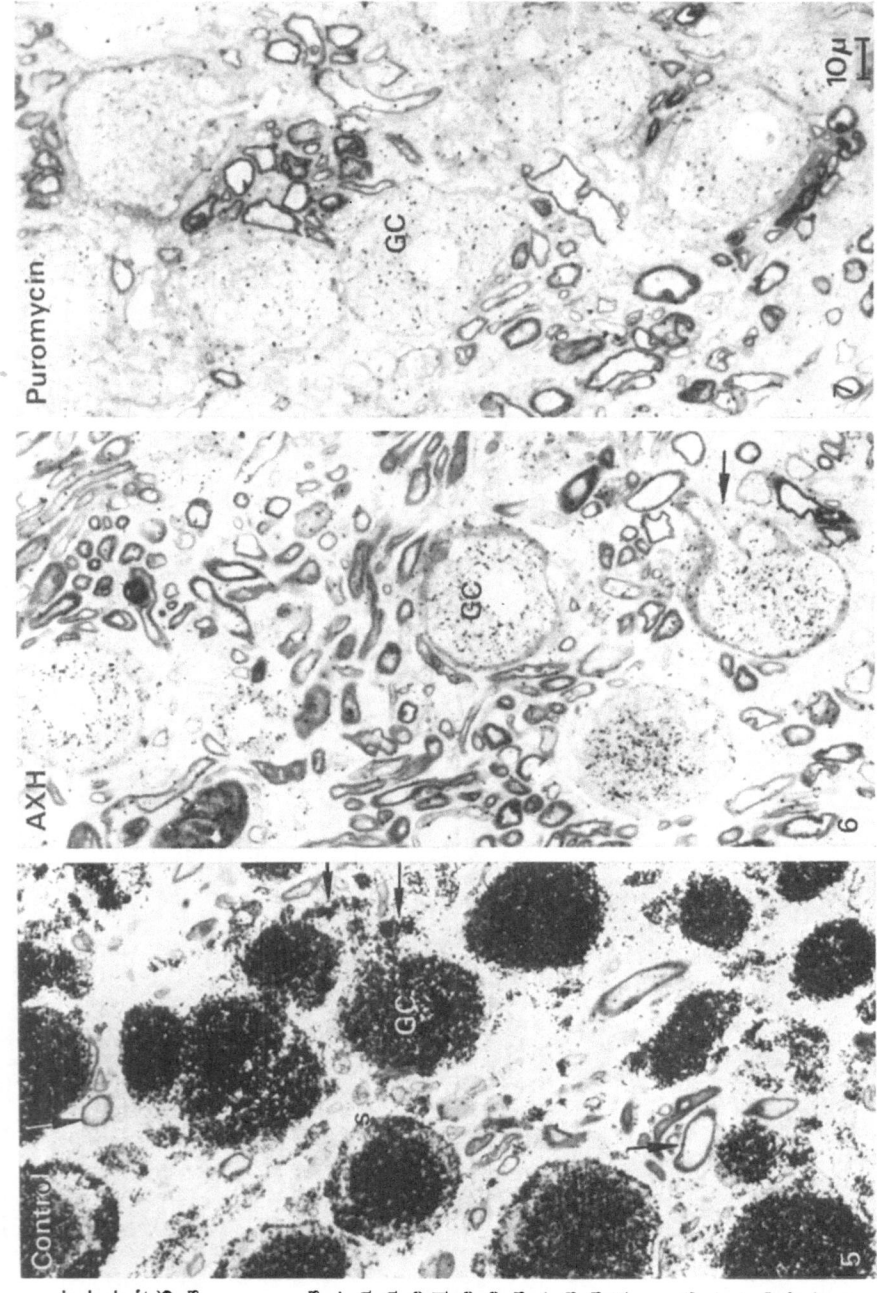

Plates III and IV. Incorporation of leucine-³H in ciliary ganglia incubated *in vitro* for 1 hour without (Figs. 5 and 8) or with inhibitors of protein synthesis (Figs. 6, 7, 9 and 10)

Fig. 5. In untreated ganglia, referred to as "control", a strong radioautographic reaction occurs over the ganglion cell bodies (*GC*), the satellite cells (*s*) and Schwann cells (*Sc*). The initial segment of the axon of ganglion cells is heavily labeled (horizontal arrow ←) whereas the preganglionic axons are free of label (vertical arrow (↓)

Fig. 6. After treatment with acetoxycycloheximide (*AXH*), the ganglion cell bodies and the initial segment of their axons (←) are weakly labeled as well as satellite and Schwann cells

Plate III

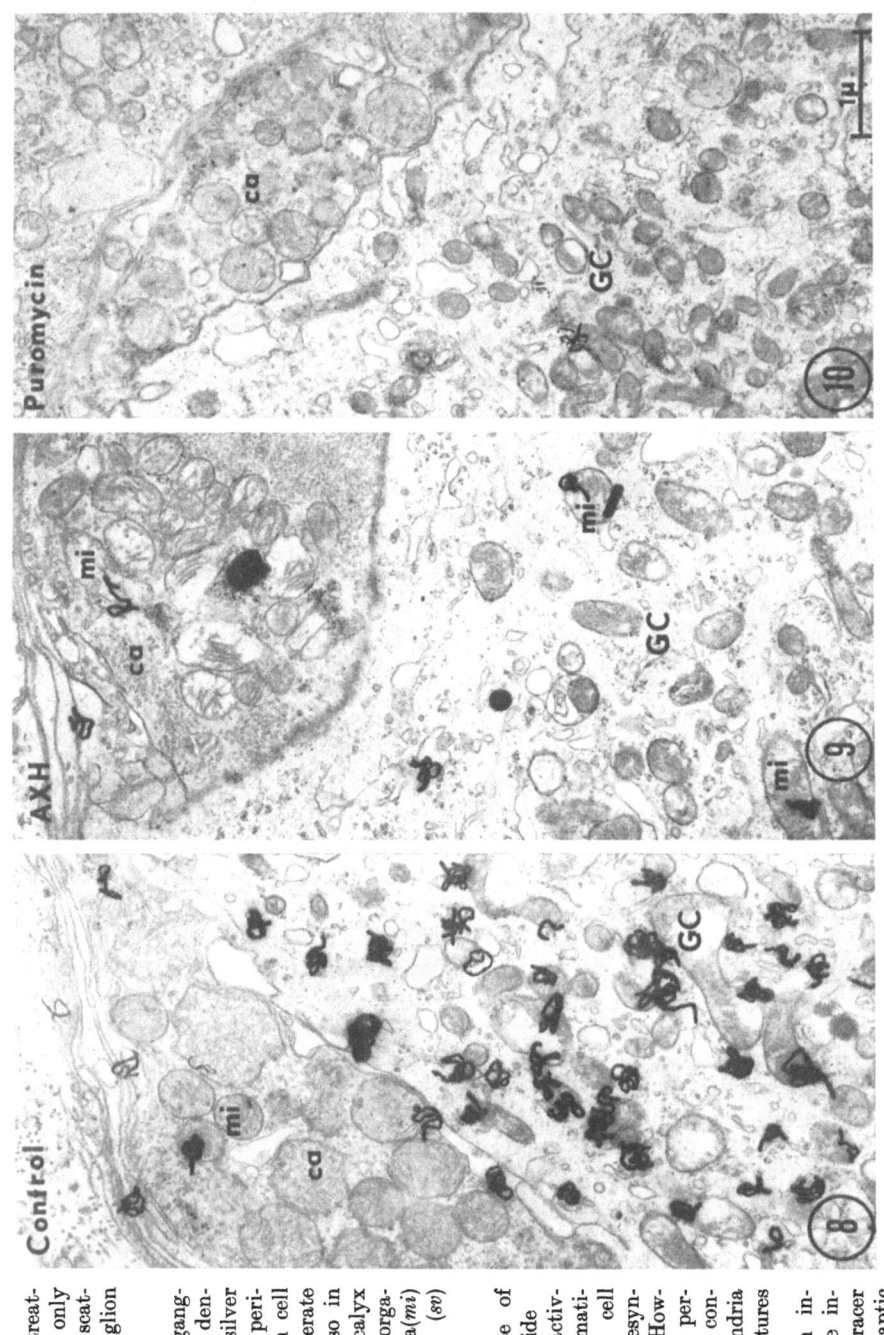

Plate IV

Fig. 7. Puromycin-treated ganglia display only a few silver grains scattered over the ganglion cell bodies

Fig. 8. Untreated ganglia (control) show a dense accumulation of silver grains over the perikaryon of ganglion cell bodies (*GC*). A moderate reaction occurs also in the presynaptic calyx (*ca*) over various organelles: mitochondria(*mi*) synaptic vesicles (*sv*) and membranes

Fig. 9. In presence of acetoxycycloheximide (*AXH*), the radioactivity decreases dramatically in ganglion cell bodies (*GC*) and presynaptic calices (*ca*). However, most of the persisting labeling is confined to mitochondria (*mi*) in both structures

Fig. 10. Puromycin inhibits strongly the incorporation of the tracer in pre- and postsynaptic structures

Table. *Concentration of radioactivity in nerve endings (calices) and perikarya of ganglion cell bodies in ciliary ganglia incubated for 1 hour with leucine-³H alone (control) or with inhibitors of protein synthesis*

	Control	Acetoxycyclo-heximide	Puromycin
Nerve endings			
Number of silver grains per 100 μ^2	49.7 ± 8.4	8.1 ± 1.3	3.8 ± 0.7
Percentage of inhibition	0	$83^0/_0$	$92^0/_0$
Perikarya of ganglion cells			
Number of silver grains per 100 μ^2	155.7 ± 27.0	13.5 ± 2.8	3.1 ± 0.5
Percentage of inhibition	0	$91^0/_0$	$98^0/_0$

(Table). When acetoxycycloheximide was added to the incubating medium, the incorporation of the label was severely impaired in nerve cell bodies and calices, except in a few mitochondria in both structures (Figs. 6 and 9, Table 1). The presence of puromycin in the incubating medium strongly inhibited the incorporation of leucine-³H in both nerve cell bodies and calices (Figs. 7 and 10) by more than 98 and 92 per cent, respectively (Table 1). Accordingly, a rapid appearance of labeled protein, sensitive to acetoxycycloheximide and puromycin, takes place in nerve endings.

Since care was taken to rule out an artifactual retention of the tracer, the incorporation of leucine-³H might correspond to a local synthesis of protein; this is probably the case for mitochondria (Figs. 8 and 9). However the lack of ribosomes in the axoplasm of nerve endings suggests other possibilities: the first one is a transfer of newly synthesized protein from the postsynaptic ganglion cell; the second one, a local synthesis of small peptides and their subsequent binding to a specific protein; the third one, the addition of leucine-³H to the NH_2-terminal group of a preformed protein. This latter mechanism has been shown to occur in Escherichia coli, thyroïd and liver cells of various mammals (Kaji, 1968; Soffer, 1970). Recently, Leibowitz and Soffer (1970) have purified the enzyme which catalyzes the transfer of amino acids from t-RNA to protein acceptors: the leucyl, phenylalanyl transfer RNA-protein transferase. This enzymatic reaction requires the presence of t-RNA, monovalent cations and is inhibited by divalent cations and by puromycin. From a theoretical point of view, we can speculate that the alteration of the biological properties of a protein either by binding a peptide or by adding an amino acid to its free α-amino group would be an efficient way to regulate the level of activity in nerve endings.

Conclusion

Radioautographic studies performed with labeled amino acids visualize the complexity of the dynamic state of protein in nerve endings. One protein fraction, at least, is replaced at a rate of 4 percent per day. On the one hand, the loss of used protein in presynaptic axon terminals seems to be balanced by the arrival of new migratory proteins, synthetized in the nerve cell bodies and conveyed along the axons at various velocities. On the other hand, the slight local incorporation of amino acids observed in nerve endings rises the question whether proteins are synthesized *in situ*; this is probably true for mitochondria. However, the configurational change of a protein by addition of an amino acid or by linkage with a peptide would be a possible mean to modulate the biological activity of presynaptic nerve endings.

Acknowledgements. The technical assistance of Mrs. J. Boyenval for the preparation of the radioautographs and of Mrs. R. Hässig for the photography has been fully appreciated.

References

Austin, L., Morgan, I. G., Bray, J. J.: The biosynthesis of proteins within axons and synaptosomes. In: Protein metabolism of the nervous system, pp. 271—287. A. Lajtha, ed., New-York: Plenum Press 1970.

Autilio, L. A., Appel, S. H., Pettis, P., Gambetti, P. L.: Biochemical studies of synapses *in vitro*: I. Protein synthesis. Biochemistry 7, 2615—2622 (1968).

Barondes, S. H.: Axoplasmic transport. Neurosci. Res. Progr. Bull. 5, 307—419 (1967).

— Axoplasmic transport. In: Handbook of neurochemistry, vol. 2, pp. 435—445. A. Lajtha, ed., New York: Plenum Press 1969.

Di Giamberardino, L.: Independence of the rapid axonal transport of protein from the flow of free amino acids. Acta neuropath. (Berl.) Suppl. V, 132—135 (1971).

Droz, B.: Protein metabolism in nerve cells. Intern. Rev. Cytol. 25, 363—390 (1969).

— Barondes, S. H.: Nerve endings: Rapid appearance of labeled protein shown by electron microscope radioautography. Science 165, 1131—1133 (1969).

— Leblond, C. P.: Axonal migration of proteins in the central nervous system and peripheral nerves as shown by radioautography. J. comp. Neurol. 121, 325—346 (1963).

Edstrom, A.: RNA and protein synthesis in Mauthner nerve fiber components of fish. In: Cellular dynamics of the neuron, pp. 51—72. S. H. Barondes, ed.. New York: Academic Press 1969.

Gordon, M. W., Deanin, G. G.: Protein synthesis by isolated rat brain mitochondria and synaptosomes. J. biol. Chem. 243, 4222—4226 (1968).

Grafstein, B.: Transport of protein by goldfish optic nerve fibers. Science 157, 196—198 (1967).

— Axonal transport: communication between soma and synapse. Advance Biochem. Psychopharmacol. 1, 11—25 (1969).

Granboulan, N., Granboulan, P.: Cytochimie ultrastructurale du nucléole. II. Etude des sites de synthèse du RNA dans le nucléole et le noyau. Exp. Cell Res. 38, 604—619 (1965).

Hendrickson, A.: Electron microscopic radioautography: Identification of origin of synaptic terminals in normal nervous tissue. Science 165, 194—196 (1969).

Hungen, K. von, Mahler, H. R., Moore, W. J.: Turnover of protein and ribonucleic acid in synaptic subcellular fractions from rat brain. J. biol. Chem. 243, 1415—1423 (1968).

Kaji, H.: Further studies on the soluble aminoacid incorporating system from rat liver. Biochemistry 7, 3844—3850 (1968).

Koenig, E.: The axon as a heuristic model for studying membrane protein-synthesizing machinery. In: Protein metabolism of the nervous system, pp. 259—267. A. Lajtha, ed., New York: Plenum Press 1970.

Koenig, H. L., Droz, B.: Transport et renouvellement des protéines dans les terminaisons nerveuses. C. R. Acad. Sci. (Paris) 270, 2579—2582 (1970).

Kopriwa, B. M., Leblond, C. P.: Improvements in the coating technique of radioautography. J. Histochem. Cytochem. 10, 269—284 (1962).

Korr, I. M., Wilkinson, P. N., Chornock, F. W.: Axonal delivery of neuroplasmic components to muscle cells. Science 155, 343—345 (1967).

Lasek, R.: Axoplasmic transport in cat dorsal root ganglion cells as studied with leucine-H³. Brain Res. 7, 360—377 (1968).

Leibowitz, M. J., Soffer, R. L.: Enzymatic modification of proteins. III. Purification and properties of a leucyl, phenylalanyl transfer ribonucleic acid-protein transferase from Escherichia coli. J. biol. Chem. 245, 2066—2073 (1970).

Morgan, I. G., Austin, L.: Synaptosomal protein synthesis in a cell free system. J. Neurochem. **15**, 41—51 (1968).

Ochs, S., Johnson, J.: Fast and slow phases of axoplasmic flow in ventral root nerve fibers. J. Neurochem. **16**, 845—853 (1969).

Schonbach, J., Cuénod, M.: Axonal transport of newly synthesized materials in the retino-tectal pathway of the pigeon. Acta neuropath. (Berl.) Suppl. V, 153—161 (1971).

Singer, M., Salpeter, M. M.: The transport of ^{3}H-histidine through the Schwann and myelin sheath into the axon, including a reevaluation of myelin function. J. Morph. **126**, 281—316 (1966).

Sjøstrand, J.: Fast and slow components of axoplasmic transport in the hypoglossal and vagus nerves of the rabbit. Brain Res. **18**, 461—467 (1970).

Soffer, R. L.: Enzymatic modification of proteins: II. Purification and properties of arginyl transfer ribonucleic acid-protein from rabbit liver cytoplasm. J. biol. Chem. **245**, 731—737 (1970).

Weiss, P., Hiscoe, H. B.: Experiments on the mechanism of nerve growth. J. exp. Zool. **107**, 315—395 (1948).

Dr. B. Droz
Département de Biologie
C.E.A. Saclay B.P. no. 2
91-Gif-sur-Yvette (France)

Acta neuropath. (Berl.) Suppl. V, 119—125 (1971)
© by Springer-Verlag 1971

Effect of Nerve Section on Protein Metabolism of Ganglion Cells and Preganglionic Nerve Endings *

H. L. Koenig

Laboratoire de Cytologie, Faculté des Sciences, Paris

B. Droz

Département de Biologie, Commissariat à l'Énergie Atomique, Saclay

Summary. Radioautographic studies of the rates of incorporation of labeled amino acids were used to study the effects of axotomy on protein metabolism in the ganglion cells and in preganglionic nerve endings of the ciliary ganglion of the chicken. Axotomized perikarya showed chromatolysis and marked depletion of labeled mitochondria, followed by a recovery period. The changes observed in the preganglionic nerve endings were interpreted as indicating an initial decrease in the amount of rapidly transported material, and an increase in the amount of slowly moving proteins, the latter corresponding to an enhanced activity of acetylcholinesterase.

Key-Words: Protein Synthesis — Nerve Endings — Radioactivity — Axonal Transport.

This paper concerns: firstly the kinetics of proteins in ganglion cell bodies after the section of their axons; secondly, the effects of postganglionic axotomy on protein metabolism and cholinesterase activities in preganglionic nerve endings.

The investigation was carried out in the ciliary ganglion of the chicken which has the following advantages: 1. The chromatolysis as well as the recovery period are very rapid, and their precise time sequence is well known (Koenig, 1965); 2. The large volume occupied by the presynaptic calices makes it possible to determine quantitatively the concentrations of radioactivity in these structures; 3. Preganglionic acetylcholinesterase activity is present in the ciliary ganglion neurons.

Experimental Procedures

The postganglionic nerve fibres of the right ciliary ganglion of chicken (ciliary nerves) were sectioned at a distance of 3—4 mm from the ganglia (Fig. 1). One day later, the operated chickens were given 4 intraperitoneal injections of a mixture of tritiated amino acids every 2 hours[1].

The chickens were sacrificed at intervals ranging from 2 to 14 days after the first injection of the series. Ciliary ganglia of the intact and operated side were removed, fixed with formaldehyde and postfixed with osmium tetroxyde. Ultrathin sections were treated for radioautography, according to the method of Granboulan and Granboulan (1965).

The radioactivity concentration of the whole perikaryon, perikaryal cell organelles and presynaptic calices, in both operated and intact ganglia, was measured at each time from a series of radioautographs by counting the number of silver grains per $100\ \mu^2$.

---

* A la mémoire de Nicole Granboulan.

1 Injected tritiated amino acids: L-glutamic acid; L-leucine; L-methionine; L histidine; DL-lysine; DL-valine; DL-phenylalanine.

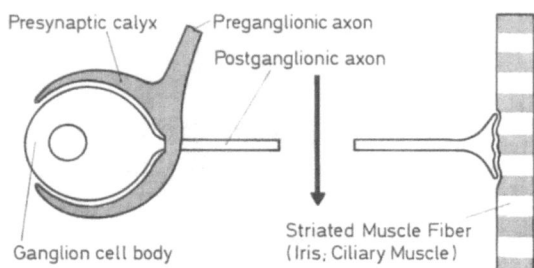

Fig. 1. Schematic drawing of a ciliary ganglion cell and its preganglionic and postganglionic axon terminals

Ganglion Cell Bodies

During the *first week* after axotomy, a chromatolytic reaction, characterized by dispersion of the Nissl substance, progressively took place in ciliary ganglion cells. Simultaneously the acetylcholinesterase activity vanished from the perikaryon (Koenig, 1965). In the whole perikaryon (Fig. 2), as well as in the Nissl substance and neuroplasm (Fig. 3), which make up 90% of the perikaryal volume, the radioactive protein disappeared at a similar rate in chromatolytic and intact cells. However the radioactivity concentration was generally at a slightly lower level in operated than in intact perikarya (Figs. 2 and 3).

In the *second week*, the labelled protein disappeared at a faster rate in axotomized cell bodies. The maximal difference was noted at 10 days after the nerve section (Figs. 2 and 3), at which time the recovery process has already started (Koenig, 1965). This period corresponds to an increased rate of synthesis (Hydén, 1958; Murray and Grafstein, 1969). Since new non-radioactive material was synthesized in our experiment, the decrease of the radioactivity concentration observed in the perikaryon might correspond either to an increased degradation of the labelled protein or, more probably, to an increased axonal transport toward postganglionic axons.

In the Golgi apparatus, the radioactivity concentration was not statistically different in operated and in intact ganglion cell bodies, at each time interval (Fig. 3).

Mitochondria. Two days after the injection, the concentration of the radioactivity was the same in mitochondria of intact and operated perikarya. By contrast, between 2 and 4 days, the concentration of the label in mitochondria dropped dramatically in axotomized cell bodies and remained later at a lower level than in intact ganglion cells (Fig. 3). The rapid disappearance of the label from the mitochondrial population in the axotomized perikarya coincides with the depletion of the oxidative mitochondrial enzymes from the nerve cell bodies and their accumulation in axons in front of the section (Friede, 1959).

Preganglionic Nerve Endings

Early Appearance of the Label in Calices. Labelled protein appears in calices early after the administration of radioactive leucine, probably by a fast transport

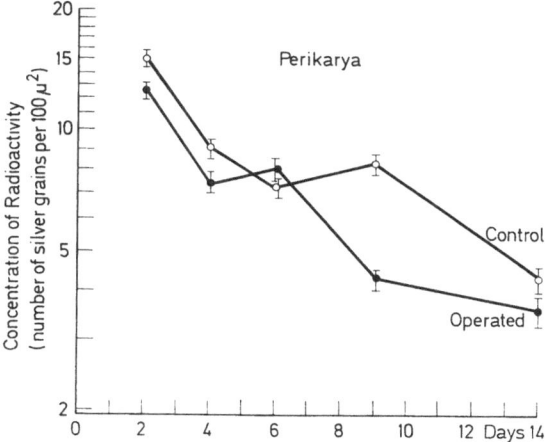

Fig. 2. Concentration of radioactivity in whole perikarya of intact (referred as control) and axotomized ganglion cells

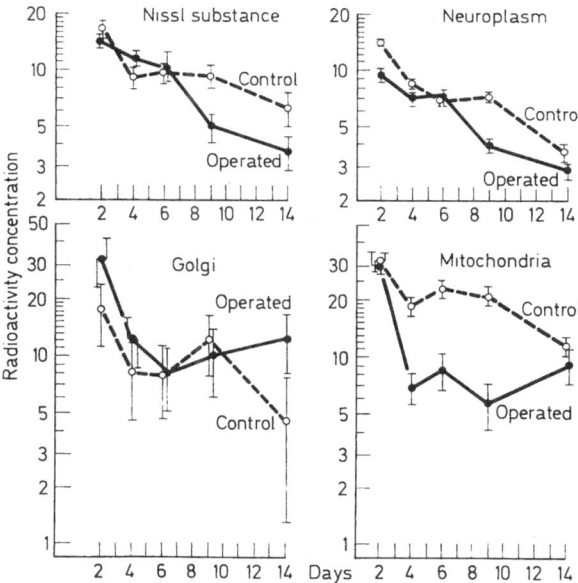

Fig. 3. Concentration of radioactivity in various cell organelles in intact and axotomized ganglion cells

along the preganglionic axons or even by a slight incorporation *in situ* (Koenig and Droz, 1970; Droz and Koenig, 1969).

To investigate whether this rapid labelling in presynaptic calices was modified after the section of postganglionic axons, the right ciliary nerves of chicken were cut 6 days before the injection of tritiated amino acids. Two hours after the injection,

Table 1. *Concentration of radioactivity in nerve endings (calices) and perikarya in intact and axotomized ganglion cell bodies 2 hours after the injection of a mixture of labeled amino acids and 6 days after the section of the right ciliary nerves. (Expressed as number of silver grains per 100μ²)*

	Intact ganglia (left side)	Operated ganglia (right side)
Nerve endings	15.8 ± 0.9	9.1 ± 0.7
Perikarya of ganglion cells	48.5 ± 1.6	51.2 ± 1.6

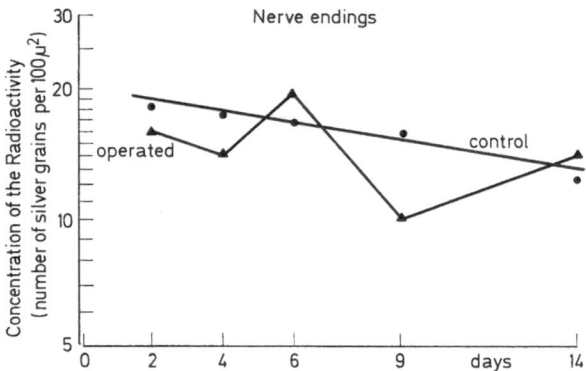

Fig. 4. Concentration of radioactivity in presynaptic nerve endings (calices) of axotomized ganglion cells as compared to the intact side.

the concentration of the label in calices was more reduced in the operated ganglion (right side) than in the intact one (left side), used as control (Table 1). Furthermore, when a labeled amino acid such as lysine-³H was injected directly into the third cerebral ventricle (Droz and Koenig, 1970), the radioactivity concentration observed 3 hours later in calices was again depressed in ganglia of the operated side.

The lower concentration of radioactivity measured in presynaptic calices of axotomized ganglion cells may be the consequence of 2 possible mechanisms: a reduced synthesis of protein in preganglionic neurons or a slackened transport of the labeled material.

In contrast, a similar incorporation of labeled amino acids was observed in the perikarya of axotomized and intact ganglion cells (Table 1).

Plate I. Acetylcholinesterase activity in ciliary ganglion neurons. Koelle method: 1 hour incubation in acetylthiocholine as substrate at pH 5.5

Figs. 5 and 6. Intact ganglion cells. Few cells show a weak preganglionic AchE activity (arrows). Note the perikaryal AchE activity. Fig. 5. ×150; Fig. 6. ×580

Figs. 7 and 8. Axotomized ganglion cells. 6 days after the ciliary nerve section. Practically all cells show a strongly enhanced preganglionic AchE activity. Note that perikaryal AchE activity vanishes. Fig. 7. ×150; Fig. 8. ×580

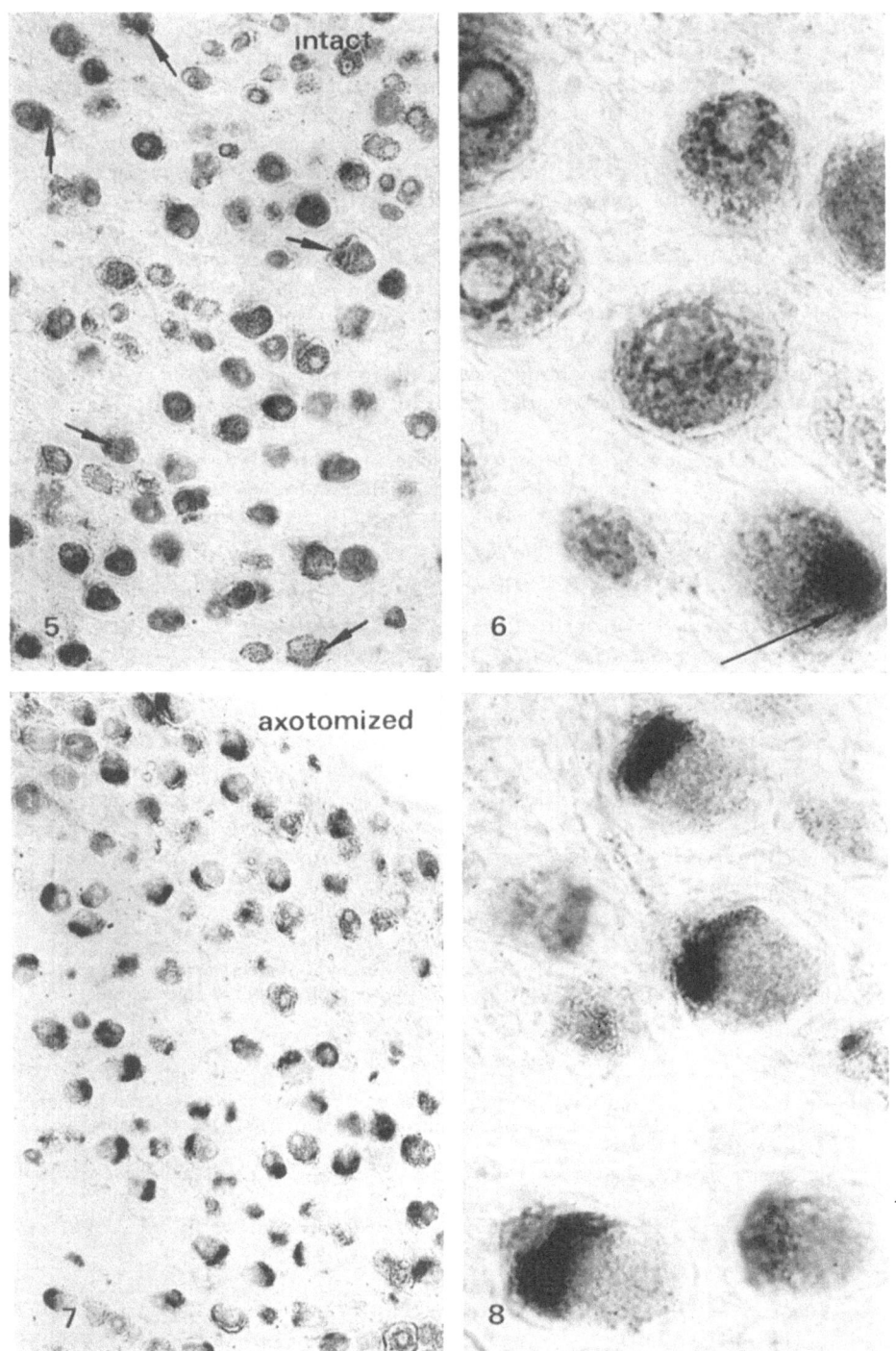

Plate I

Disappearance of Labeled Protein from Calices. When the radioactivity concentration in calices of the axotomized side was measured at various time intervals, the time curve showed a rather serrated aspect which contrasted with the regular rate of disappearance of the label on the intact side (Fig. 4).

The peak observed at 6 days in the operated side corresponds, probably to a late arrival of labelled protein. It must be noted that this peak coincides with an enhanced activity of acetylcholinesterase in preganglionic calices.

Preganglionic Acetylcholinesterase Activity. The histochemical method of Koelle, as used by Couteaux and Taxi (1952), visualizes an acetylcholinesterase activity in ganglion cells and their axons as well as in preganglionic calices[2]. The acetylcholinesterase activity was generally weak in most calices (Figs. 5 and 6) (Szentagothaï *et al.*, 1954; Taxi, 1961; Koenig, 1965). However, 5—7 days after the section of the postganglionic nerve fibers, the presynaptic acetylcholinesterase activity was strongly enhanced in all calices (Figs. 7 and 8) (Taxi, 1961; Koenig, 1965).

The simultaneous rise of the acetylcholinesterase activity and labelled protein in calices, 5—7 days after the section of the ciliary nerves, might result from an increased accumulation of material slowly transported down the preganglionic axons.

Conclusions

Radioautographs performed after injection of labeled amino acids allowed us to investigate quantitatively the effects of the section of postganglionic nerves on protein metabolism in the ciliary ganglion of the chicken.

The perikarya of axotomized ganglion cells show first a chromatolytic process and a dramatic depletion of labeled mitochondria, than a recovery period.

The preganglionic nerve ending, connected with the axotomized ganglion cells, display, 6 days after nerve section: 1. a late arrival of slowly moving protein and an enhanced acetylcholinesterase activity 2. a decreased amount of rapidly transported material. Thus, the section of an axon modifies protein dynamics of presynaptic neurons and the metabolic effect observed in preganglionic nerve endings would therefore reflect a transneuronal modulation.

Acknowledgements. The technical assistance of Mrs. J. Boyenval for the preparation of the radioautographs and of Mrs. P. Cloup for the photography is being appreciated.

References

Couteaux, R., Taxi, J.: Recherches histochimiques sur la distribution des activités cholinestérasiques au niveau de la synapse myoneurale. Arch. Anat. micr. Morph. exp. **41**, 352—392 (1952).

Droz, B., Koenig, H. L.: The turnover of proteins in axons and nerve endings. In: Cellular dynamics of the neuron, pp. 35—50. S. H. Barondes, ed., New York: Academic Press 1969.

— — Dynamic condition of protein in axons and axon terminals. Acta neuropath. (Berl.) Suppl. V, 109—118 (1971).

2 The enzyme activity was inhibited by DFP (3×10^{-6} M), a specific inhibitor of AchE; but was maintained after Mipafox treatment (4×10^{-6} M), an inhibitor of ChE. (Pecot-Dechavassine, 1961). Furthermore, incubations with butyrylthiocholine as substrate gave negative results.

Friede, R.: Transport of oxidative enzymes in nerve fibers. A histochemical investigation of the regenerative cycle in neurons. Exp. Neurol. 1, 441—466 (1959).

Granboulan, N., Granboulan, P.: Cytochimie ultrastructurale du nucléole. II. Etude des sites de synthèse du RNA dans le nucléole et le noyau. Exp. Cell Res. 38, 604—619 (1965).

Hydén, H.: Biochemical changes in glial cells and nerve cells at varying activity. In: Biochemistry of the central nervous system, vol. III, pp. 64—89. F. Brück, ed., New York Pergamon Press 1958.

Koenig, H. L.: Relations entre la distribution de l'activité acétylcholinestérasique et celle de l'ergastoplasme dans les neurones du ganglion ciliaire du Poulet. Arch. Anat. micr. Morph. exp. 54, 937—964 (1965).

— Droz, B.: Transport et renouvellement des protéines dans les terminaisons nerveuses C. R. Acad. Sci. (Paris) 270, 2579—2582 (1970).

Kung, S. H.: Incorporation of tritiated precursors in the cytoplasm of normal and chromatolytic sensory neurons as shown by autoradiography. Brain Res. 25, 656—660 (1971).

Murray, M., Grafstein, B.: Changes in the morphology and amino acid incorporation of regenerating Goldfish optic neurons. Exp. Neurol. 23, 544—560 (1969).

Pécot-Dechavassine, M.: Etude histochimique, pharmacologique et biochimique des cholinestérases des muscles striés chez les Poissons, les Batraciens et les Mammifères. Arch. Anat. micr. Morph. exp. 50, 341—438 (1961).

Szentagothaï, J., Donhoffer, A., Rajkovits, K.: Die Lokalisation der Cholinesterase in der interneuronalen Synapse. Acta histochem. 1, 272—281 (1954).

Taxi, J.: La distribution des cholinestérases dans divers ganglions du système nerveux autonome des Vertébrés. Bibl. anat. (Basel) 2, 73—89 (1961).

Dr. H. L. Koenig
Laboratoire de Cytologie
Faculté des Scienes
12 rue Cuvier
Paris (5è) France

Acta neuropath. (Berl.) Suppl. V, 126—131 (1971)

Some Observations on the Experimental Production of Acute Neuroaxonal and Synaptosomal Dystrophy *

HAROLD KOENIG

Neurology Service, VA Research Hospital and Department of Neurology,
Northwestern University Medical School, Chicago

Summary. Fluorocitrate, and fluoroacetate block the Krebs cycle in neural tissue, cause convulsive seizures, and produce interesting neuropathological lesions, notably a swelling of neuronal and glial mitochondria and neuroaxonal and synaptosomal dystrophy. Axonal ballooning is a consequence of convulsive seizures coupled with inhibition of the Krebs cycle. Mg^{++} suppresses the convulsive seizures produced by fluorocitrate and prevents axonal ballooning. Strychnine convulsions do not cause neuroaxonal dystrophy. However, Mg^{++} does not prevent mitochondrial swelling or axonal dystrophy. Fluorouracil produces similar neuropathological lesions, apparently because it is degraded partly to fluoroacetate. Numerous agents with diverse biological actions also produce dystrophic changes in axons and nerve endings. These include: cyanide, arsenious oxide, ouabain, puromycin, parabenzoquinone, malonate, succinate, 3-acetylpyridine, desoxypyridoxine, methionine sulfoximine, antimycin A, iminodiproprionitrile, plasmocide, pyrathiamine, cupric sulfate, Trypan blue. Electron microscopic examination showed that the following agents also caused mitochondrial swelling: cyanide, iminodiprionitrile, plasmocide, 3-acetylpyridine, methione sulfoximine, puromycin and Trypan blue. It is proposed that a swelling of perikaryal mitochondria is the common basis for the increased disgorgement of lysosomes, mitochondria and other cytoplasmic constituents occurring in neuroaxonal and synaptosomal dystrophy.

Key-Words: Dystrophy, Neuroaxonal — Dystrophy, Synaptosomal — Electron Microscopy — Mitochondria, Neuronal — Mitochondria, Glial.

Introduction

In an earlier investigation Koenig (1967, 1969a) observed that fluorocitrate (FC), a convulsant and a potent inhibitor of the Krebs cycle which blocks the aconitase-catalyzed interconversion of citrate and isocitrate (Peters, 1957), produces interesting neuropathological lesions in cat spinal cord, including an acute neuroaxonal dystrophy. When injected into the lumbar theca in cat, FC produces dramatic spinal cord convulsions and induces neurons to expel multitudinous lysosomes, mitochondria, and other cytoplasmic constituents into their axons. After convulsive seizures commence, spectacular axonal balloons develop owing to obstruction of axonal flow by "log jams" of extruded organelles. A swelling of neuronal mitochondria occurred as an early event in FC-poisoned tissues and was implicated as a major causal factor in the disgorgement of cytoplasmic material into axons. Mitochondrial swelling had been noted together with axonal dystrophy in certain other experimental injuries, e.g., x-irradiation (Andres, 1963; Forsmann *et al.*, 1966) and poisoning by plasmocide (D'Agostino, 1967), and cyanide (Hirano *et al.*, 1967; Hager *et al.*, 1960). However, these two lesions had not previously been causally linked. Subsequently, Koenig (1969b,

* These studies were supported by the Veterans Administration, and by grants from the National Multiple Sclerosis Society (MS-512-B-7) and NIH (NS 05509, NS 06838 and NS 01456).

and unpublished observations) found that a number of metabolic inhibitors with different modes of action, when injected into the lumbar theca of cat, cause mitochondrial swelling in spinal neurons and dystrophic changes in their axons. This report summarizes some of these results.

Material and Methods

Drugs were injected intrathecally in cat under an L-7 laminectomy performed under pentobarbital anesthesia. The animal was kept in the head-up position reduce rostral flow of drug. Lumbosacral spinal cord was fixed *in situ* by vascular perfusion with phosphate-buffered $4^0/_0$ paraformaldehyde or cacodylate-buffered $4^0/_0$ glutaraldehyde, and processed for histological, cytochemical and in some instances ultrastructural studies. Further experimental details are described in an earlier publication (Koenig, 1969a).

Results

Fluorocitrate. Fluorocitrate was given to cats in a dose of $3-50$ µg of the active isomer by injection into the lumbar subarachnoid space. After a latent period of $1-2$ hrs convulsive movements appear in the tail, hindlimbs, and trunk, culminating in a remarkable clonic-tonic seizure disorder of the (thoraco)lumbosacral spinal cord which may persist for many hours. In routine paraffin sections structural changes become evident in gray matter only after convulsive seizures have been present for a time, usually $4-6$ hrs after a 10 µg dose of FC. These include blurring of fragmentation of Nissl bodies, swelling and diminished basophilia of nucleoli, clumping of neuronal and glial chromatin, spongy state of neuropil. Fixed-frozen sections stained for acid phosphatase activity reveal a notable dislocation of lysosomal particles into axons long before the aforementioned structural lesions become discernible. In FC-poisoned spinal cord, implantation cones and emergent axons of gray matter are rendered conspicuous by a localized accumulation of reactive lysosomes within $15-60$ min of drug injection, and axons both myelinated and unmyelinated, in neuropil acquire increased numbers of lysosomes. After convulsive seizures commence, axonal balloons or dilatations develop, usually $3-4$ hrs after a small dose, or $1-2$ hrs after a large dose (30 to 50 µg) of FC, and subsequently increase in size and numbers. Axonal balloons usually occur in the initial segment of the axon which is without birefrigent myelin when viewed in the polarizing microscope. Many myelinated axons distal to balloons as well as axons without balloons, also contain abundant enzyme product. Restricted during the early hours to the neuropil, intraaxonal reaction product extends distally to the root exit zone by 24 hrs after a small dose (6 µg) of FC. Axonal balloons also are well demonstrated in preparations stained for the lysosomal hydrolases, β-glucuronidase, and acid esterase, and for the mitochondrial enzymes, nicotinamide adenine dinucleotide diaphorase, lactate dehydrogenase, and malate dehydrogenase.

The principal ultrastructural changes observed in the electron microscope during the latent period preceding convulsions are: (1) a swelling of mitochondria in the perikaryon and dendrites of neurons, and in glia, and (2) the appearance of abnormal numbers of mitochondria, dense bodies, neurofibrils, and other structures within some axons and nerve endings. Mitochondria within axons and nerve endings are unaltered early, possibly because these structures are impermeable to FC; later some of these are swollen. After convulsions commence, the mitochondrial swelling and the axonal abnormalities become more marked and more widespread and axonal balloons develop. Axonal balloons occur in nonmyelinated or thinly myelinated portions of axons. They are stuffed with various structures among which the following can be identified: mitochondria, many of which are swollen and degenerating; dense and multilamellated lysosome-like bodies; vesicles and other membranous structures; and neurofibrils. Nerve endings frequently acquire these structures also. Other fine structural lesions are: dissociation of polyribosomes in neurons and glia, swelling of endoplasmic reticulum, clumping of nuclear chromatin, loosening and disorganiation of compact myelin, and astrocytic swelling.

Fluoroacetate. Fluoroacetate (FA) is a potent convulsant when given systemically. We found that FA, when injected into the lumbar cistern of the cat, causes epileptiform seizures and neuropathological lesions indistinguishable from FC. However, the minimum effective dose, 1.5 to 2 mg, is 300 to 400 times greater than that of FC. This seems to be a direct effect of FA on nervous tissue, as it is largely confined to that portion of the neural axis close to the injection site. It seems likely, therefore, that FA is converted to the toxic derivative, FC, to a limited extent in cat spinal cord.

Fluorocitrate $+ Mg^{++}$. $MgCl_2$, 5 mg/kg, given intrathecally prevents the development of FC seizures in cat spinal cord and rat brain (Patel, Koenig, and Szabo, unpublished observations). Mg^{++} also completely suppresses FC seizures after they are fully developed. This finding afforded an opportunity to assess the role of seizure activity on the evolution of the neuropathological lesions produced by FC. Treatment of FC-poisoned spinal cord of cat with Mg^{++} did not prevent the swelling of neuronal and glial mitochondria, nor was the efflux of lysosomes and mitochondria into axons and nerve endings discernibly altered. In light microscopic sections reacted for acid phosphatase activity, the axons were heavily stained and stood out boldly in the otherwise unstained neuropil. However, axonal balloons did not develop during a period of four hours of FC poisoning, provided that convulsions were prevented by Mg^{++}. Thus, as inferred earlier (Koenig, 1969a), convulsive activity plays a significant role in facilitating the development of axonal ballooning, but is not involved in the intraaxonal extrusion of cytoplasmic organelles.

Strychnine. To test the potential role of convulsive activity itself on the dystrophic process, we used strychnine, 1 mg, intrathecally in cat. Within a minute after injection, the hindquarters are thrown into violent convulsive spasms which gradually moderate but persist for the duration of the experiment, 4 hrs. $MgCl_2$, 5 mg/kg intrathecally, also suppresses strychnine seizures. Histopathological examination of strychnine-treated spinal cord with and without Mg^{++} failed to reveal significant lesions. In particular, acid phosphatase reacted sections showed no indication of an increase in intraaxonal lysosomes over control tissues, nor were axonal balloons in evidence. We may deduce from these observations that persistent convulsions *per se* do not enhance the entry of lysosomes, and inferentially other cytoplasmic organelles, into axons.

Fluorouracil. The pyrimidine analog fluorouracil has been used extensively in the chemotherapy of malignant neoplasms. Recently, Riehl and Brown (1964) described an acute neurological disorder which developed in about 2% of patients

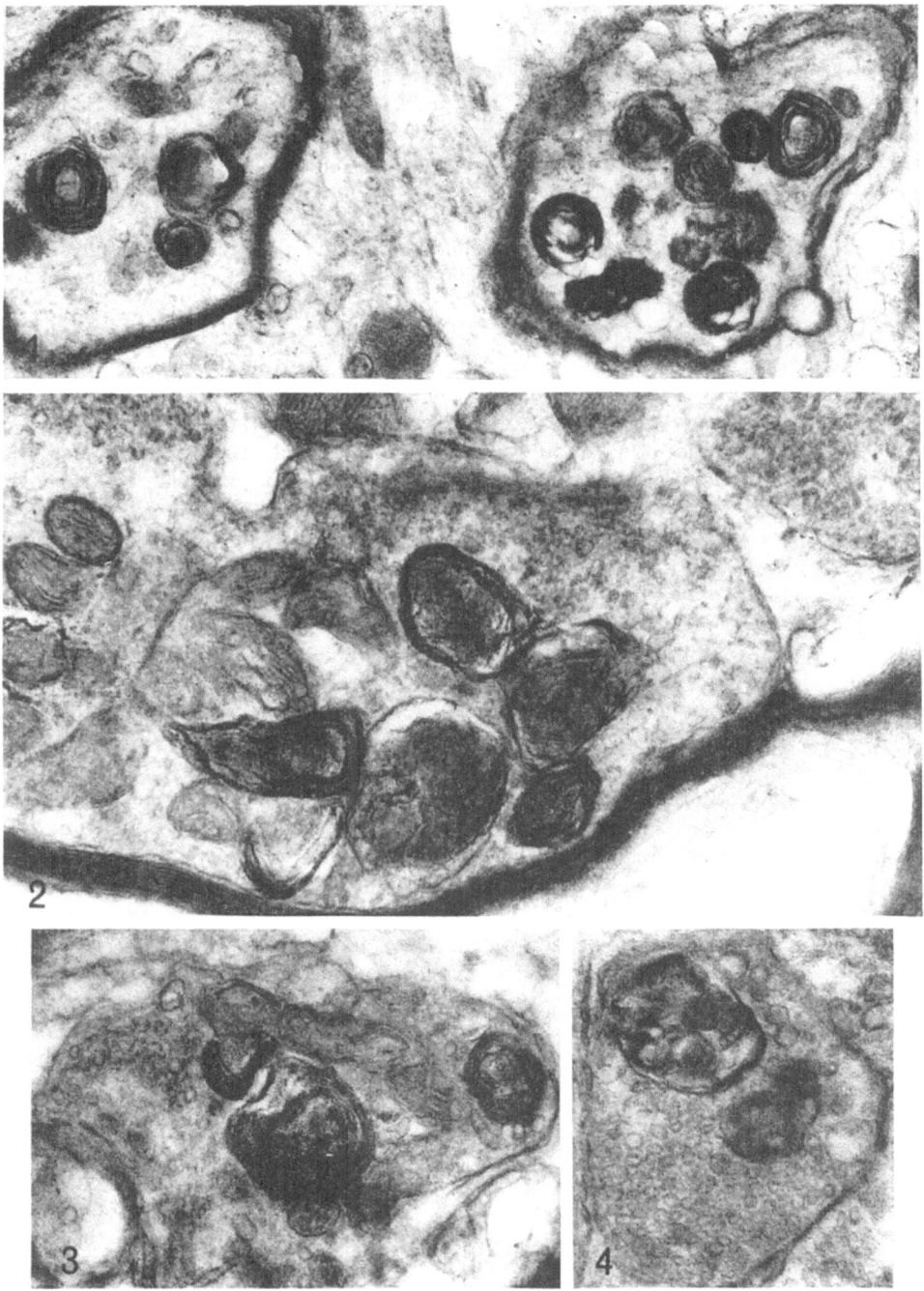

Figs. 1 and 2. Fluoracil (30 mg/kg, 24 hrs). Cat cerebellum. Fig. 1. Dystrophic axons, ×34,000;
Fig. 2. Dystrophic nerve ending, ×46,000

Fig. 3. D,L-Methionine sulfoximine (15 mg, 5 hrs), cat spinal cord. Dystrophic nerve ending,
×46,000

Fig. 4. Puromycin (10 mg, 2 days), cat spinal cord. Dystrophic nerve ending, ×46,000

during the course of treatment with fluorouracil. This disorder featured an abrupt onset, severe disability involving mentation, cerebellar, vestibular, and pyramidal tract functions, and rapid reversibility after stopping or reducing the dose of fluorouracil. Neuropathological examination of one patient who died while being treated with fluorouracil without overt neurotoxicity revealed marked chromato-lytic changes in neurons of the olivary and dentate nuclei and a loss of neurons in the granular layer of the cerebellum. Riehl and Brown (1964) found that fluoroura-cil also is neurotoxic to the cat and produces neuropathological lesions similar to those seen in their human patient.

Recently I noted a marked similarity between the neuronal lesions produced in cat by fluorouracil and those produced by FC (Koenig, 1969a). This observation suggested the possibility that fluorouracil might be degraded to FA, a potent convulsant and rat poison, in extra-neural tissues. Fluoroacetate undergoes metabolic conversion to FC, an inhibitor of the Krebs cycle which acts by blocking aconitase, the enzyme which catalyzes the reversible interconversion of citrate and isocitrate. We have since shown that fluorouracil, given intravenously to cats in doses commonly used for man, causes a substantial elevation in citrate level in several tissues, including blood and brain, indicating a block in the Krebs cycle (Koenig and Patel, 1969, 1970). Alpha-fluoro-β-alanine, a major breakdown product of fluorouracil in man and other species, produces similar elevations in tissue citrate levels concomitant with the development of convulsive seizures and ataxia. A comparable increase in blood citrate levels was found in two human patients on fluorouracil chemotherapy, suggesting that this agent in therapeutic doses may interfere with the Krebs cycle in man.

The neuropathological changes produced by a single dose of FU (20—45 mg/kg) occur to varying degrees throughout the CNS, but are particularly marked in the cerebellar cortex and the dentate and olivary nuclei. In general, the cytopathologic effects closely resemble those produced by FC and FA. However, they tend to be less severe than those produced by a large dose of FC (Figs. 1, 2). Increased num-bers of lysosomes and mitochondria regularly appear in axons and nerve endings but axonal balloons have not been seen after a single dose of FU.

Other Agents which Produce Acute Neuroaxonal Dystrophy. Diverse inhibitors of cell respiration or oxidative phosphorylation and other cytotoxic agents have been tested for their ability to produce neuroaxonal dystrophy in cat spinal cord. These included: puromycin (10 mg), potassium cyanide (0.1—0.2 mg), arsenious oxide (0.5 mg), oubain (1 mg), parabenzoquinone (2 mg), malonate (5 mg), succi-nate (5 mg), 3-acetylpyridine (2 mg), desoxypyridoxine (2 mg), methionine sulf-oximine (15 mg), antimycin A (5 mg), iminodiproprionitrile (IDPN) (15 mg), plasmocide (2—10 mg), pyrothiamine (2 mg), cupric sulfate (0.1 mg), Trypan blue (0.05 mg). Drugs were injected into the lumbar cistern and cats killed 2—5 hrs later by vascular perfusion with phosphate buffered cold paraformaldehyde or glutaraldehyde. Aldehyde-fixed frozen sections were stained for acid phosphatase activity by Gomori's lead glycerophosphate method. In all experimental tissues the axonal hillocks and axons in the spinal gray matter were generally more conspicuous than in control tissues due to increased members of reactive lysosomes.

In a small number of experiments, tissues were also examined by electron microscopy. Neuronal mitochondria were found to be moderately swollen and increased numbers of mitochondria and lysosomes were present in some axons and nerve endings. The agents which produced these changes were: cyanide, IDPN, plasmocide, 3-acetylpyridine, methionine sulfoximine, puromycin and Trypan blue (Figs. 3, 4).

Discussion

The author had proposed earlier (Koenig, 1969a) that the FC-induced swelling of neuronal mitochondria may initiate the efflux of cytoplasmic constituents into the axon, and provide the propulsive force for their distal migration. Mitochondria collectively occupy a substantial portion of the neuronal perikaryon, perhaps $10-15\%$ of the total volume. Therefore, a rapid expansion of the mitochondrial compartment would necessarily result in a displacement of a comparable volume of cytoplasmic material into the axon. This inference is, of course, based on the reasonable assumption that the shift of water from the neuroplasm into mitochondria is accompanied by an entry of water into the perikaryon from extraneuronal sources to maintain osmotic equilibrium.

It is clear that the advent of the epileptic state initiates a second phase in the dystrophic process which is associated with a further swelling of neuronal mitochondria and an augmented expulsion of cytoplasmic material into axons. Thus, prevention of FC seizures blocked the development of axonal balloons but did not markedly reduce either the mitochondrial swelling or the disgorgement of lysosomes and mitochondria into axons.

A number of agents with diverse biological effects can elicit an increased disgorgement of perikaryal constituents into axons and nerve endings. The one other effect which these agents seem to exert in common is a swelling of neural mitochondria. We suggest that these two events are causally related. These observations are consistent with the hypothesis advanced earlier (Koenig, 1969a) that mitochondrial swelling, however induced, may be of general importance as a mechanism for the production of neuroaxonal and synaptosomal dystrophy.

Acknowledgements. I acknowledge the valuable contributions of Mrs. B. S. Newson and Mr. C. T. Hughes to the electron microscopic aspects of this study. I am also indebted to Misses G. T. Ronga, S. M. Koenig, and L. E. Koenig, and Mrs. D. L. Thomas for the light microscopic preparations, and to Mr. E. Washington for aid in carrying out the animal experiments.

Bibliography

Andres, K. H.: Z. Zellforsch. **61**, 1 (1963).
D'Agostino, A. N.: Neurology (Minneap.) **14**, 114 (1967).
Forssmann, W. G., Tinguely, H., Posternak, J. M., Rouiller, Ch.: Z. Zellforsch. **72**, 325 (1966).
Hager, H., Hirschberger, W., Scholz, W.: Aerospace Med. **31**, 379 (1960).
Hirano, A., Levine, S., Zimmerman, H. M.: J. Neuropath. exp. Neurol. **26**, 200 (1967).
Koenig, H.: In: Brain damage in the fetus and newborn from hypoxia or asphyxia. (L. S. James, and R. E. Meyers, eds.), p. 36. Columbus, Ohio: Ross Laboratories 1967.
— Science **164**, 310 (1969a).
— J. Neuropath. exp. Neurol. **28**, 173 (1969b).
Riehl, J. L., Brown, W. J.: Neurology (Minneap.) **14**, 961 (1964).
Peters, R. A.: Advanc. Enzymol. **18**, 113 (1957).
— Patel, A.: Trans. Amer. Neurol. Ass. **94**, 290 (1969).
— — Arch. Neurol. (Chic.) **23**, 155 (1970).

Harold Koenig
Neurology Service, VA Research Hospital
Northwestern University Medical School
Chicago, Illinois 60611/U.S.A.

Acta neuropath. (Berl.) Suppl. V, 132—135 (1971)
© by Springer-Verlag 1971

Independance of the Rapid Axonal Transport of Protein from the Flow of Free Amino Acids

L. Di Giamberardino

Départment de Biologie, Commissariat à l'Énergie Atomique, Saclay, France

Summary. The level of TCA-precipitable and TCA-soluble radioactivity was measured in the optic nerve and optic tectum of goldfish after injecting tritiated leucine into one eye. It was demonstrated that protein synthesized in the retina is transported down the nerve to the contralateral optic tectum, at a rate of 50—70 mm/day. This rapid transport of protein cannot be accounted for by a transport of free amino acid. It was demonstrated that free amino acid is able to reach the optic nerve but unable to reach the contralateral optic tectum.

Key-Words: Axonal Transport — Radioactivity — Protein Synthesis.

It is now widely accepted that protein synthesized in the neuron cell body can be transported down the axon to the axon terminal at velocities of 50 to 500 millimeters per day (for a review see Grafstein, 1969; Barondes, 1969).

Most of the experimental evidence for this theory was obtained by injecting labeled amino acids near the neuron cell bodies and analysing the time course of the appearance of labeled protein along the nerve or at the axon terminals. In such experiments, a wave of labeled protein seen to move along the nerve, or an accumulation of labeled protein at the axon terminals, would be taken as evidence of transport of protein. However, these results can as well be interpreted not as a somatofugal transport of protein, but as a transport of free amino acid from the point of injection followed by synthesis of protein *in situ*.

To answer this argument and give a direct evidence that flow of amino acids and rapid transport of protein are two independent phenomena, two experiments were performed in the optic system of the goldfish.

Time Course of the Appearence of TCA-precipitable and TCA-soluble Radioactivity in the Optic Nerve and Optic Tectum of Goldfish

In the first experiment the level of TCA-precipitable and TCA-soluble radioactivity in the optic nerve and optic tectum of goldfish was measured at intervals of 3, 6 and 12 hours after injecting tritiated leucine into the right eye (Fig. 1).

The following results were obtained.

1. The TCA-precipitable radioactivity in the right optic nerve was consistently about 10 times greater than in the left optic nerve (Fig. 1 A).

2. The TCA-soluble radioactivity in the right optic nerve was 10, 7 and 4 times greater than in the left optic nerve, respectively at 3, 6 and 12 hours after the injection (Fig. 1 B).

3. The accumulation rate of the TCA-precipitable radioactivity in the left optic tectum, connected to the injected eye, starting from 3 hours after the injection, was 4 times faster than in the right optic tectum (Fig. 1 C).

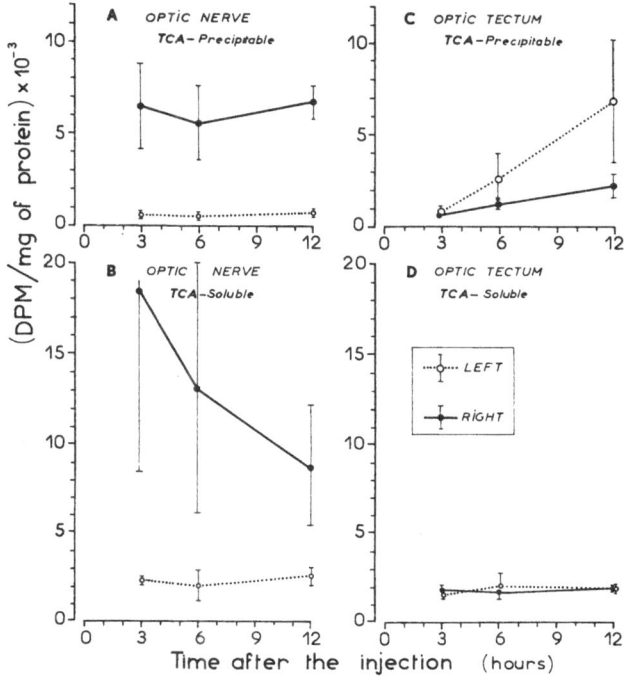

Fig. 1. Distribution of TCA-precipitable and TCA-soluble radioactivity in the optic nerve and optic tecta of goldfish after injecting 20 μCi of ³H-L-Leucine (35 Ci/mM, 10 Ci/ml; CEA, France) into the vitreous humor of the right eye. The nerves and tecta were homogenized in water, treated for one hour with TCA (10⁰/₀, 0°C). The TCA-precipitable fraction was resuspended in 0.1 N-NaOH. The protein concentration was assayed with the Lowry methods. The radioactivity was measured placing 0.2—0.5 ml of sample in 10 ml Bray's scintillator. Efficiency was measured with an internal standard of ³H-water. Data are expressed as dpm per mg of protein in the TCA-precipitable fraction. Each point is the average of 3—4 fish with standard deviation

4. The TCA-soluble radioactivity in the left optic tectum (Fig. 1 D). never exceeded the background level (we call background the TCA-soluble and the TCA-precipitable radioactivity found in the left optic nerve and in the right optic tectum, which is probably due to an uptake and redistribution of free leucine by the blood stream followed by local incorporation).

These results indicate that after injection into the right eye free leucine reached the right optic nerve, either intra- or extraaxonally, to be actively incorporated into TCA-precipitable material in surrounding meninges, glial cells and possibly axonal mitochondria. Yet free leucine, even though largely available to the right optic nerve, did not seem to reach the left tectum. As reported by McEwen and Grafstein (1968), who in a similar experiment also did not find any difference between the TCA-soluble radioactivity of the two tecta, it is "... extremely unlikely that free leucine could enter the optic tectum from the nerve and be immediately incorporated into protein without being detected first as free amino acid in the tectum". This view is reinforced by the fact that the amount of amino acid incorporated locally in the nerve endings is exceedingly small (Droz and Koenig, 1971).

Thus it can be concluded that at least $^3/_4$ of the TCA-precipitable radioactivity detected in the left optic tectum at 12 hours after the injection, corresponds to protein synthesized outside the tectum and transported there by a rapid transport mechanism. The other $^1/_4$ can be accounted for by local background incorporation.

Site of Synthesis of the Rapidly Transported Material

The results of the previous experiment clearly show that an extra-tectal, TCA-precipitable material is rapidly transported to the optic tectum. However the origin of the rapidly transported material remains to be established. Indeed, on the ground of the results reported above, two hypothesis concerning the site of synthesis may be proposed. 1. This material might have been synthetized in the retina and then transported to the contralateral optic tectum at a velocity of 50—70 mm/day, or else 2. it may have been synthesized all along the optic nerve and then transported to the optic tectum at a much lower velocity (tentatively 25—35 mm/day). To assess whether the retina or the optic nerve was the site of synthesis of the rapidly transported material, a second experiment was performed.

The right optic nerve of goldfish was cut at the eyeball 10 min after injecting tritiated leucine into the right eye. After 12 hours the fish were killed and the radioactivity measured as in the previous experiment.

The following results were obtained (Table).

Table. *Level of radioactivity in the optic nerve and optic tectum of goldfish after transection of the optic nerve. The right optic nerve was transected at the eyeball 10 min after injecting 20 μCi ³H-L-Leucine into the vitreous humour of the right eye. The fish were killed 12 hours after the injection and treated as in Fig. 1. The data are in dpm/mg prot. Averages were made on three fish. The standard deviation is reported*

	Optic nerve		Optic tectum	
	Right	Left	Right	Left
TCA-prec.	4963 ± 2900	584 ± 178	1325 ± 516	1089 ± 247
TCA-sol.	11851 ± 1104	1486 ± 508	1298 ± 513	1540 ± 1200

1. The TCA-precipitable and the TCA-soluble radioactivity in the distal trunk of the transected nerve (right) were about ten times greater than in the left nerve.

2. The TCA-precipitable as well as the TCA-soluble radioactivity in the left optic tectum, connected to the transected nerve, were identical to the TCA-precipitable and TCA-soluble radioactivity in the right optic tectum.

The first result indicate that the transection of the optic nerve at the eyeball did not prevent the migration and the incorporation of free leucine into the distal trunk of the transected nerve. Indeed free leucine could have reached the distal trunk either within the optic nerve (in the 10 min between the injection and the transection), or from outside the nerve, e.g. by leakage into the optic cavity, after the transection of the nerve. The second result demonstrate that the transection of the nerve completely prevented the appearence of the rapidly transported material in the left optic tectum. Since the transection of the nerve should not impair the mechanism of rapid transport of protein (Ochs and Ranish, 1970), this result excludes the possibility of the optic nerve being the site of synthesis of the rapidly transported material. Therefore it can be concluded that the rapidly transported material is synthesized only in the retinal ganglion cells and from there transported to the synaptic endings of the contralateral optic tectum (McEwen and Grafstein, 1968; Schonbach and Cuénod, 1970).

Conclusion

The experiments described in this communication directly confirm that proteins synthesized in the neuron cell body are rapidly transported down the axon to the axon terminal. Independently from the rapid axonal transport of protein free amino acids can invade the nerve, extraaxonally or even from outside the nerve, and be incorporated locally. The possibility that free amino acids can migrate rapidly inside the axons and be incorporated in the axon and at the nerve ending cannot be completely ruled out, but seems rather improbable and would be completely independent from the rapid axonal flow of protein.

Acknowledgement. This work was started at the Department of Biophysics, The Johns Hopkins University, Baltimore, in the laboratory of Dr. Marcus Jacobson and completed at the Department de Biologie, Commissariat à l'Energie Atomique, Saclay, in the laboratory of Dr. Bernard Dorz. The author wish to express his appreciation to Dr. Marcus Jacobson and Dr. Bernard Droz for their support and encouragement. The author is a Long Term EMBO Fellow.

Bibliography

Barondes, S.: Axoplasmic transport. In: Handbook of neurochemistry, vol. II, pp. 435. A. Lajtha, ed. New York-London: Plenum Press 1969.

Droz, B., Koenig, H. L.: The dynamic condition of protein in axons and axon terminals. Acta neuropath. (Berl.), Suppl. V, 109—118 (1971).

Grafstein, B.: Axonal transport: communication between soma and synapse, pp. 11—26. Recent advances in biochemical psychopharmacology. E. Costa and P. Greengard, eds. New York: Raven Press 1969.

McEwen, B. S., Grafstein, B.: Fast and slow component in axonal transport of protein. J. Cell Biol. **38**, 494—508 (1968).

Ochs, S., Ranish, N.: Metabolic dependence of fast axoplasmic transport in nerve. Science **167**, 878 (1970).

Schonbach, J., Cuénod, M.: Axonal transport of newly synthesized materials in the retinotectal pathway of the pigeon. Acta neuropath. (Berl.), Suppl. V, 153—161 (1971).

Dr. L. Di Giamberardino
Departement de Biologie
CEA, Saclay
B.P. no 2-91-Gif-Sur-Yvette, France

Acta neuropath. (Berl.) Suppl. V, 136—143 (1971)

Acetylcholinesterase in Mammalian Peripheral Nerves and Characteristics of its Migration

Liliana Lubińska

Department of Neurophysiology, Nencki Institute of Experimental Biology
Warsaw, Poland

Summary. The survey of various peripheral nerves of dogs suggests a correlation between the size of motor units and AChE activity of the nerve. Nerve fibres innervating a large number of muscle fibres exhibit a higher AChE activity than those innervating only a few muscle fibres.

Most nerves exhibit a slight longitudinal proximodistal gradient of AChE activity.

In transected nerves, axonal AChE migrates in both directions. Characteristics of migration were determined by studying the process of accumulation of the enzyme near the site of transection in the central and peripheral stumps and in isolated nerve segments.

About 15% of AChE content of the nerve is migrating by "fast" transport: 10.5% in the cellulifugal and 4.5% in cellulipetal direction. The respective velocities of translocation are 260 mm/day and 134 mm/day.

The fate of migrating AChE is discussed.

Key-Words: Acetylcholinesterase — Peripheral Nerve — Axonal Transport.

AChE in axons is found at two intracellular locations, at the surface membrane and in the axoplasm. In the latter it is usually connected with tubules of the smooth endoplasmic reticulum (Brzin, Tennyson, and Duffy, 1966; Novikoff, Quintana, Villaverde, and Forschirm, 1966; Schlaepfer and Torack, 1966; Kokko, Mautner, and Barnett, 1969). Gruber and Zenker (personal communication) found also the reaction products dispersed in the axoplasm.

In normal mammalian peripheral nerves the Schwann cells do not contain AChE (Cavanagh, Thompson, and Webster, 1954; Tewari and Bourne, 1960; Koelle, 1951 and others) so that it is practically confined to axons if one disregards the contribution of the enzyme from erythrocytes in nerve capillaries.

AChE in Various Peripheral Nerves

A survey of AChE activity, expressed in nmole of AThCh split/mg protein/ 2 hours, in peripheral nerves of dogs (Lubińska, Niemierko, Oderfeld, and Szwarc, 1963) has shown a rather wide scatter of activity in various mixed somatic nerves. Thus AChE activity in nerve to big muscles of fore- and hind limbs was 820—930, in the hypoglossal 750, in the phrenic 480, whereas in zygomatic and buccal branches of the facial it was 290 to 380. Since in large muscles of the limbs a single axon innervates well over a hundred muscle fibres whereas in facial muscles the innervation ratio is of the order of 1:10, there seems to be a trend for axons supplying a large number of end plates to exhibit a higher AChE activity than axons innervating a few end plates only. It should be noted that the facial is practically a purely motor nerve whereas the mixed nerves to limbs contain a large proportion of sensory fibres. The actual difference in AChE activity between motor axons in the two groups of nerves is therefore probably larger than that shown by analyses. The relationship between the size of motor units and the level of AChE activity in their axons has not, however, been investigated in detail.

The cervical vago-sympathetic trunk of the dog has an activity of 2250 and the cervical sympathetic of cat 4770 nmole of AThCh slit/mg protein/2 h. Is this very high activity of sympathetic axons due to axolemmal or axoplasmic AChE? There seem to be no pertinent electron microscopic data. But sympathetic fibres are much thinner than average somatic fibres and there is, therefore, much more axolemmal material per unit volume of sympathetic than of somatic fibres. It might therefore be tentatively surmised that it is the axolemmal AChE which accounts mainly for the high activity of sympathetic fibres.

Sensory nerves (lingual, radial superficial, saphenous) have an activity of 360 to 650. It is possible that this relatively high activity of sensory nerves is to some extent due to admixture of sympathetic fibres in the nerve trunks.

Gradients of AChE Activity

AChE activity is not uniformly distributed along the nerve trunks. It decreases with the distance from cell bodies. In nerves which do not start from plexuses and run as separate trunks from the exit from the vertebrae to the beginning of branching above the entry into the muscle, which may therefore be analyzed over most of their length, a regular linear decrease of AChE activity is observed (Lubińska, Niemierko, Oderfeld, and Szwarc, 1962). Thus in the nerve to levator scapulae, the activity decreases but about 3.6% of the value of the uppermost part along every 10 mm of the nerve and in the phrenic this gradient corresponds to 1.8%. Proximodistal gradients of activity were found also in most nerves in which for anatomical reasons only a part of axonal length was available for analyses. In the dog these gradients ranged from 0.4 to 7.2% per 10 mm. The total protein content does not change along the nerve and fibre diameters remain constant along unbranched parts of axons. It may be assumed therefore that the gradient of AChE activity corresponds to actual changes of concentration of the enzyme along the axons. Several other substances exhibit proximo-distal gradients of concentration along nerves (for ref. see Lubińska, 1964) and gradients in the reverse direction were described in the tractus gracilis by Friede and Knoller (1964) for lactic, succinic, malic and glucose-6-phosphate dehydrogenase and probably cytochrome oxidase.

Migration of AChE in the Axons

It is generally assumed that in mature neurons AChE is formed almost exclusively in the perikarya and a part of it passes into the axons and is carried down the axonal pathway to the nerve endings. It has not been possible, as yet, to study the character of axonal migration of AChE in intact nerves by radioactive tracers as it was done for many proteins synthesized in the cell bodies. Information about the transport of AChE in the axons could nevertheless be obtained by studying transected or crushed nerves in which changes of AChE activity, easily detected and measured, permit to determine the characteristics of its migration.

Histochemical Findings. In crushed nerves AChE activity increases on both sides of the crushed region, the depth of staining increasing with time (Zeleńa and Lubińska, 1962).

In nerves crushed in two places, several millimetres apart, the increase is seen on the distal side of the distal lesion and on the proximal side of the proximal lesion. When, however, the distance between the two crushes is long, four sites of increased activity appear, one on each side of each lesion.

The shape of the stained region of axons differs according to its site. In the dog proximally to the crush it is thick, elongated, usually rounded up toward the lesion and decreasing progressively in the intensity of staining and diameter away from it. On the distal side, the terminal, stained portion forms a rounded head continuing by a thin tail (Fig. 1, inset). Similar results were obtained in crushed nerves of rats, dogs and rabbits.

The increase of activity on the proximal side of the crush was observed for many enzymes (for review see Lubińska, 1964, and Friede, 1966). It was interpreted by various authors either as a sign of a local reaction of injuried fibres or as a damming of the proximo-distal flow of axoplasm according to Weiss' theory (Weiss and Hiscoe, 1948).

The fact that the appearance of increased AChE activity at the ends of a segment isolated between two crushes depends on its length suggests strongly that it is not a local reaction but a phenomenon in which the undisturbed part of axons is also involved. We tentatively interpreted it as a result of translocation of AChE along the axons and its arrest near the site of the crush. The increase of activity on both sides of the lesion was considered as indication that the enzyme moves in the axons both in the proximo-distal and disto-proximal directions.

Quantitative Results. These hypotheses were tested by quantitative analysis of the behaviour of AChE in transected nerves.

In order to keep as close as possible to the conditions prevailing in undisturbed nerves, the duration of experiments had to be kept relatively short. This was determined by following considerations.

1. The distal part of a severed nerve is destined to degenerate. Although its AChE activity remains unchanged for about four days in dog nerves, there are indications that the mechanism of transport is affected much earlier.

2. The perikaryal reaction to axonotmesis includes, among other features, a marked decrease in AChE activity (Schwarzacher, 1958; Fredricsson and Sjöqvist, 1962; Flumerfelt and Lewis, 1969, and others). The axonal AChE being formed in the perikaryon the course of accumulation on the proximal side of the lesion should be studied before the decreased amount of AChE from the reacting perikaryon is discharged into the axon, or, more exactly, before this diminished amount reaches the vicinity of the lesion.

To be on the safe side of these limitations the duration of experiments was confined to the initial 20 h after transection.

The experiments were made on transected peroneal nerves of dogs. AChE activity increased progressively near the cut ends. The changes in size of these terminal pools of AChE were used as basis for calculation of velocity and of the amount of enzyme migrating in each direction. For details of experimental procedure and statistical analysis of results, see Lubińska and Niemierko (1971).

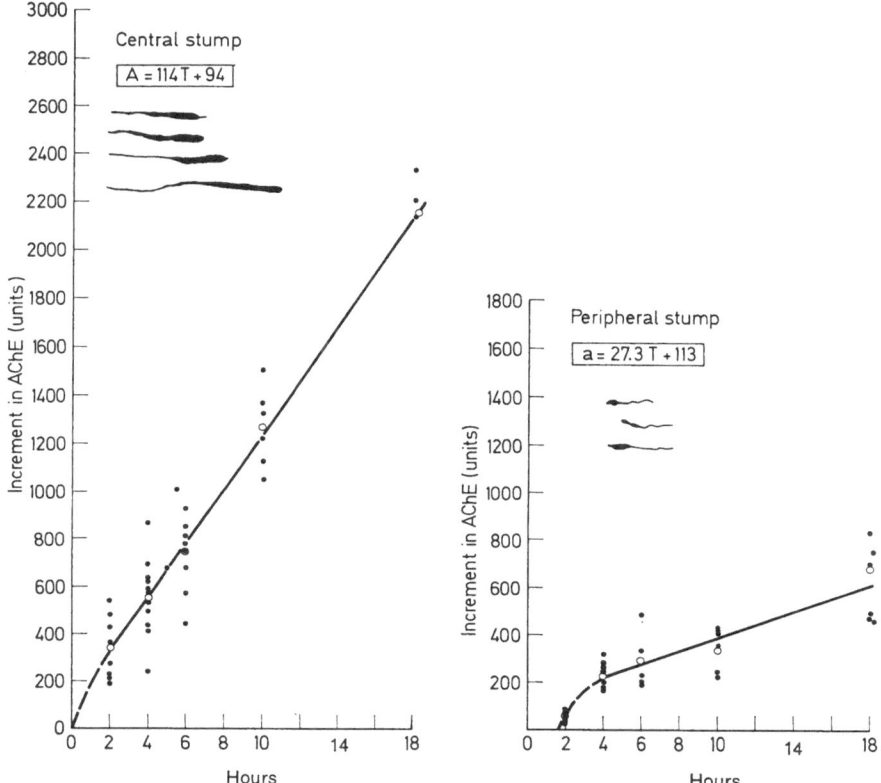

Fig. 1. Time course of increase of the terminal pools of AChE in the central and peripheral stumps. Dots—results of individual experiments, circles—means for a given time interval. The regression equation for accumulation in the central stump (A) was calculated for time interval 2—18 h, that for the peripheral stump (a) for interval of 4—18 h. The approximate course of the initial non-linear increase, somewhat delayed in the distal stump, is shown by dashed lines. The characteristic shape of the histochemically stained terminal part of axons in the central and peripheral stump is shown in the upper left hand corner of each graph (from Zelená and Lubińska, 1962).

The size of the terminal pools of AChE increases linearly with time at the ends of the central and peripheral stumps (Fig. 1) of transected nerves, except at the very beginning when the increase is faster. After this initial period, attributable to the direct effect of nerve injury, a steady amount of 114 units is added each hour to the pool on the proximal side and of 27 units to the pool on the distal side (100 units per mm corresponding to the normal control level of AChE activity in the investigated nerve).

In order to decide whether the slower increase of the terminal pool of AChE at the end of the peripheral stump is due to a slower velocity of translocation or to a smaller amount of AChE migrating in the cellulipetal direction, or to both these factors, a series of experiments was made on nerve segments of variable

L. Lubińska:

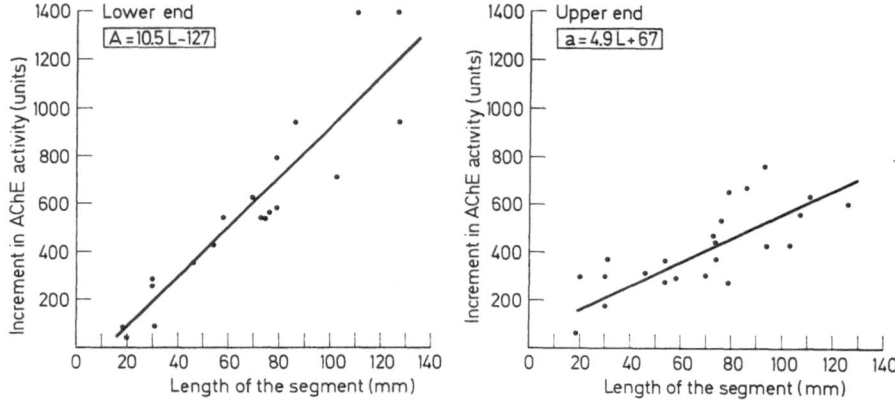

Fig. 2. Influence of length of the isolated segment on the final size of pools of AChE above the distal transection (*A*) and below the proximal transection (*a*). 22 h after transection. Dots—results of individual experiments. Straight lines show regression of size of pools on length of segments. (For details of statistical analysis see Lubińska and Niemierko, 1971)

length isolated by two transections from the cell bodies and from the terminal portion of axons and the innervated periphery.

In such segments the total AChE content remains unchanged (Lubińska, Niemierko, Odenfeld-Nowak, and Szwarc, 1964) whereas AChE accumulates at both ends of the segment.

The course of accumulation above the distal transection is similar to that seen in the central stump. Below the proximal transection it is similar to that of the distal stump, so that the polarity of transport exhibited by nerves with a single transection is preserved. The process of accumulation proceeds for a certain time, dependent on the length of the segment and then it is arrested. The final size of terminal pools when the accumulation is completed is proportional to the length of axons (Fig. 2).

By combining the equations showing the dependence of size of the terminal pools of AChE on time elapsed after transection and on the length of axons involved, both the velocity of migration and the amount of AChE migrating in each direction may be calculated.

As seen in Table 1, where these results are summarized, the movements of AChE in transected axons occur both in cellulifugal and cellulipetal directions. Though both fall within the range of "fast" transport, their characteristics are different. In the cellulipetal direction the flux is smaller and the velocity slower. If Schmitt's (1969) hypothesis that fast transport is brought about by interaction between the moving particles and microtubules (or neurofilaments) is correct, the present results would suggest that gliding down the microtubules is faster than climbing up and that the difference is due either to a certain polarity of surface organization of microtubules or to different properties of AChE-containing particles moving in the ascending and descending stream.

Table 1. *Characteristics of bidirectional migration of AChE in transected peroneal nerves of dogs*

	Cellulifugal direction	Cellulipetal direction
Velocity, in mm/24 h	260	134
Amount of migrating AChE, in % of total AChE content of the nerve	10.5	4.5

The characteristic shape of the histochemically stained region in the terminal part of axons, distinct on the proximal and distal side of the lesion, suggests the possibility that migration in each direction occurs in spatially segregated layers of axoplasm as, for instance, in the tentacles of *Tocophrya* described by Rudzinska (1967). The axons lack, however, the ultrastructural organization underlying the segregation in tentacles.

Only about 15% of AChE content of axons is moving by fast transport. The remainder is either immobile or moving very slowly. It is tempting to surmise that axolemmal AChE is relatively stabile whereas AChE in the axoplasm is migrating. However, experimental data supporting such hypothesis are as yet lacking.

The question to what extent the characteristics of migration obtained on transected nerves are valid for normal intact nerves was discussed in detail elsewhere (Lubińska and Niemierko, 1971, see also Ochs in this volume).

The Fate of Migrating AChE

AChE activity studied in nerve trunks does not provide direct information about its fate in the entire neurons. Both perikarya and the terminal parts of axons are anatomically intimately intermingled with other cellular elements so that it is practically impossible in mammals to obtain samples of a homogeneous population of whole neurons for biochemical analyses.

What inferences concerning the fate of AChE in the neurons may then be drawn from a quantitative study of AChE activity and its migration in the axonal portion of nerve cells?

It is seen from the data described here that the amount of AChE arriving per unit time to the nerve endings is about four times as large as that leaving the endings by transport in the cellulipetal direction.

This would result in a daily increase of over 2100 units of AChE at the endings. Since there are no indications of a leakage of this enzyme into the intercellular space or to the innervated cells, a tremendous increase of AChE in nerve terminals with increasing age of the animal should be apparent. No such increase was ever reported in mature animals, indicating the existence of degradation of AChE at the nerve endings, compensated for by continual arrival of fresh amounts of the enzyme brought by axoplasmic migration.

The hypothesis of metabolic degradation of AChE at nerve endings is to some extent corroborated by the fact, quoted at the beginning of this paper, that axons innervating a large number of end plates have a higher AChE content than axons innervating only a few end plates. This suggests that a more intense axonal supply is needed to maintain a steady amount of AChE at the numerous nerve endings of the large motor units.

The existence of a linear gradient of AChE along nerves in spite of the absence of tapering of fibres in nerve trunks (Rexed, 1944; Quilliam, 1956; Causey, 1948; Thiel, 1957) and the constant amount of bulk proteins along the nerve seems to indicate that a fraction of AChE is in some way used up in its travel along the nerve trunk and never reaches the endings.

Although there is a general consensus that enzyme molecules are not degraded by their metabolic activity it is difficult to escape such conclusion for AChE on the basis of its behaviour in peripheral nerves.

Similar questions would probably arise in connection with other migratory axonal enzymes unless the "circulation" is complete and the same amount of enzyme arrives at the endings by proximo-distal migration as leaves them by ascending transport. With non-enzymic material a catabolic degradation along the lines hypothesized initially by Weiss and Hiscoe (1948), could probably take care of the problem. At present only transmitters and other substances known to leak out at nerve endings or through the surface membrane of axons would not pose the baffling problem of their ultimate fate.

Acknowledgements. My sincere thanks are due to Professor Stella Niemierko, co-author of most of the work on which the present paper is based, for helpful discussion and to Professors L. Wojtczak and W. Drabikowski who warned me that enzymes are not degraded during their metabolic activity.

References

Brzin, M., Tennyson, V. M., Duffy, P. E.: Acetylcholinesterase in frog sympathetic and dorsal root ganglia. A study by electron microscope cytochemistry and microgasometric analysis with the magnetic diver. J. Cell Biol. **31**, 215—242 (1966).

Causey, G.: The effect of pressure on nerve fibres. J. Anat. (Lond.) **82**, 262—270 (1948).

Cavanagh, J. B., Thompson, R. H., Webster, G. R.: The localization of pseudo-cholinesterase activity in nervous tissue. Quart. J. exp. Physiol. **39**, 185—197 (1954).

Flumerfelt, B. A., Lewis, P. R.: Changes in the hypoglossal nucleus following axotomy. J. Anat. (Lond.) **104**, 587 (1969).

Fredricsson, B., Sjöqvist, F.: A cytomorphological study of cholinesterase in sympathetic ganglia of the cat. Acta morph. neerl.-scand. **5**, 140—166 (1962).

Friede, R. L.: Topographic Brain Chemistry. New York: Academic Press 1966.

— Knoller, M.: Proximo-distal increase of enzymatic activity in the dorsal spinal tracts. J. Neurochem. **11**, 679—686 (1964).

Koelle, G. B.: The elimination of enzymatic diffusion artifacts in the histochemical localization of cholinesterases and survey of their cellular distributions. J. Pharmacol. exp. Ther. **103**, 153—171 (1951).

Kokko, A., Mautner, H. G., Barnett, R. J.: Fine structural localization of acetylcholinesterase using acetyl-B-methylthiocholine and acetylselenocholine as substrates. J. Histochem. Cytochem. **17**, 625—640 (1969).

Lubińska, L.: Axoplasmic streaming in regenerating and in normal nerve fibres. Ed. M. Singer and J. P. Schadé, Progr. Brain Res. Vol. 13, pp. 1—71, Amsterdam: Elsevier 1964.

— Niemierko, S.: Velocity and intensity of bidirectional migration of acetylcholinesterase in transected nerves. Brain Res. **27**, 329—342 (1971).

— — Oderfeld, B., Szwarc, L.: Decrease of acetylcholinesterase activity along peripheral nerves. Science **135**, 368—370 (1962).

— — — — The distribution of acetylcholinesterase in peripheral nerves. J. Neurochem. **10**, 25—41 (1963).

— — — — Behaviour of acetylcholinesterase in isolated nerve segments. J. Neurochem. **11**, 493—503 (1964).

Niemierko, S., Lubińska, L.: Two fractions of axonal acetylcholinesterase exhibiting different behaviour in severed nerves. J. Neurochem. 14, 761—769 (1967).

Novikoff, A. B., Quintana, N., Villaverde, H., Forschirm, R.: Nucleoside phosphatase and cholinesterase activities in dorsal root ganglia and peripheral nerve. J. Cell Biol. 29, 525—546 (1966).

Ochs, S.: The dependence of fast transport in mammalian nerve fibres on metabolism. Acta neuropath. (Berl.) Suppl. V, 86—96 (1971).

Quilliam, T. A.: Some characteristics of myelinated fibre populations. J. Anat. (Lond.) 90, 172—187 (1956).

Rexed, B.: Contributions to the knowledge of the postnatal development of the peripheral nervous system in man. Acta psychiat. neurol., Suppl. 33, 1—206 (1944).

Rudzinska, M. A.: Ultrastructures involved in the feeding mechanism of suctoria. Trans. N.Y. Acad. Sci., Ser. II, 29, 512—525 (1967).

Schlaepfer, W. W., Torack R. M.: The ultrastructural localization of cholinesterase activity in sciatic nerve of the rat. J. Histochem. Cytochem. 14, 369—378 (1966).

Schmitt, F. O.: Fibrous proteins and neuronal dynamics. Ed. S. H. Barondes, Symposia of the International Society for Cell Biology, Vol. 8. New York: Academic Press 1969.

Schwarzacher, H. G.: Der Cholinesterasegehalt von motorischen Nervenzellen während der axonalen Reaktion. Acta anat. (Basel) 32, 51—65 (1958).

Tewari, H. B., Bourne, G. H.: Histochemical localization of specific and nonspecific cholinesterases in myelinated nerves. Exp. Cell Res. 21, 245—248 (1960).

Thiel, W.: Morphologische Ergebnisse an einzelnen markhaltigen Nervenfasern und ihre funktionelle Bedeutung. Acta anat. (Basel) 31, 156—192 (1957).

Weiss, P., Hiscoe, H. B.: Experiments on the mechanism of nerve growth. J. exp. Zool. 107, 315—395 (1948).

Zelená, J., Lubińska, L.: Early changes of acetylcholinesterase activity near the lesion in crushed nerves. Physiol. bohemoslov. 11, 261—268 (1962).

Prof. Liliana Lubińska
Nencki Institute of Experimental Biology
Pasteura 3, Warsaw 22 (Poland)

Acta neuropath. (Berl.) Suppl. V, 144—152 (1971)

Role of Slow Axonal Transport in Nerve Regeneration *

BERNICE GRAFSTEIN

Department of Physiology, Cornell University Medical College, New York

Summary. After section of the optic tract in goldfish, axonal outgrowth begins 6—8 days after the cut and is accompanied by an increase in the slow component of axonal protein transport. Application of colchicine to intact or cut tracts decreases the rate of the transport in the optic nerve at points upstream from the injection. The colchicine treatment may also inhibit axonal outgrowth in the cut tracts, but in some cases outgrowth occurs even when the transport rate is decreased, Therefore, the increase in transport rate observed during regeneration is not a prerequisite for axonal outgrowth, but may be the consequence of such outgrowth.

Key-Words: Nerve Regeneration — Axonal Transport — Protein — Axonal Outgrowth.

In the adult goldfish, the cut axons of the retinal ganglion cells are capable of vigorous regeneration (Attardi and Sperry, 1963). After section of the optic tract, restoration of vision takes about 3 weeks, and the advance of the regenerating fibers has been found to be about 0.2 mm per day (Grafstein and Murray, 1969). During regeneration the ganglion cells do not show the typical chromatolytic changes seen in some regenerating mammalian nerve cells (Bodian and Mellors, 1945), but do become enlarged and hyperchromic. The earliest change in the cell body, beginning 3—4 days after the cut, is an increase in nucleolar material leading to an increase in protein synthesizing capacity (Murray and Grafstein, 1969). A few days later there is an increase in the rate of the slow component of protein transport along the intact portion of the axons. This rate is normally about 0.4 mm per day (Grafstein, 1967; McEwen and Grafstein, 1968), but rises to a maximum of about 3 times normal at approximately the time that the new axons reconnect with the tectum (Grafstein and Murray, 1969). Presumably this increased rate is important in providing materials for laying down new axoplasm. In the present study, the morphology of the axons at the cut nerve tip was examined in order to determine how the increase in slow protein transport was related to axonal outgrowth, and how both the outgrowth and transport rate were affected when colchicine was applied to the site of the cut.

Methods

Goldfish of 6—8 cm body length (10—12 cm to tip of tail) were used, maintained at a temperature of 21—23°C. The optic tract on one or both sides was cut intracranially close to the optic tectum. The length of an average optic axon is about 12 mm, including 3 mm within the eye, 4 mm in the optic nerve, 3 mm in the optic tract and 2 mm in the tectum. The tract section

* This work was supported by Grant no. NS 09015 from the National Institute for Neurological Diseases and Stroke. I am indebted to Miss Roberta Alpert for preparation of the histological material.

removed the terminal 3—4 mm, i.e. about 30% of the total length. For determinations of axonal transport rate, 3—6 µCi of ³H-leucine (specific activity 5 Ci/mM) were injected into the posterior chamber of each eye. Three days after the injection, each animal was killed and the head was fixed in Bouin's solution with the optic nerves stretched in the orbit to keep them straight. The distribution of radioactive protein in the optic nerve between the eyeball and the chiasma was determined by a liquid scintillation counting technique previously described (Grafstein and Murray, 1969). The length of optic tract from the chiasma to the level of the cut was embedded in paraffin, and longitudinal sections were cut at 15 µ, then stained with Bodian's silver technique (Bodian, 1936). For the experiments involving intracranial injections, 10 µl of either colchicine solution or normal saline were injected through the midline of the skull by means of a microliter syringe with the tip of the needle extending about 3 mm into the skull cavity.

Results

1. Morphology of the Cut Optic Nerve Fibers

In the normal goldfish all the optic axons are myelinated and most are in the 0.5—1 µ diameter range, although there are an appreciable number between 3 and 7 µ (Grafstein and Seeman, unpublished results). Twenty-four hours after the optic tract was sectioned, axons of all sizes showed enlargements at their cut tips. These were obviously not "growth cones" (Cajal, 1928), since they developed so early after the cut and did not advance from the point at which they were initially observed. They were most likely formed by the extrusion of axoplasm from the cut ends of the fibers (Lubińska, 1964). Only the tips of small-size fibers extended right to the level of the cut (Fig. 1 A; see also Fig. 8 in Guth and Windle, 1970), while the end-bulbs on the largest-size fibers typically occurred in a narrow band across the nerve about 300—500 µ back from its tip (Fig. 1 A). The bulbs were evident on both sides of the cut but were more prominent on the retinal side. The following description is confined to events on the retinal side.

The bulbs on the small-size fibers began to disappear 3 days after the section (Fig. 2). Apparently they underwent fragmentation, since their disappearance was accompanied by an appreciable increase in the amount of fragmented debris at the edge of the cut (Fig. 1 B, Fig. 2). The bulbs on the large-size fibers did not disappear at the same time. They were still present 2 weeks after the operation (Fig. 2), although they had begun to look "frayed". By about 3 weeks their original smooth outline (Fig. 1 C), was completely lost, leaving a tangled knot of neurofibrils and in this configuration they were found to persist as late as 2 months after the section (Fig. 1 D), with no evidence of axonal outgrowth. Occasionally, large fibers could be seen with a regenerating collateral emerging about 20 µ behind the end-bulb, but this was rare, and it is likely that many of the largest-size fibers remained permanently disconnected from the tectum. At no time during the regeneration was there any obvious enlargement of the fibers attached to the end-bulbs as might be expected from "damming" of the axoplasm behind the bulb (Weiss and Hiscoe, 1948). Neither was there any obvious decrease in the diameter of the axons in regions closer to the cell body, such as has been reported by Kreutzberg (1971) for mammalian motor nerve. Except for the terminal 500 µ, the nerve looked normal.

The first signs of axonal outgrowth appeared in the small-size fibers 3—4 days after the cut. The new axons were very small in diameter, and collected into characteristic dense bundles which were easily recognizable (Fig. 1 B), although growth cones were never seen. In the 3—4 day period, such bundles occurred only

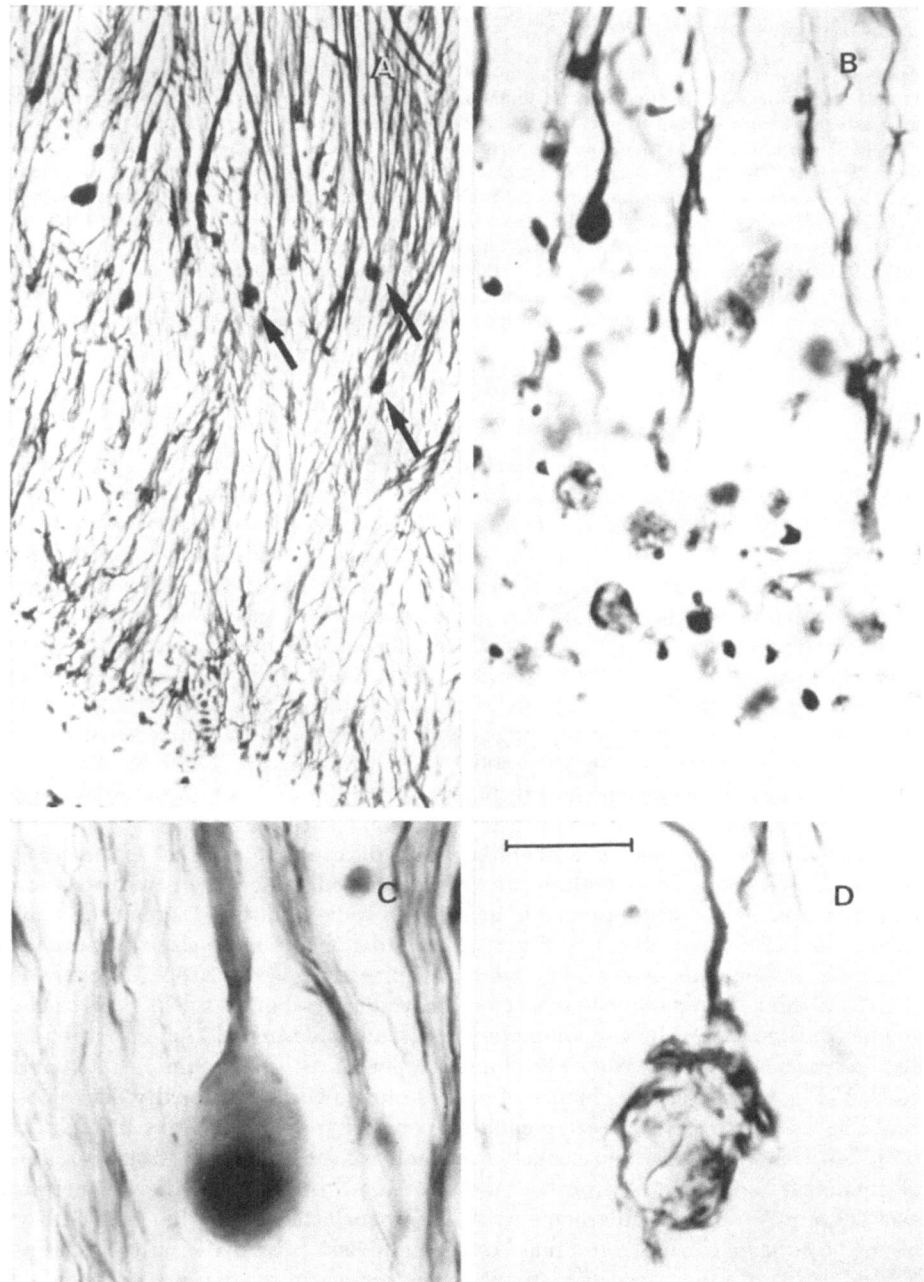

Fig. 1 A—D. Morphological features of cut goldfish optic axons. Bodian silver stain. A Retinal side of cut in optic tract two days after operation. Cut passes diagonally at lower left. Arrows point to some of the end-bulbs on large-size fibers. In most preparations these bulbs occurred about twice as far back from cut. 400×; B Retinal side of cut 4 days after operation. Note large amount of fragmented material adjacent to cut edge. Axon at upper left still retains its end-bulb. In center and at right are small bundles of axons which have lost their end-bulbs and are beginning to collect together in an early stage of regeneration. 1600×; C End-bulb on large-size axon 2 days after cut. 1600×; D Reticulated end-bulb on large-size fiber 66 days after cut. 1600×. Horizontal bar indicates 40 μ for Fig. 1 A, 10 μ for Fig. 1 B—D

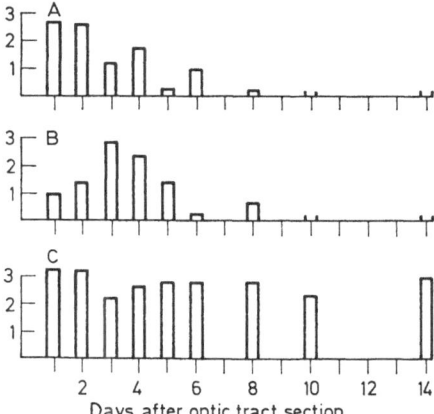

Fig. 2 A—C. Time course of end-bulb changes in axons on retinal side of cut optic tract. A Small fiber bulbs: incidence of end-bulbs on small-size fibers; B Fragmentation: incidence of fragmented material at edge of cut. C Large fiber bulbs: incidence of end-bulbs on large-size fibers. Numerical values were assigned as follows: 1 rare; 2 readily detectable but not typical of most regions of cut tip; 3 characteristic of most regions of tip; 4 extremely well developed. Values for each time-point represent an average for 3—9 preparations. The columns open at the top indicate a value of zero

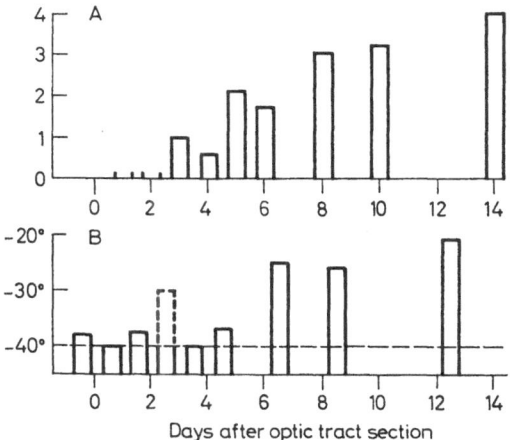

Fig. 3 A and B. Comparison of time of axonal outgrowth and change in rate of slow protein transport after section of goldfish optic tract. A Grade of outgrowth was assigned numerical values as follows: 1 rare; 2 readily detectable in some regions of the nerve tip; 3 characteristic of most regions; 4 well advanced past the original line of section. Values represent average of 3—9 preparations for each time point. The columns open at the top indicate a value of zero. B Rate of slow transport was measured as the slope angle of the semilogarithmic plot of the distribution of radioactive protein in the nerve. A 3-day interval between isotope injection and sacrifice was used and values have been plotted at the mid-point of each interval. Negative values indicate slopes below the horizontal. Each value is the average of 5—11 preparations. The broken line represents the average value obtained in 39 normal nerves. The value for the interval with mid-point $2^1/_2$ days appears to be elevated but this is probably not significant (see text). The maximum level attained in the time period shown in this diagram represents a transport rate between 2 and 3 times normal

very rarely. By 5—6 days they were generally readily detectable, but involved only a fraction of the nerve fiber population (Fig. 3 A). By 8 days after the cut, the bundles were a characteristic feature throughout most of the nerve tip, although they seldom extended for more than 50—100 μ. The picture was essentially the same at 10 days and by 14 days the bundles had advanced several hundred microns beyond the line of the cut, usually bridging the gap to the degenerating stump.

2. Protein Transport in the Intact Portion of the Nerve

It has been shown that the distribution of radioactive protein along the optic nerve following the injection of labelled amino acid into the eye can be used to measure the rate of slow protein transport in the nerve (Grafstein and Murray, 1969). The distribution follows an exponential curve, so that a semi-logarithmic plot of the radioactivity gives a straight line. The slope of this line changes with time after the injection (Grafstein, 1967), and this change occurs more rapidly in regenerating nerve, indicating a more rapid rate of transport (Grafstein and Murray, 1969). Thus, at any time after the injection, the difference between the slopes obtained in the normal and regenerating nerves provides an index of the difference in their rates of transport (Fig. 4 A). However, since it is necessary to wait several days after the injection for this difference in the slopes to become detectable, an instantaneous comparison of the rates cannot be made. The minimum interval that has been found to be satisfactory is 3 days, and Fig. 3 B shows the slope angles of the distributions obtained with injections made at various times after optic tract section, using a 3-day interval between injection and sacrifice. As has previously been shown (Grafstein and Murray, 1969), measurements made in the 5—8 day interval (mid-point $6^1/_2$ days) were elevated, whereas measurements made in the 3—6 day interval (mid-point $4^1/_2$ days) were normal. Apparently there was an increase in protein transport beginning between 6 and 8 days after the cut. In the present study it was found that prior to this, the transport rate remained normal. The value obtained in the 1—4 day interval (mid-point $2^1/_2$ days) appeared to be elevated, but the validity of this finding is doubtful, since the values for overlapping periods, i.e. 0—3 days (mid-point $1^1/_2$ days) and 2 to 5 days (mid-point $3^1/_2$ days), did not show a corresponding change. It is possible that some degree of artefact was introduced by the accumulation of rapidly transported protein at the cut (Livett et al., 1968). Therefore it appears that the transport rate in the regenerating nerves was not significantly changed until 6—8 days after the section, which, as shown above, corresponds to the time when most of the small-size fibers began their outgrowth.

3. Effect of Intracranial Application of Colchicine

Colchicine can arrest axonal outgrowth (Pinner-Poole and Campbell, 1969; Seeds et al., 1970) and has been found to block axonal transport. Usually fast transport is seen to be affected (Kreutzberg, 1969; Dahlström, 1968) but slow transport can also be inhibited (Karlsson and Sjöstrand, 1969; Fernandez et al., 1970; James et al., 1970). In order to examine more closely the correlation described above between outgrowth and the increase in the rate of slow transport, the effects of cholchicine on these two parameters were examined.

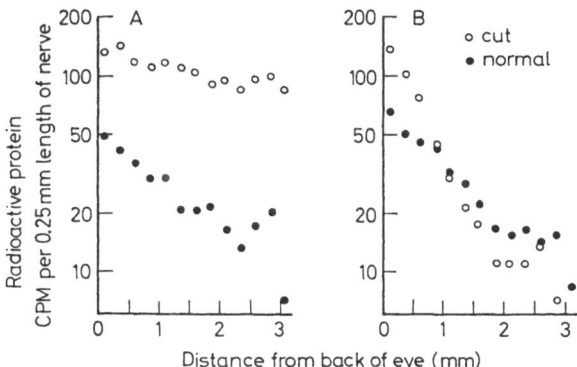

Fig. 4A and B. Examples of distributions of radioactive protein in normal optic nerve (•) and regenerating nerve (o) in the same animal 3 days after injection of tritiated leucine into each eye. Five days before this injection an intracranial injection was made of (A) 10 μl saline or (B) 6 μg colchicine in 10 μl saline. One optic tract had been cut 5 days before the intracranial injection. Note steep slopes of distributions in nerves treated with colchicine, especially cut nerve

The experiments were performed in animals in which one optic tract had been sectioned. The colchicine was applied to both optic tracts by intracranial injection at a time when outgrowth was just beginning in the cut tract, 5 days after the cut had been made. Eight days later, when profuse outgrowth over a distance of several hundred microns would have been expected, no outgrowth was observed in any of 5 animals which had received a 6 μg dose of colchicine. If we estimate the volume of distribution as 100 μl, this would represent an effective concentration of 0.2 mM. In these cases, the rate of transport in the cut nerves was reduced, below normal, as indicated by the slope of the distribution of radioactive protein in the nerves (Fig. 4). The average slope angle was $-71° \pm 4$ (S.D.) in the cut nerves after colchicine treatment, as compared with an average value of $-33° \pm 9$ for uncut nerves without colchicine. Transport in the uncut nerves in the colchicine-treated animals was also reduced, although not so severely. The average slope angle in these nerves was $-54° \pm 6$. With a 3 μg dose of colchicine, outgrowth was not blocked in any of 5 animals examined, but transport rate was reduced in 3 of the 5 to about the same degree as with the higher dose. These effects were not produced by interference with retinal protein synthesis resulting from the leakage of colchicine into the eye, since the incorporation of labelled amino acid into protein was the same in the retinas of both the colchicine-treated animals and those that had received intracranial injections of saline. The results of this experiment show that although colchicine interferes with both outgrowth and protein transport, the dose required to reduce the rate of transport is lower than that required to block outgrowth. Since outgrowth can occur when transport is blocked, the increase in transport rate that is normally associated with outgrowth is apparently not a prerequisite for such outgrowth.

It is interesting to note that in the regenerating nerves, the level of radioactivity just behind the eye was about twice normal in both the nerves treated with saline and those treated with colchicine (Fig. 4), indicating a higher level of incorporation of the injected label. Evidently the colchicine treatment did not interfere with the development of the increased rate of protein synthesis that is characteristic of the regenerating ganglion cells (Murray and Grafstein, 1969).

Discussion

In general, the characteristic features of the cut goldfish optic axons can be recognized in classical descriptions of cut mamalian peripheral nerve (Cajal, 1928): the cut fibers developed end-bulbs at their terminations; the bulbs on the large-size fibers occurred further back from the cut than those on the small-size fibers; the bulbs that persisted beyond the early states of regeneration were converted into knots of neurofibrils. However, the fish nerve presented a more uniform and stereotyped picture, with very little cellular debris and relatively little infiltration by phagocytic elements into the stump of the retinal side of the cut. This small degree of disturbance may be in part responsible for the highly efficient regeneration that is characteristic of this system.

The differences between the responses of the small-size and large-size fibers in the fish nerve were particularly striking. The large-size fibers were apparently more susceptible to the traumatic effects of cutting, or to the conditions of local anoxia in the region of the cut, since their cut tips are retracted for a considerable distance. In subsequent changes leading to dissolution of the end-bulbs, the large fibers appeared to be less susceptible than the small ones, since the large-fiber bulbs persisted appreciably longer. It is possible that the local increase of proteolytic activity characteristic of the cut axon (Holtzman and Novikoff, 1965) was not adequate in the large fibers to deal with the larger volume of accumulated axoplasm in the end-bulb. Whatever the mechanism, it appears that dissolution of the end-bulb is a pre-requisite for outgrowth of the regenerating axonal sprouts, since it was only in the fibers from which the end-bulbs were rapidly removed that outgrowth appeared.

The reticulated appearance that the end-bulbs on the large-size fibers took on after several weeks was very similar to that described by (Cajal, 1928, Figs. 84 and 86) as a stage in the degeneration of "gigantic balls" at the ends of fibers that have been arrested in their outgrowth. In some cases the altered end-bulbs resembled the helicoidal "nervous spools" that Cajal described at the tips of myelinated fibers at long intervals after nerve section. His view was that these structures were formed by axonal outgrowth ("continuation of the assimilative process") confined within a "digestive chamber" or pocket of Schwann cells. It is not clear whether the reticulated bulbs seen in the present preparation arose from such continued outgrowth of the axon within a confined space, or whether they represented a modification of the original end-bulb in which the neurofibrillar skeleton was exposed by the dissolution of the surrounding axoplasm. The latter seems to be the more reasonable proposal, since the reticulated structure did not obviously increase in size or complexity after its initial appearance at about 3 weeks after the cut. In any case, since the reticulated appearance developed so late, we must assume that any outgrowth of the large-size axons, even within the confines of the end-bulb, was similarly delayed if not completely absent.

It is interesting to note, therefore, that all the retinal ganglion cells, including the "giant" cells from which the large fibers presumably arise, underwent the nucleolar increase and cellular hypertrophy that are the typical consequences of axotomy in this preparation (Murray and Grafstein, 1968; Grafstein and Murray, unpublished results). Apparently the cell body reaction developed in these neurons independently of the progress of axonal outgrowth. This, together with the fact that outgrowth in most of the optic fibers began about a week after the cut whereas the cell body changes began at 3—4 days, tends to contradict Watson's proposal (1969) that outgrowth may serve as a "signal" for the cell body changes (Cragg, 1970).

What of the relationship between axonal transport and outgrowth? An increase in transport rate and the beginning of outgrowth are closely related in time, occurring about a week after the cut. It is unlikely, however, that the increased transport is a prerequisite for outgrowth, since outgrowth sometimes occurred when the rate of transport had been reduced below normal by the application of colchicine.

An alternative hypothesis which suggests itself is that axonal sprouting, occurring as a purely local response of the cut axon tip, is in turn the circumstance that leads to an increase in protein transport. In this view, the transport is seen as being regulated by the "demand" established by conditions existing at the peripheral end of the axon, rather than at the cell body where the materials for transport are produced. In line with this hypothesis, it is possible that colchicine acts by changing conditions in the terminal part of the axon to inhibit transport in the part close to the cell body. Fernandez et al. (1970) have also demonstrated that colchicine produces such an "upstream" effect on slow transport in crayfish nerve cord. It is not yet clear how much of this effect, if any, is related to the action of colchicine on the neurotubules (Schmitt, 1968).

A point that remains puzzling is the fact that the rate of transport was initially unchanged after tract section which amputated about 30% of the axonal volume. One would expect a corresponding decrease in the rate or amount of materials transported if steady state conditions were to be rapidly re-established. It is hard to believe that after the end-bulbs disintegrated and before outgrowth began, soluble material continued to leak out of the free ends of the axons in the amount that was normally supplied by axonal transport. This point will need further careful examination in any analysis of how transport is regulated.

References

Attardi, D. G., Sperry, R. W.: Preferential selection of central pathways by regenerating optic fibers. Exp. Neurol. 7, 46—64 (1963).

Bodian, D.: A new method for staining nerve fibers and nerve endings in mounted paraffin sections. Anat. Rec. 65, 89—97 (1936).

— Mellors, R. C.: The regenerative cycle of motoneurons, with special reference to phosphatase activity. J. exp. Med. 81, 469—487 (1945).

Cragg, B. G.: What is the signal for chromatolysis? Brain Res. 23, 1—21 (1970).

Dahlström, A.: Effect of colchicine on transport of amine storage granules in sympathetic nerves of rat. Europ. J. Pharmacol. 5, 111—113 (1968).

Fernandez, H. L., Huneeus, F. C., Davison, P. F.: Studies on the mechanism of axoplasmic transport in the crayfish cord. J. Neurobiol. 1, 395—409 (1970).

Grafstein, B.: Transport of protein by goldfish optic nerve fibers. Science **157**, 196—198 (1967).
— Murray, M.: Transport of protein in goldfish optic nerve during regeneration. Exp. Neurol. **25**, 494—508 (1969).
Guth, L., Windle, W. F.: The enigma of central nervous regeneration. Exp. Neurol. Suppl. **5**, 1—43 (1970).
Holtzman, E., Novikoff, A. B.: Lysosomes in the rat sciatic nerve following crush. J. Cell Biol. **27**, 651—669 (1965).
James, K. A. C., Bray, J. J., Morgan, I. G., Austin, L.: The effect of colchicine on the transport of axonal protein in the chicken. Biochem. J. **117**, 767—771 (1970).
Karlsson, J.-O., Sjöstrand, J.: The effect of colchicine on axonal transport of protein in the optic nerve and tract of the rabbit. Brain Res. **13**, 617—619 (1969).
Kreutzberg, G.: Neuronal dynamics and axonal flow. IV. Blockage of intra-axonal enzyme transport by colchicine. Proc. nat. Acad. Aci. (Wash.) **62**, 722—728 (1969).
—, Schubert, P.: Volume changes in the axon during regeneration. Acta neuropath. (Berl.) **17**, 220—226 (1971).
Livett, B. G., Geffen, L. B., Austin, L.: Proximo-distal transport of [14C] noradrenaline and protein in sympathetic nerves. J. Neurochem. **15**, 931—939 (1968).
Lubińska, L.: Axoplasmic streaming in regenerating and in normal, nerve fibers, pp. 1—66. In: Mechanisms of neural regeneration, M. Singer and J. P. Schadé (eds.). Progr. Brain Res., Vol. 13. Amsterdam: Elsevier 1964.
McEwen, B. S., Grafstein, B.: Fast and slow components in axonal transport of protein. J. Cell Biol. **38**, 494—508 (1968).
Murray, M., Grafstein, B.: Changes in the morphology and amino acid incorporation of re-generating goldfish optic neurons. Exp. Neurol. **23**, 544—560 (1969).
Pinner-Poole, B., Campbell, J. B.: Effects of low temperature and colchicine on regenerating sciatic nerve. Exp. Neurol. **25**, 603—615 (1969).
Ramón y Cajal, S.: Degeneration and regeneration of the nervous system, Vol. I. (Trans. R. M. May). Cambridge: Oxford University Press 1928.
Schmitt, F. O.: The molecular biology of neuronal fibrous proteins. Neurosci. Res. Progr. Bull. **6**, 119—144 (1968).
Seeds, N. W., Gilman, A. G., Amano, T., Nirenberg, M. W.: Regulation of axon formation by clonal lines of a neural tumor. Proc. nat. Acad. Sci. (Wash.) **66**, 160—167 (1970).
Watson, W. E.: The response of motor neurones to intramuscular injection of botulinum toxin. J. Physiol. (Lond.) **202**, 611—630 (1969).
Weiss, P., Hiscoe, H. B.: Experiments on the mechanism of nerve growth. J. exp. Zool. **107**, 315—395 (1948).

Bernice Grafstein, Ph. D.
Dept. of Physiology
Cornell University Medical College
New York N.Y. 10021, U.S.A.

Acta neuropath. (Berl.) Suppl. V. 153—161 (1971)
© by Springer-Verlag 1971

Axoplasmic Streaming and Proteins
in the Retino-Tectal Neurons of the Pigeon *

J. Schonbach and M. Cuénod

Brain Research Institute, University of Zürich, Switzerland

Summary. Time course studies based on the biochemical and autoradiographic detections of labelled proteins after intraocular injection of tritiated leucine have been made to analyse the origin and the fate of newly synthesized macromolecules in the retino-tectal neurons of the pigeon. Some of them migrated intra-axonally at a rate of 20—500 mm/day, and seemed to be largely destined to renew some synaptic materials, possible some components of vesicles and mitochondria. The largest portion of the migrating proteins moved at a rate of about 1 mm/day, and was found mainly in the soluble and microsomal fractions. It was probably destined to renew some elements of the axon; however it reached also the terminals. Some data suggested that the rapid phase of axoplasmic flow might be subdivided.

Key-Words: Radioactivity — Axonal Transport — Protein — Nerve Terminals.

In their general organization, the protoplasms have long been deemed to be fundamentally alike, and protoplasmic movement is recognized as one of the major functions of life (Jahn and Bovee, 1969). Studies of this phenomenon in the nerve cell were hampered by the inaccessibility of neurons to direct *in vivo* observation. Indirect experimental approaches had to be devised, and those involving radioactive tracers were the most fruitful.

The application of radioactive amino-acids near the neuronal perikaryon, first initiated by Taylor and Weiss (1966), contributed largely to the recent wealth of data on the behavior of neuronal proteins, especially their axoplasmic translocation. A preferential labelling of the neuroplasmic precursor pools allowed Grafstein (1967) to demonstrate the rapid appearance of newly synthesized proteins in regions rich in synaptic endings. She interpreted her observations as the consequence of a fast intra-axonal transport of proteins. Similar data were obtained by many groups using different systems (see Grafstein, 1969, for a review, and other papers in this symposium), strengthening the concept of a biphasic, unidirectional axoplasmic streaming. Still, most of the evidence was circumstantial and more refined techniques were needed to test this concept.

We decided to use the retino-tectal system of the pigeon which presents many advantages: the two optic ways are completely crossed (Cowan *et al.*, 1961) providing an exactly symmetrical control on the same animal; the system is short and can be entirely visualized in histological preparations; the tectal organization facilitates identification of those regions containing axon terminals; the optic lobe is big enough to be fractionated into subcellular elements; the precursor can be easily introduced, in an exactly reproducible manner, into the

* Supported by grants nr. 4806, 4356 and 3.137.69 from the Swiss National Fund for Scientific Research, and grant nr. 47 from the Hartmann-Müller foundation.

vitreous humor of one eye; the avian retina is avascular and the labelled amino-acid reaches the ganglion cells in a physiological way.

We tried to answer the following questions: is there indeed a fast axoplasmic flow of protein? What is the destination of the rapidly moving molecules and which cellular components are involved? Is the fast flow a homogeneous entity or can it be subdivided? What are the differences between the rapid and slow phases? Is there a bi-directional axoplasmic flow as suggested by Lubińska (1964)?

Material and Methods

More than 100 pigeons, Columba livia, were used in this study. They were injected in the right eye with an aqueous solution of ^{3}H-l-leucine and sacrificed at different times after injection, ranging from 15 min up to 3 months. One series was used for subcellular fractionation and biochemical detection of radioactivity in the retinae, optic tracts and optic lobes; a second series was used for light microscopic autoradiographic studies of the optic pathways. In each case the injected dose was 30 μCi. Seven animals were used for electron microscopic autoradiographic studies. In these experiments, the injected dose was 500 μCi. Detailed descriptions of the technical procedures and references will be found elsewhere (Cuénod and Schonbach, 1970; Schonbach and Cuénod, 1970; Schonbach et al., 1971).

Results and Comments

1. *Is there a Rapid Phase of Axoplasmic Flow?* Or, are the diverse reports of rapidly migrating molecules misinterpretations of a local synthetic process linked to extra-ocular diffusion of the labelled compound? Our data are summarized in Fig. 1, 2, 3, and 4, showing the temporal evolution of the left-right differences of the protein specific activities in the optic pathways and the optic lobe sub-cellular fractions, and of the left-right differences of the grain counts over chiasma and tectal layers (classification of Cajal, 1911).

It can be seen that subcellular fractions of the layer 1 (containing retino-tectal axons), the layer 5 (rich in retino-tectal terminals), and the optic lobe showed more label then the contralateral controls as soon as 2 to 3 h after injection. The difference was maximum at about 12 hto 1 day after injection.

The early presence of radioactive proteins far from the retina in regions known to be connected with it, was not in itself proof of fast axoplasmic transport. The radioactivity of the control side could be attributed to local labelling by blood-borne leucine because of the complete crossing of the optic nerves. In the same way, significant diffusion of tritiated leucine in the extracellular space of the experimental side was ruled out by the observation, at all times after injection, of identical counts over experimental and control layers 8 and 14 which do not contain any element coming from the retina (Schonbach and Cuénod, 1970). Furthermore the acid-soluble radioactivity was always the same on both sides, which eliminated a possible intra-axonal diffusion of the precursor (Cuénod and Schonbach, 1970). Thus, it was highly probable that we were observing an intra-axonal migration of proteins synthesized in the ganglion cell perikarya. Incorporation of the precursor into the retinal proteins was found to be at maximum very soon after injection, between 30 min and 4 h, being located in the ganglion cells (Cuénod and Schonbach, 1971; Schonbach and Cuénod, 1971). The labelling of the ganglion cells decreased thereafter. Electron microscopic autoradiographs

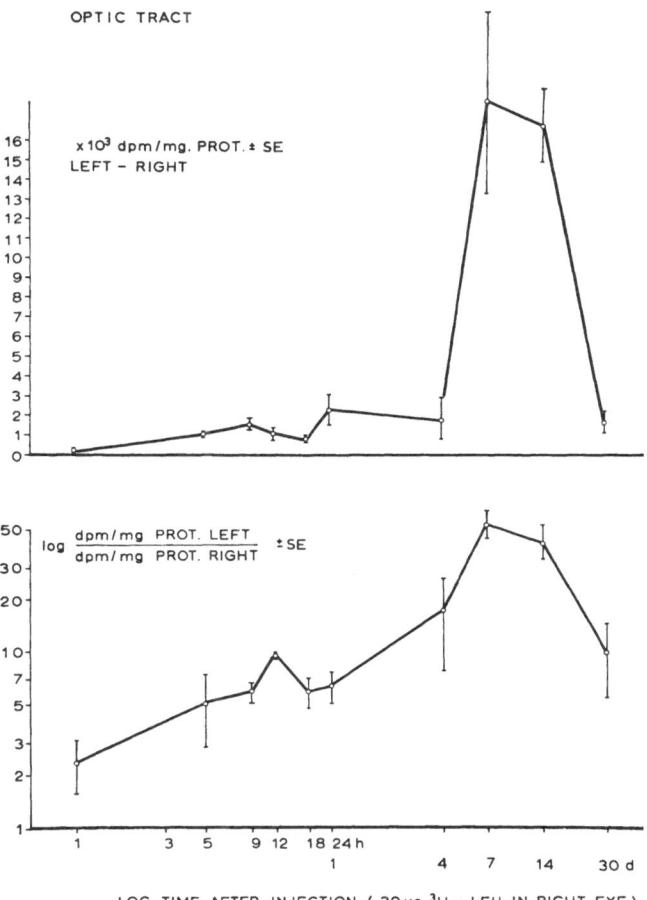

Fig. 1. Temporal evolution of the specific activity of the proteins in the optic tracts after injection of 30 µCi of ³H-l-leucine in the right eye. Upper curve: left-right, lower curve, left/right. Time in log

of the tectal layer 1, 12 h after injection, confirmed that the newly-synthesized protein were located intra-axonally. Seventy per cent of the grains were observed over the axons (Schonbach *et al.*, 1971).

2. *What is the Destination of the Fast Flow, and which Cellular Components are Involved?*

Biochemical and autoradiographic techniques showed (Fig. 2 and 4) that the synaptosomes and the tectal layer 5 were the most labelled structures in the optic lobe during the early period following precursor injection. The localization of the newly-synthesized proteins in axon terminals was confirmed by electron microscopic autoradiographs of the tectal layer 5 and 12 h after injection. Sixty-seven per cent of the grains were detected over synaptic endings (Fig. 8), although

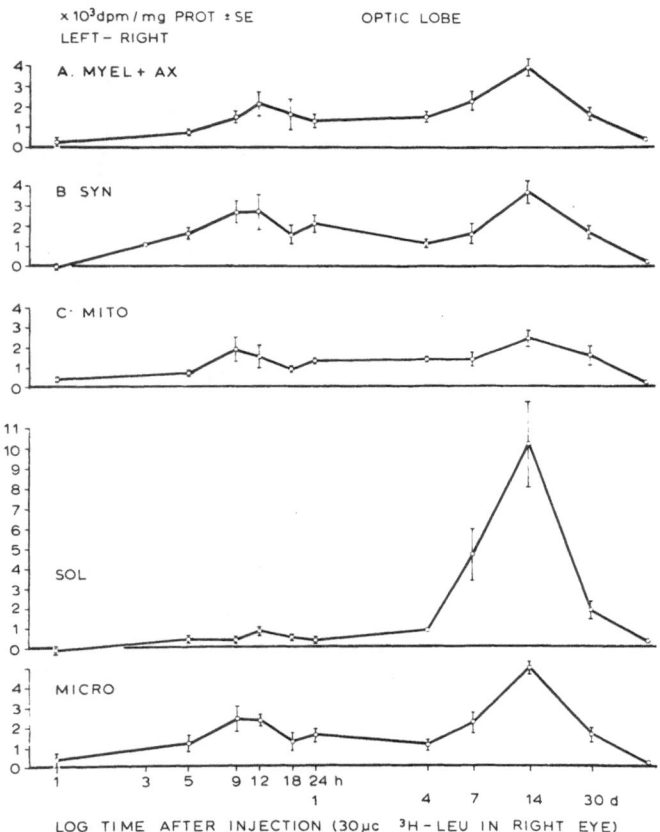

Fig. 2. Temporal evolution of the difference of the specific activity of the proteins between left and right tectal subcellular fractions, after injection of 30 µCi of ³H-l-leucine in the right eye. Time in log

the axon terminals occupied only 15 to 25% of the total area examined in tectal layer 5 (Schonbach et al., 1971). We also attempted to determine which synaptic elements were labelled. Although the resolution of the technique did not allow direct determination of the precise origin of the radiations, we could indirectly observe that the grain distribution over the endings was compatible with a labelling of the synaptic mitochondria and vesicles, but not of the outer-membranes.

The grain distribution over the axons of layer 1 was also studied to see if specific axonal components were labelled. Any labelling of the neurofilaments was dismissed at this stage. However axonal grains were often associated with elements of agranular endoplasmic reticulum (Fig. 7) and their localization was also compatible with a labelling of the axolemma.

We concluded that a majority of the rapidly migrating newly-synthesized proteins were probably destined to renew components of the synaptic endings.

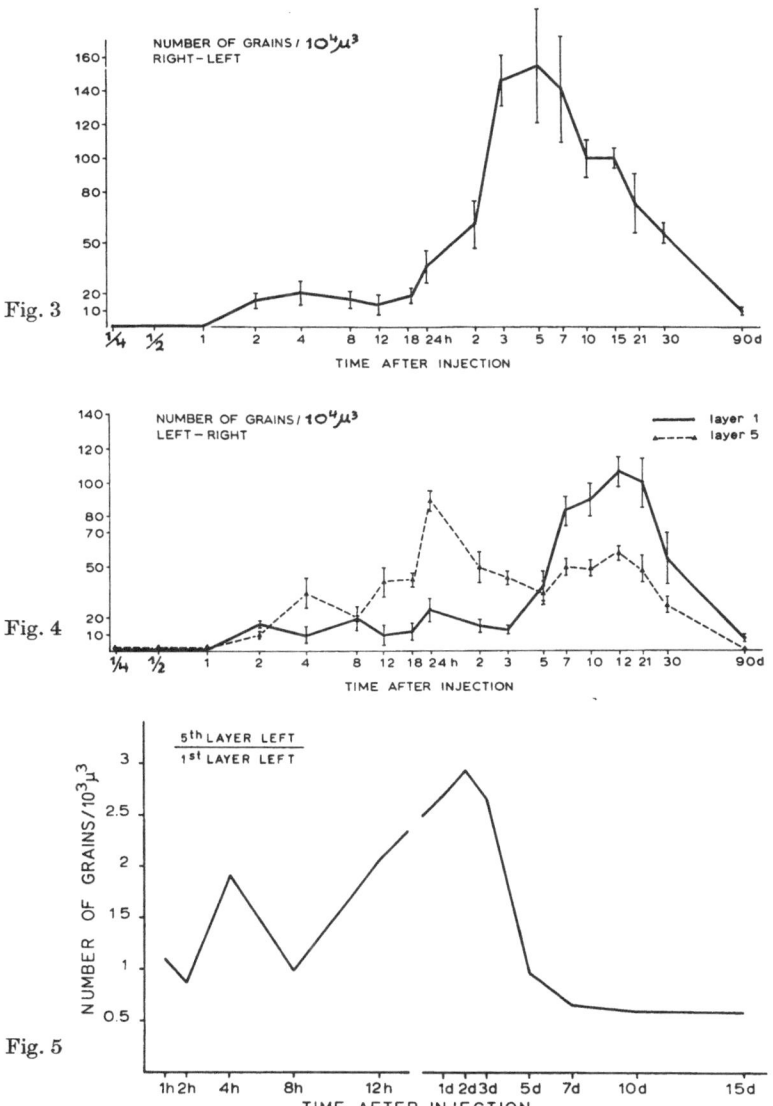

Fig. 3

Fig. 4

Fig. 5

Fig. 3. Temporal evolution of the difference of the grain counts between right and left sides over the optic chiasma, after injection of 30 µCi of ^{3}H-l-leucine in the right eye ($\pm$ SD). Time in log

Fig. 4. Temporal evolution of the difference of the grain counts between left and right tectal layers 1 and 5 after injection of 30 µCi of ^{3}H-l-leucine in right eye. ($\pm$ SD). Time in log

Fig. 5. Temporal evolution of the ratio between the grain counts over left tectal layers 5 and 1, after injection of 30 µCi of ^{3}H-l-leucine in the right eye

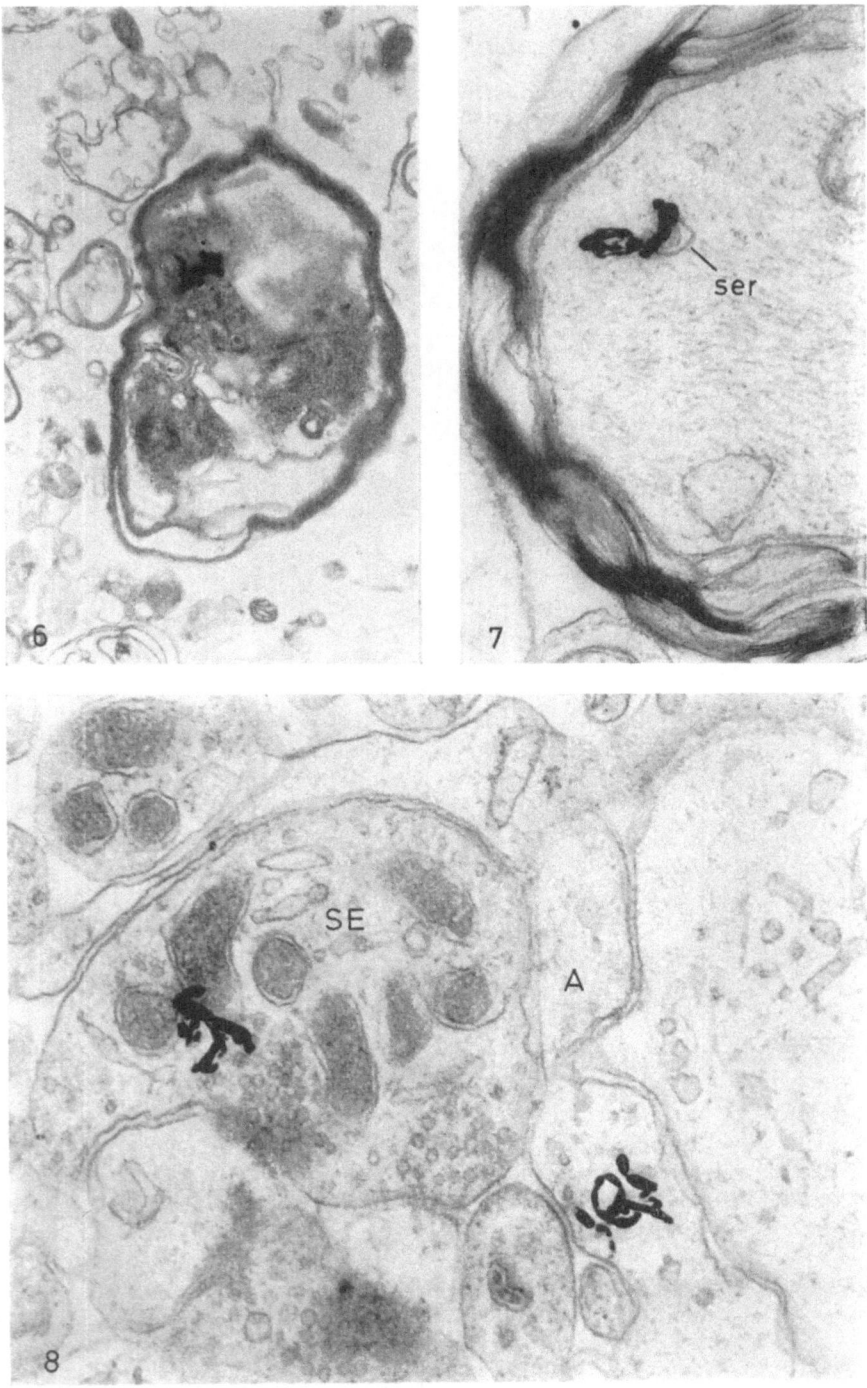

Figs. 6—8

3. *Is the Rapid Phase of Axoplasmic Flow a Homogenous Entirely?*

As we noticed large discrepancies in the literature between the reported speeds of rapid intra-axonal migration, we tried to determine if any observations in our study would speak in favor of a pluri-phasic phenomenon.

The biochemical and autoradiographic approaches gave indirect evidence that the rapid phase may be subdivided into two separate components. It was found that the left/right ratio of the protein specific activities of the optic lobe synaptosomal fractions was lower at 9 hours after injection than at 6 and 12 hours after injection (Cuénod and Schonbach, 1971). The left/right ratio of the grain counts over tectal layer 5 was also lower at 8 h than at 4 and 12 h. Another argument was given by the autoradiographic data on the repartition of the radioactivity among the tectal layers. This is summarized in Fig. 5 which shows the evolution of the grain count ratio between experimental layers 5 and 1. The two peaks observed at 4 and 24 h after injection, might be interpretated as the translocation of two separate populations of molecules. The first one would migrate at a rate of 100—500 mm/day and the second at a rate of 20—60 mm/day. Although our data are not conclusive, the possible subdivision of the rapid phase of axoplasmic flow must be kept in mind.

4. *What are the Differences between the two Phases of Axonal Flow?*

The two phases could be differentiated by their speed of migration, the rapid phase advancing at a rate of 20—500 mm/day, and the slow phase at a rate of 1—2 mm/day.

There was also a conspicuous quantitative difference between the two phases: the specific activity of the proteins was seven times higher during the late period in the optic tract than at the first day after injection, and the grain counts were also much higher over chiasma and layer 1 during the slow phase.

The repartition of the radioactivity among the subcellular fractions also differed between the two phases: synaptosomal, axonal, mitochondrial and microsomal fractions were the main labelled elements in the early phase; soluble and microsomal fractions in the late phase. Our data indicated that the slow phase of axoplasmic flow may reach the synaptic ending. However it was evident that the slowly migrating proteins were mainly destined to renew axonal material, and that only a small portion reached the terminals.

5. *Is there a Bidirectional Axoplasmic Flow?*

To test this hypothesis, we took advantage of the presence in the avian retina of centrifugal fibers (Cowan and Powell, 1963) whose origin is located in the

Fig. 6. E. M. autoradiograph of the subcellular fraction A (myelin) of the left optic lobe, 12 h after injection of 500 μCi of ^{3}H-l-leucine in the right eye. Two grains are localized over the protoplasm of an axonal fragment. ×6000

Fig. 7. E. M. autoradiograph of an axon in the left tectal layer 1, 12 h after injection of 500 μCi of ^{3}H-l-leucine in the right eye. A grain is localized over a profile of axoplasmic smooth-surfaced endoplasmic reticulum (ser). ×18,000

Fig. 8. E. M. autoradiograph of left tectal layer 5, 12 h after injection of 100 μCi of ^{3}H-l-leucine in the right eye. A grain is localized over a synaptic ending (SE), another one is localized over an axonal profile. ×18000

isthmo-optic nucleus. A preferential labelling of this nucleus was searched for
with light microscopic autoradiography.

The grain concentrations were always similar on the experimental and control
sides, and never higher than the physiological background dependant on blood-
borne leucine. However as the synthetic capacity of the terminals is low, our
observation does not dismiss completely the hypothesis of a backward flow.

General Comments

Time course studies based on the detection of labelled proteins after injection
of the radioactive precursor in the vicinity of the neuronal perikaryon, allowed
us to analyse the origin and the fate of the newly-synthesized molecules. Some of
them migrated rapidly at a rate of 20—500 mm/day, and seemed to be largely
destined to renew synaptic materials, possibly components of vesicles and mitochondria. The largest portion of the migrating proteins, moved at a rate of about
1 mm/day, and was found mainly in the soluble and microsomal fractions. It was
probably destined to renew elements of the axon; however it also reached the
terminals. Some data suggested that the rapid phase of axoplasmic flow might be
subdivided into several components. We could not find any observations favoring
the hypothesis of a bidirectional axoplasmic flow.

A comparison of our data with the observations of other groups working on
different systems allowed us to formulate the following hypothesis, which, in
some regards, is similar to ideas advanced by Barondes (1966), Droz (1967) and
Grafstein (1969): the rapid phase of axoplasmic flow might involve the agranular
endoplasmic reticulum which may be considered as derived from the Golgi apparatus; this membraneous organelle, functioning as a packaging unit, would carry
newly-synthesized proteins such as enzymes to their destination in axolemma,
mitochondria and synaptic vesicles; on the other hand, the slow phase would be
composed of non-membrane bound, water soluble macromolecules forming a pool
destined to renew structural elements of the axons such as microtubules, neurofilaments and possibly the apparently ubiquitous structural proteins of plasmatic
and endoplasmatic membranes (Green et al., 1968).

Our data are also pertinent to the problem of the origin of synaptic vesicles.
The simultaneous presence of radioactivity in agranular endoplasmic reticulum
and synaptic vesicles may favor the theory of their perikaryal origin, but other
interpretations are possible as well. Furthermore it is likely that unknown local
conditions in the axon endings are necessary for the formation of the vesicles.
It is not possible to state how the proteins coming from the cell body may participate in this process.

The main axoplasmic constituents, tubules and filaments, which are probably
renewed by slowly transported proteins, have been implicated in the propelling
mechanisms. The involvement of the tubules has been conjectured on the basis
of experiments using colchicine (see other papers in this symposium). Boesch and
Cuénod in our laboratory have also shown that colchicine interferes with the rapid
phase of axoplasmic flow, without giving gross quantitative modifications of the
retinal protein synthesis. The colchicin-binding protein of mammalian brain
which is thought to be the main constituent of microtubules, is rich in acidic

amino-acids (Weisenberg *et al.*, 1968). Histochemical observations using ruthenium red (Tani and Ametani, 1970) revealed that the neurotubules are probably negatively charged at their periphery. This would create an electrostatic field which could interact with the surface charges of organelles thus generating electrokinetic forces. This could be a possible mechanism for the saltatory movements of axoplasmic organelles (Burdwood, 1965).

References

Barondes, S. H.: On the site of synthesis of the mitochondrial proteins of nerve endings. J. Neurochem. **13**, 721—727 (1966).

Burdwood, W. O.: Rapid bidirectional particle movement in neurons. J. Cell Biol. **27**, 115 A (1965).

Cajal, S. Ramon y: Histologie du système nerveux, Vol. II, p. 197, Reimpres. 1955 Instituto Ramon y Cajal, Madrid 1911.

Cowan, W. M., Adamson, L., Powell, T. P. S.: An experimental study of the avian visual system. J. Anat. (Lond.) **95**, 545—563 (1961).

— Powell, T. P. S.: Centrifugal fibres in the avian visual system. Proc. roy. Soc. B **158**, 232—252 (1963).

Cuénod, M., Schonbach, J.: Synaptic proteins and axonal flow in the pigeon visual pathway. J. Neurochem. (in print) (1971).

Droz, B.: Synthèse et transfert des protéines cellulaires dans les neurones ganglionnaires. Etude radioautographique quantitative en microscopie électronique. J. Microscopie **6**, 201—228 (1967).

Grafstein, B.: Transport of protein by goldfish optic nerve fibers. Science **157**, 196—198 (1967).

— Axonal transport: communication between soma and synapse. Advanc. Biochem. Psychopharm. **1**, 11—25 (1969).

Green, D. E., Haard, N. F., Lenaz, G., Silman, H. I.: On the non-catalytic proteins of membrane systems. Proc. nat. Acad. Sci. (Wash.) **60**, 227—284 (1968).

Jahn, T. L., Bovee, E. C.: Protoplasmic movements within cells. Physiol. Rev. **49**, 793—862 (1969).

Lubińska, L.: Axoplasmic streaming in regenerating and in normal nerve fibres. Progr. Brain Res. **13**, 1—71 (1964).

Schonbach, J., Cuénod, M.: Axoplasmic migration of proteins in the avian visual system. An autoradiographic study. Exp. Brain Res. (in print) (1971).

— Schonbach, Ch., Cuénod, M.: Rapid phase of axoplasmic flow and synaptic proteins. An electron microscopical autoradiographic study. J. comp. Neurol. **141**, 485—488 (1971).

Tani, E., Ametani, T.: Substructure of microtubules in brain nerve cells as revealed by ruthenium red. J. Cell Biol. **46**, 159—165 (1970).

Taylor, A. C., Weiss, P.: Demonstration of axonal flow by the movement of tritium-labeled protein in mature optic nerve fibers. Proc. nat. Acad. Sci. (Wash.) **54**, 1521—1572 (1965).

Weisenberg, R. C., Borisy, G. G., Taylor, E. W.: The colchicine-binding protein of mammalian brain and its relation to microtubules. Biochemistry **7**, 4466—4479 (1968).

Dr. Jacques Schonbach
Pharmakologisches Institut der Universität
Gloriastraße 32
CH-8006 Zürich, Schweiz

Acta neuropath. (Berl.) Suppl. V, 162—170 (1971)

Different Modes of Substance Flow in the Optic Tract *

HINRICH RAHMANN

Zoologisches Institut der Universität, Münster. i. W., Germany

Summary. Investigations of the modes of transport of different labelled substances in the optic tract of vertebrates following intra-ocular application of the substances were reported. Nerve cells of the optic system are capable of selecting those substances which are
a) conveyed by intra-axonal flow after their uptake and incorporation into macromolecular compounds (proteins, small amounts of RNA, serotonine; chlorpromazine),
b) conveyed by extra-axonal flow to the site of their utilization (glucose, palmitic acid, methamphetamine), and
c) not conveyed at all, but are retained at the site of injection (amino acids, noradrenaline, trypan blue, diaminoacridine).

Key-Words: Axonal Transport — Radioactivity — Protein — Amines, Biogenic.

Introduction

Inspired by the investigations of Taylor and Weiss in 1965, the optic tract of vertebrates has been used frequently as a model for the analysis of neuronal transport phenomena. The simple structure of the optic system of lower vertebrates, in particular of teleosts, is especially suitable for such investigations, because there is a complete crossing of both nerves in the optic chiasm. The optic nerves and the chiasm are separated by a relatively thick pia mater and an avascular arachnoid from the neighboring tissue, but the area of contact between the two optic nerves in the chiasm and the site of their entry into the brain are deficient of leptomeninges (Polyak, 1957). These anatomical features render the optic system particularly suitable for investigations of both intra-axonal and extra-axonal transport phenomena. Also, new prospects are opened concerning the nerve cell's ability to select the substances to be taken up.

Based on our findings, I like to give a survey of investigations on neuronal transport mechanisms in the optic system up to the time of this symposium.

Material and Methods

Animals. Our investigations were made on *Carassius carassius*, a close relative of C. auratus, which has been used by Grafstein (1967) in her studies.

Tracers. The following tritium labelled compounds were used: ^{3}H-histidine and ^{3}H-uridine as precursors of proteins, or RNA respectively, ^{3}H-glucose to label polysaccharides and ^{3}H-palmitic acid to label lipids. ^{3}H-methamphetamine and ^{35}S-chlorpromazine were the psychotropic drugs used; trypanblue and acridine orange served as colour tracers. To bypass the blood-stream, these substances were injected into the eye with a glass capillary.

Processing of the Optic Tracts. 8 h to 51 days after the application of the tracers, the fish were decapitated. Their eyes, optic nerves and brains were put into the fixatives required for the preservation of proteins, RNA (Bouin's solution), lipids (formalin), or carbohydrates (Gendre). Tissue of animals treated with psychotropic drugs was frozen in liquid nitrogen and

* Supported by the Deutsche Forschungsgemeinschaft.

cut in a cryostate. Fixation of all other tissues was followed by paraplast embedding. Sections were cut 10 µm thick; to prove a specific labelling of the various macromolecular compounds, adjacent sections were treated with protease, RNase, diastase, pyridine or TCA before being subjected to the autoradiographic process.

Autoradiography. Autoradiographs were prepared using Agfa-dipping emulsion Nuc 7.15. Displacement of water-soluble compounds was avoided by using cryostate sections. The autoradiographs were exposed for 21 to 70 days. Grains counts were made in retina, optic nerve, chiasm, and optic tectum.

Scintillation Counting. In addition to autoradiographic investigations, the total radioactivity of the tissue and that of tissue fractions was determined by liquid scintillation counting. The optic tract was cut into 4 pieces, which were weighed, treated with TCA and dissolved by immersion in soluene (Packard). Counts were obtained using a Packard scintillation spectrometer (model 3320).

Results

1. Intra-axonal Flow of Substances

The intra-axonal flow of substances, postulated by Weiss and coworkers (Weiss and Hiscoe, 1948) was demonstrated clearly in experiments using injection of labelled protein precursors into the eye.

For example, after the unilateral, intra-ocular application of ^{3}H-histidine (Rahmann, 1967, 1968a), autoradiographic studies of the optic system of Carassius revealed a flow of labelled proteins in the injected visual system only (Fig. 1a and b) The flow could be followed over a distance of more than 1 cm. This technique also permitted the exact identification of primary visual pathways in the optic tectum.

Intra-axonal flow of proteins has been described, up to this symposium, in optic tracts of mammals, amphibians, and fish (Tab. 1). Different speeds of transport were found to exist, as was observed for peripheral nerves as well. Moreover,

Table 1. *Intra-axonal flow of substances in the tractus opticus of vertebrates*

Compound	Animal	Rate of transport	Authors
Protein	Mice	1 mm/day	Taylor and Weiss (1965)
Protein	Rabbit	1.5 resp. 110—150 mm/day	Karlsson and Sjöstrand (1968) Sjöstrand and Karlsson (1969)
Protein	*Carassius au.*	0.4 resp. >40 mm/day	Grafstein (1967), McEwen and Grafstein (1968)
Protein	*Carassius car.*	1—3 resp. 5 mm/day	Rahmann (1967, 1968a)
Protein	Bullfrog	10—22 mm/day	Goldberg and Koiani (1967)
RNA	*Carassius car.*	1—2 mm/day	Rahmann and Wolburg (1971)
RNA	Rat	—	Casola et al. (1968)
RNA	Rat	—	Peterson et al. (1968)
Serotonine	Rat	—	O'Steen and Vaughan (1968)
Chlorpromazine	*Carassius car.*	1—2 mm/day	Rösner (1971)

Sjöstrand and Karlsson (1969) showed that the specific radioactivity of the high-speed protein component (110—150 mm/day) is linked mainly to the structural proteins of the microsomal fraction, whereas most of the radioactivity of slow-transport components (1.5—2 mm/day) is in soluble proteins.

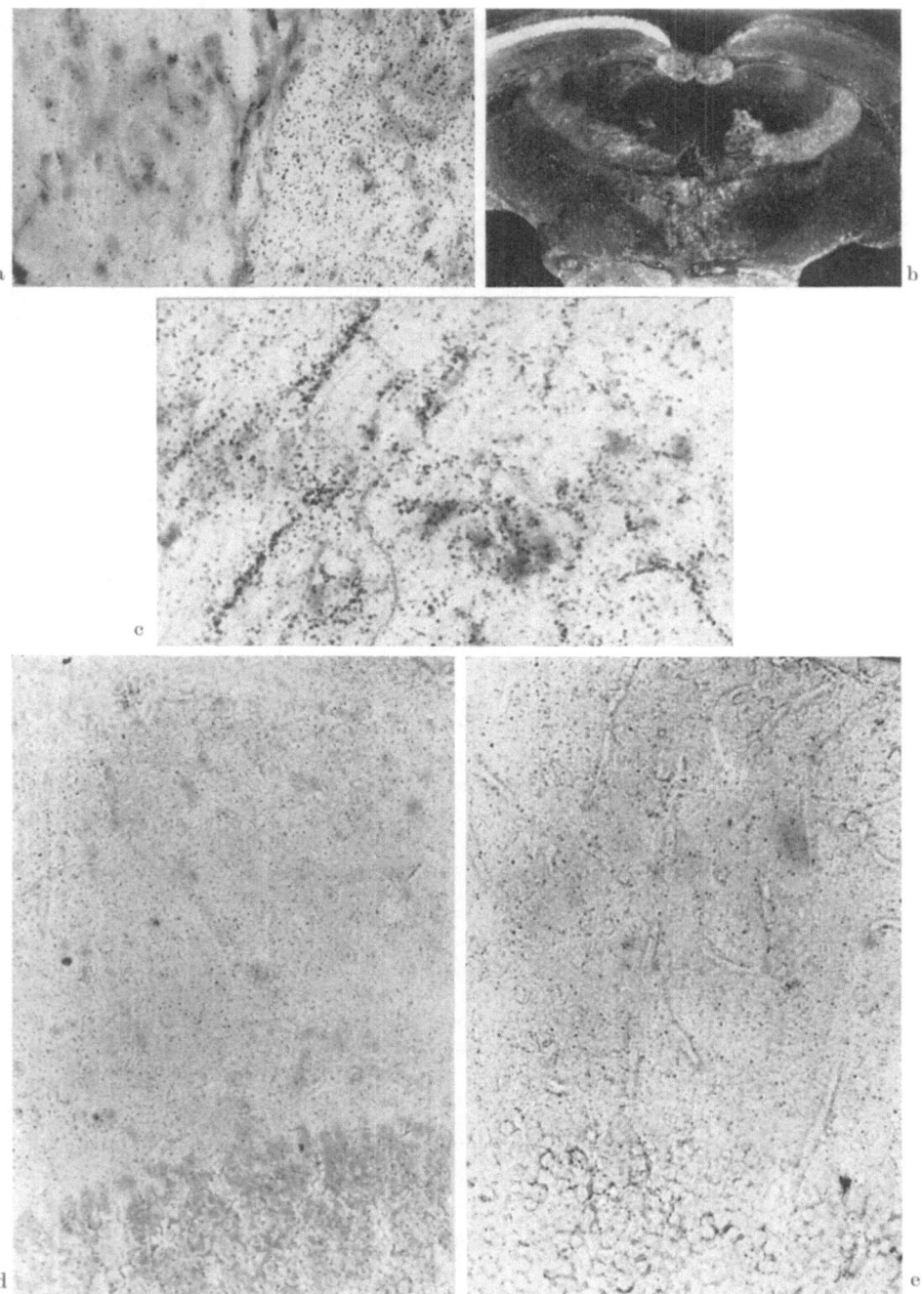

Fig. 1 a—e. Autoradiographs showing the distribution of labelled proteins and lipids, respectively, in different sections of the optic tract of *Carassius*, following unilateral intra-ocular application of ³H-histidine and ³H-palmitic acid. a and b intra-axonal flow of labelled proteins,
limited to the injected system; a chiasm (high power photograph); b low power photograph
of mesencephalon and optic tectum, with visual layers at the upper left;   c—e extra-axonal
flow of ³H-palmitic acid in the injected as well as in the system originally not injected;
   c chiasm;   d and e ipsilateral and contralateral optic tectum showing uniform labelling

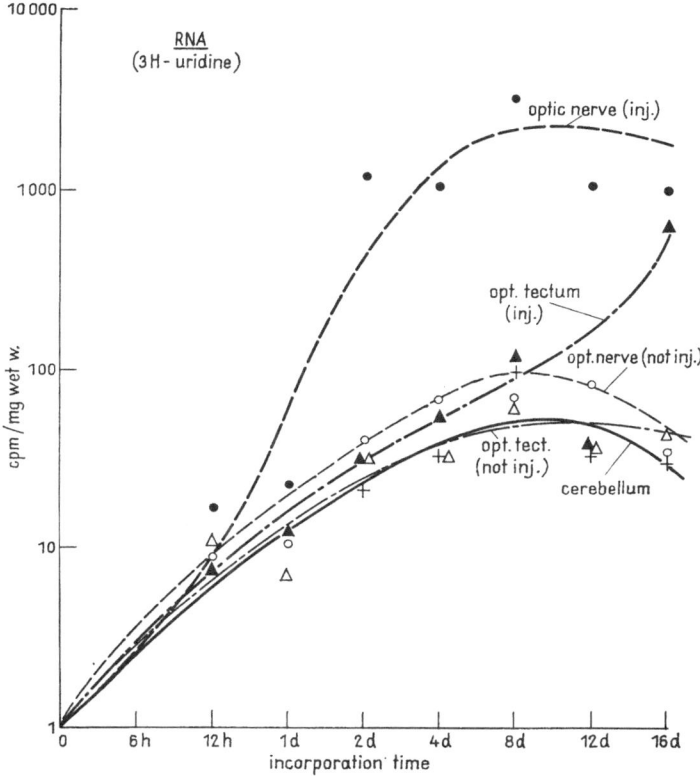

Fig. 2. Labelling (cpm/mg wet weight) following unilateral, intra-ocular application of ³H-uridine in section of the optic nerve between eyeball and chiasm, in optic tectum and in cerebellum of *Carassius*, after 6 h to 16 days. Increase in labelling (following TCA-treatment) limited to structures belonging to the injected eye indicates intra-axonal flow of RNA

Thus, the available data show that upon intra-ocular application amino acids are rapidly incorporated into proteins by the perikarya of the retinal cells; it is in the form of proteins only that they are conveyed within the axon. To a certain degree, the behavior of RNA-precursors appears to be similar (Peterson *et al.*, 1968; Casola *et al.*, 1969; Rahmann and Wolburg, 1971): Following unilateral intra-ocular injection of ³H-uridine, a slow increase of RNase-sensitive, TCA-resistant labelling was observed in the injected optic tract of *Carassius* by auto-radiographic and biochemical techniques (Fig. 2 and 3). These experiments revealed that the portion of the optic nerve next to the eyeball was labelled after 2 days; after a delay of 16 days a substantial increase in radioactivity could be detected in the contralateral hemisphere of the tectum, indicating a speed of transport of 1—2 mm/day. The labelling of the corresponding portions of the non-injected system as well as that of the cerebellum was only slight, resulting from a distribution of the isotopes by the blood stream.

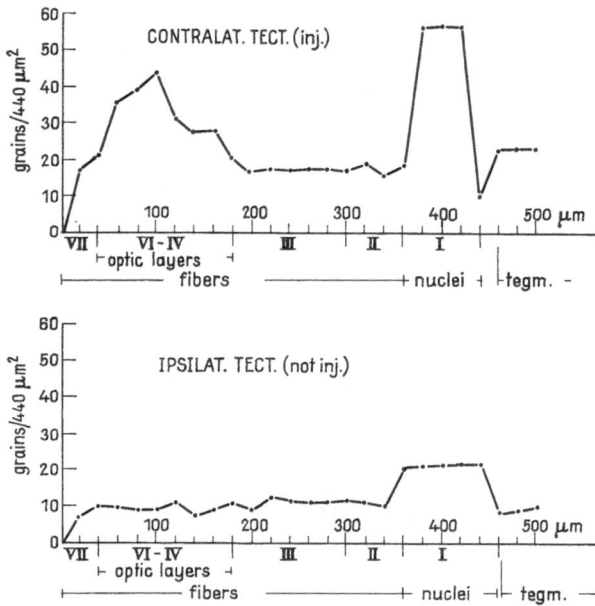

Fig. 3. Labelling (grain counts in autoradiographs) of optic layers limited to contralateral tectum 12 days after unilateral, intra-ocular application of ³H-uridine indicating intra-axonal flow of RNA

At present one cannot decide whether this flow of macromolecular uridine components represents a flow of free RNA or of RNA in neuronal mitochondria, which are also known to migrate by axonal flow (Nakai, 1956, 1964; Weiss and Pillai, 1965). To answer this question, we initiated experiments with acetoxycyclo-heximide and ethidium bromide, two agents known to inhibit specifically the synthesis of cytoplasmic or mitochondrial RNA, respectively (Wolburg, in prep.).

In addition to the intra-axonal flow of proteins and small amounts of RNA, an intra-axonal transport of ³⁵S-chlorpromazine could also be demonstrated in the optic tract of teleosts by my coworker Rösner (1970a). Biochemical methods indicated, however, that the drug appeared to be adsorbed to proteins transported at a rate of 1—2 mm/day.

The experiments of O'Steen and Vaughan (1968), who injected 5-HTP into the eye, do not permit a definite conclusion as to whether this substance itself is transported within the axon or whether it has to be converted to serotonine first.

2. Extra-Axonal Flow of Substances

Apart from the intra-axonal flow reported above, we were particularly interest-ed in the possibility of an extra-axonal flow of substances in the optic tract. Following unilateral, intra-ocular application of various compounds we were able to demonstrate in Carassius that certain compounds are not only taken up by the retinal layer to be used as precursors of macromolecular compounds, but appear to be transported also by the extra-cellular fluid of the optic tract. Upon arrival at the chiasm they invade the extra-cellular spaces of the non-injected system. Thus, the label is not confined to the terminations of the optic fibers, as for labelled proteins; instead, all layers of both hemispheres of the optic tectum and the tegmentum are labelled.

To illustrate these findings, Fig. 1 c—d shows incorporation of ^{3}H-palmitic-acid in different portions of the optic tract 4 days after unilateral intra-ocular application of the tracer (Rahmann, 1970a). Similar distribution patterns were found after injection of ^{3}H-glucose (Rahmann, 1968b) and methamphetamine (Rösner, 1970b) (Tab. 2). Thus it was established that various compounds travel by extra-axonal flow at a speed of more than 40 mm/day to the site of their utilization. In

Table 2. *Extra-axonal flow of substances in the tractus opticus of vertebrates*

Compound	Animal	Rate of transport	Author
Glucose	*Carassius car.*	>40 mm/day	Rahmann (1968b)
Palmitic acid	*Carassius car.*	>40 mm/day	Rahmann (1970)
Methamphet- amine	*Carassius car.*	>40 mm/day	Rösner (1970)

this way ^{3}H-palmitic acid is conveyed to the site of synthesis, which takes place throughout the whole length of the nerve cells, whereas ^{3}H-glucose is mainly conveyed to the nerve fiber terminals, where it is used to synthesize glycogen (see Rahmann, 1970b).

As mentioned before, a certain amount of ^{3}H-uridine injected into the eyeball is incorporated into macromolecular RNA which is conveyed within the axon. In addition, a flow of TCA-soluble, ^{3}H-uridine-labelled compounds was demonstrated in the optic tract (Rahmann and Wolburg, 1971). Soon after the unilateral, intra-ocular injection of ^{3}H-uridine, the labelling of RNA plus TCA-soluble compounds was as intense in the ipsilateral hemisphere of the tectum as it was in the contralateral hemisphere. The total amount of radioactivity in either hemisphere was distinctly higher than the degree of labelling in the cerebellum, caused by distribution of the tracer through the blood. Labelling of the portion of the optic nerve next to the injected eyeball was substantially higher than that of the corresponding section next to the non-injected eye. These results suggest an extra-axonal flow of soluble ^{3}H-uridine compounds. However, they were obtained by comparing the labelling of the section of the optic tract next to the eyeball only with the labelling of the tectum. Therefore, further investigations with special regard to the pretectal sections are required to show, whether or not an extra-axonal flow of ^{3}H-uridine really exists.

The extra-axonal transport in the optic tract may be compared with transport in the endoneuronal spaces of peripheral nerves, as demonstrated for various low molecular compounds by Weiss *et al.* (1945).

Table 3. *No flow of substances in the optic tract of vertebrates*

Compound	Animal	Author
Amino Acids	*Carassius aur.*	McEwen and Grafstein (1968)
Noradrenaline	*Carassius aur.*	McEwen and Grafstein (1968)
Diaminoacridine	Mammals	Rodriguez-Peralta (1966)
Trypan blue	*Carassius car.*	Rahmann (1968a)

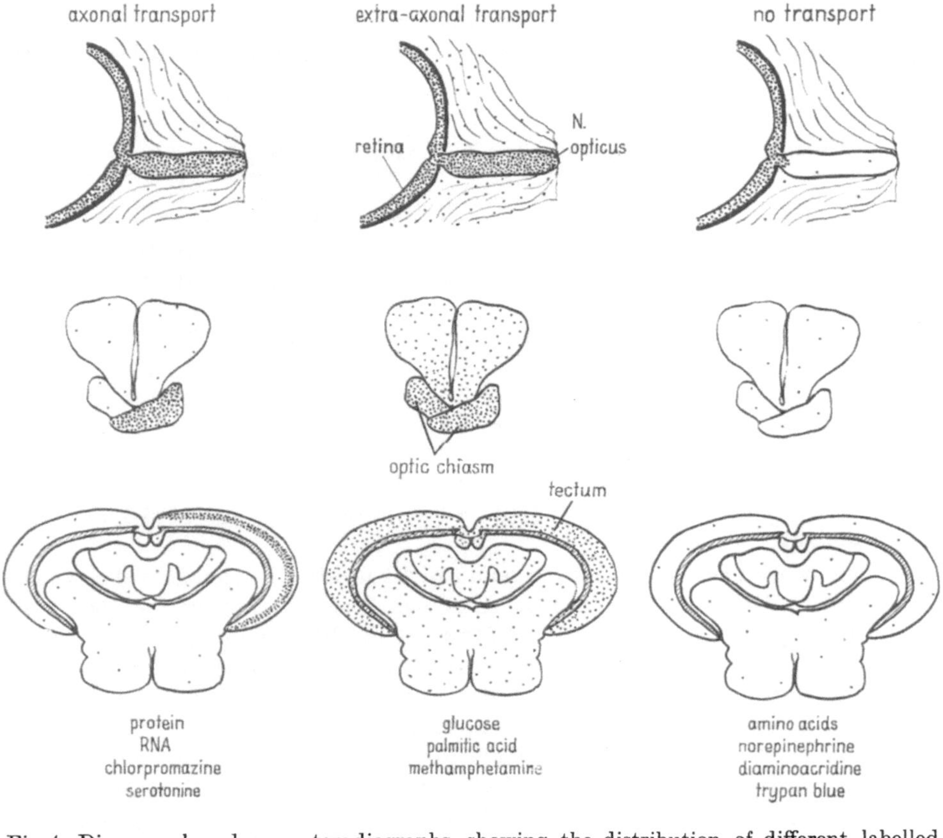

Fig. 4. Diagram, based on autoradiographs, showing the distribution of different labelled compounds following unilateral, intra-ocular application

3. Substances Showing no Redistribution

Apart from substances conveyed either by intra-axonal or by extra-axonal flow in the optic tract of vertebrates, there are other compounds not conveyed after intra-ocular application (Tab. 3). For instance, McEwen and Grafstein (1968) reported, that free amino acids (leucine or cycloleucine), injected into the eye, do not arrive in the contra-lateral hemisphere of the tectum. Neither is ³H-noradrenaline transported by the cholinergic optic nerve. Moreover, it was shown that macromolecular foreign compounds, such as trypan blue (Rahmann, 1968a) or diaminoacridine (Rodriguez-Peralta, 1966) are not transported in the optic nerve.

Discussion

The results of these experiments (Fig. 4) show that the nerve cell possesses a quite sensitive capacity for selecting compounds for uptake. The selection mechanism is apparently located in the cell membranes of the perikarya. There the decision is made which compounds are to be taken up by the cell body to be utilized *in situ*; which compounds are to be conveyed by extra-axonal flow to the site of their utilization; and which compounds are not to be used at all. The mechanism by which this selection is achieved is unknown. Apparently the uptake or rejection of the various compounds depends not only on molecular size or electrical charge. It seems more likely, that various mechanisms of active transport are present in the membranes of the perikaryon and fibers.

In my opinion, the experiments demonstrate, how suitable a model the optic nerve of lower vertebrates is for the investigation of the selection mechanisms available to the nerve cell. Further investigations are urgently required.

References

Casola, L., Davis, G. A., Davis, R. E.: Evidence for RNA in rat optic nerve. J. Neurochem. **16**, 1037—1041 (1969).

Goldberg, S., Koiani, M.: zit. in McEwen, B. S., and B. Grafstein (1968).

Grafstein, B.: Transport of protein by goldfish optic nerve fibers. Science **157**, 196—198 (1967).

Karlsson, J. O., Sjöstrand, J.: zit. in J. Sjöstrand, and J. O. Karlsson (1969).

McEwen, B. S., Grafstein, B.: Fast and slow components in axonal transport of protein. J. Cell Biol. **38**, 494—508 (1968).

Nakai, J.: Dissociated dorsal root ganglia in tissue culture. Amer. J. Anat. **99**, 81—129 (1956).

— The movement of neurons in tissue culture. In: R. D. Allen and N. Kamiya (eds.). Primitive motile systems in cell biology. New York: 1964.

O'Steen, W. K., Vaughan, G. M.: Radioactivity in the optic pathway of the rat after intraocular injection of tritiated 5-hydroxy-tryptophan. Brain Res. 8, 209—212 (1968).

Peterson, J. A., Bray, J. J., Austin, L.: An autoradiographic study of the flow of protein and RNA along peripheral nerve. J. Neurochem. **15**, 741—745 (1968).

Polyak, S.: The vertebrate visual system, ed. by H. Klüver. Chicago: Univ. Press 1957.

Rahmann, H.: Darstellung des intra-neuronalen Proteintransports vom Auge in das Tectum opticum und die Cerebrospinalflüssigkeit von Teleostiern nach intra-ocularer Injektion von ³H-Histidin. Naturwissenschaften **54**, 174—175 (1967).

— Sytheseort und Ferntransport von Proteinen im Fischhirn. Z. Zellforsch. **86**, 214—237 (1968a).

— Transportweg von ³H-Glucose und Syntheseort von Polysacchariden im Zentralnervensystem von Teleosteern. Exp. Brain Res. **6**, 32—48 (1968b).

— Transport von ³H-Palminsäure im ZNS von Teleosteern. Z. Zellforsch. **110**, 444—456 (1970a).

— Entstehungsorte und Verbleib von Syntheseprodukten im Zentralnervensystem von Vertebraten. Zool. Anz. Suppl. **33**, 430—460 (1970b).

— Wolburg, H.: Intra-axonaler Transport von ³H-Uridin-Verbindungen im Tractus opticus von Teleosteern. Experientia (Basel), (im Druck) (1971).

Rodriguez-Peralta, L. A.: Hematic and fluid barriers in the optic nerve. J. comp. Neurol. **126**, 109—122 (1966).

Rösner, H.: Untersuchungen zur Wirkung von Chlorpromazin im ZNS von Teleosteern II. — Aufnahme und Verteilung von 35S-Chlorpromazin sowie Bindung an Neuroplasmakomponenten. Neuropharmacology (im Druck), (1971).
— Radioaktive Tracerstudien zum Einbau und zur Wirkungsweise von Methamphetamin und Chlorpromazin im ZNS von Teleosteern. Dissertation, Univ. Münster 1970.
Sjöstrand, J., Karlsson, J. O.: Axoplasmic transport in the optic nerve and tract of the rabbit: a biochemical and radioautographic study. J. Neurochem. 16, 833—844 (1969).
Taylor, A. C., Weiss, P.: Demonstration of axonal flow by the movement of tritium-labelled protein in mature optic nerve fibers. Proc. nat. Acad. Sci. (Wash.) 54, 1521—1527 (1965).
Weiss, P., Hiscoe, H. B.: Experiments on the mechanism of nerve growth. J. exp. Zool. 107, 315—395 (1948).
— Pillai, A.: Convection and fate of mitochondria in nerve fibers. Axonal flow as vehicle. Proc. nat. Acad. Sci. (Wash.) 54, 48—56 (1965).
— Wang, H., Taylor, A. C., Edds, Mac V., Jr.: Proximo-distal fluid convection in the endoneurial spaces of peripheral nerves, demonstrated by colored and radioactive (isotope) tracers. Amer. J. Physiol. 143, 521—540 (1945).

Prof. Dr. Hinrich Rahmann
Zoologisches Institut der Universität
BRD-4400 Münster i. W.
Hindenburgplatz 55
Deutschland

Acta neuropath. (Berl.) Suppl. V, 171—178 (1971)

A Symmetrical Double-Label Method
for Studying the Rapid Axonal Transport of Radioactivity
from Labelled D-Glucosamine in the Goldfish Visual System

David S. Forman

The Rockefeller University, New York, U.S.A.

Summary. After radioactive D-glucosamine is injected into the eye of the goldfish, labelled macromolecules are axonally transported to the optic tectum. These labeled macromolecules, presumably glycoproteins, move mainly in the rapid component of axonal transport. Labelled chloroform-methanol extractable and acid-soluble materials are also transported. After subcellular fractionation by differential centrifugation, the labelled transported macromolecules are found in particulate fractions, while the acid-soluble transported radioactivity is concentrated in the high-speed supernatant. A symmetrical double-labelling technique is described which is useful in studies of axonal transport with precursors like glucosamine that produce significant background labelling.

Key-Words: Axonal Transport — Radioactivity — Glucosamine.

Introduction

The biosynthesis of glycoproteins has been studied in many laboratories, but there has been little consideration of the role which axonal transport may play in glycoprotein metabolism in the neuron. Dr. Bernice Grafstein of the Cornell University Medical College, Dr. Bruce McEwen of the Rockefeller University, and I have examined this question in the visual system of the goldfish, which has proved to be convenient for studies of axonal transport (Grafstein, 1967; McEwen and Grafstein, 1968; Elam et al., 1970; Elam and Agranoff, 1971. See also B. Grafstein, H. Rahmann, and L. di Giamberardino, these proceedings). Our findings have been reported in detail elsewhere (Forman et al., 1971) and will therefore only be summarized here.

D-glucosamine is a useful precursor for studies of glycoprotein synthesis. Glucosamine is converted to N-acetylglucosamine, N-acetylgalactosamine, and sialic acids (Davidson, 1969) which are incorporated into the carbohydrate moieties of glycoproteins and glycolipids (Roseman, 1968; Barondes, 1968; Ginsburg and Neufeld, 1969). When labeled glucosamine is injected into the goldfish eye, radioactivity is transported to the optic tectum. More than half of the transported radioactivity is in macromolecules which are precipitated by trichloroacetic acid (TCA), and remain in the TCA precipitate after extraction with chloroform-methanol, 1:1. Unlike the results of similar experiments with labelled amino acids, TCA-soluble and chloroform-methanol extractable radioactivity are also transported. The transported materials labelled by glucosamine move in the rapid component of axonal transport. Whereas most of the transported radioactivity in amino-acid-labelled proteins moves in the slow component of axonal transport (McEwen and

Grafstein, 1968), little or none of the radioactivity from glucosamine can be found moving with the slowly transported proteins. The transported labeled macro-molecules also resemble rapidly transported proteins in being mainly particulate; only a few per cent of the transported glucosamine label is incorporated into soluble protein. Inhibition of protein synthesis in the retina with the drug acetoxy-cycloheximide prevents the appearance of labelled macromolecules in the tectum. Both axonal transport and local synthesis (Barondes, 1968; Barondes and Dutton, 1969) may have roles in nerve ending glycoprotein metabolism.

The chemical nature of the transported materials must be determined before their significance can be evaluated. Research is now in progress on the chemical analysis of each of these components. The transported, labelled macromolecules are apparently glycoproteins. Some of this glycoprotein may be the sulfated muco-polysaccharide proteins which are rapidly transported in the goldfish visual system (Elam et al., 1970). The labelling of chloroform-methanol extractable materials is not surprising, since glucosamine would be expected to label ganglio-sides (Burton et al., 1963). The TCA-soluble transported radioactivity presumably represents small molecules.

The chemical analysis of these materials is hampered by the relatively high level of "background" labelling. After an injection of isotope into the right eye, axonally transported radioactivity moves through the right optic nerve (which crosses at the chiasma to become the left optic tract) to the left optic tectum, where the retinal ganglion cell axons terminate. However, some isotope also leaves the eye and is carried in the blood stream to the brain where it is locally incorporated in both tecta. It is therefore necessary to subtract the "background" level of radioactivity measured in the right tectum, which is due only to local incorporation, from the level in the left tectum (which contains both transported and locally incorporated radioactivity) in order to calculate the amount of radio-activity which has been transported. When labelled glucosamine is the injected isotope, the background of radioactivity which arrives via the bloodstream is usually a significant fraction of the total radioactivity in the left tectum (for typical values, see Table 2). Nevertheless, in simple experiments it is easy to reliably measure the amount of transported radioactivity as the difference between the tecta. In experiments with many steps, the possibility increases that un-controllable experimental factors such as unequal recoveries could introduce differences between samples from the left and right tecta, producing invalid estimates of transported radioactivity. This problem is most acute in continuous systems such as density gradients, gel electrophoresis, etc., where the collection of perfectly corresponding fractions cannot be assured. A similar problem arises in examining optic tracts, which are so small that the dissection of symmetrical samples for comparison is difficult. These problems are not unique to transported radioactivity from glucosamine, but apply as well, for example, to transported proteins labeled with radioactive leucine.

One approach to the calculation of transported radioactivity in the presence of background labelling is to use symmetrical double-labeling. In the experiments described below I injected ^{3}H-glucosamine into the right eye, and ^{14}C-glucosamine into the left eye of the same fish. Transported ^{3}H is then calculated as left minus right, while transported ^{14}C is calculated as right minus left. If the results from

both isotopes agree closely, once can have confidence that spurious differences
have not been introduced, and that the calculations of transport are valid.

Methods

Six large (8—12 cm) pond-raised goldfish *(Carassius auratus)* were used in each experiment.
They received a 5 μL. injection of D-glucosamine-6-³H (1160m Ci/mMole, New England Nuclear
Corp.) in the right eye and of D-glucosamine-1-¹⁴C (52 mCi/mMole, New England Nuclear
Corp.) in the left eye 24 h before sacrifice. For the measurement of radioactivity in whole
tecta and tracts (Table 2), the tissues were immersed overnight in cold 10⁰/₀ trichloroacetic
acid containing 1 mM glucosamine to precipitate labelled macromolecules, and the precipiᵗates
were extracted with chloroform-methanol (1:1, v/v) to remove lipids. The lipid-free precipitates
were dried, weighed, and dissolved in Soluene-100 (Packard Instrument Corp.) for scintillation
counting in a toluene scintillator. TCA-soluble radioactivity was measured in Bray's scintillator (Bray, 1960). These methods are described in detail elsewhere (Forman *et al.*, 1971).

In the cell fractionation experiments, pooled tecta or tracts from the left or right sides
were gently homogenized in 1.4 ml of 0.32 M sucrose using a Dounce homogenizer (Kontes
Glass Co.). After samples were taken for scintillation counting and protein determination,
1.0 ml of the homogenate was centrifuged in a Lourdes Model A-2 "Betafuge" at $1100 \times g_{av}$
for 10 min. The pellet was resuspended in 1.0 ml 0.32 M sucrose and spun again at $1100 \times g_{av}$
to give a pellet which is designated the "N" fraction. The combined supernatants were spunat
$16,000 \times g_{av}$ for 20 min to give a pellet ("P_2") and a supernatant which was in turn sedimented
at $110,000 \times g_{av}$ for 120 min in a Spinco Model 40 rotor in a Spinco Model L Ultracentrifuge.
The final pellet is designated the M fraction, and the supernatant is the "S" fraction. The
temperature was 0—4° C throughout the fractionation. The pellets were suspended in distilled
water, and macromolecules in samples of the fractions were precipitated with 10⁰/₀ TCA containing 1 mM D-glucosamine. The TCA precipitates were dissolved in Soluene-100 for scintillation counting or in 0.5 N NaOH for protein analysis by the method of Lowry *et al.* (1951). The
TCA supernatants were extracted three times with diethyl ether to remove the TCA, concentrated by evaporation, and counted in Bray's scintillator (Bray, 1960). Efficiency of counting
was measured by the Packard Automatic External Standard, and calculations of ³H and ¹⁴C
disintegrations per minute were made using a computer program written by Dr. Brian Poole
of the Rockefeller University (Packard Program Library No. 09672). Note that in the cell
fractionation experiments, the lipid was not removed from the TCA precipitate, which therefore includes labeled lipids as well as macromolecules.

Results

The results of the differential centrifugation experiments are presented in
Fig. 1 and Table 1. For both tracts and tecta, transported ³H is calculated as the
concentration of radioactivity (dpm/mg protein) of the left side minus the value
of the right side, while transported ¹⁴C is calculated as right minus left. In order to
compare the results obtained with ³H and ¹⁴C glucosamine, the radioactivities
have been converted to relative values by dividing the concentration of radioactivity in each fraction by the concentration in the homogenate. In the tecta,
the three particulate fractions (N, P_2, and M) have about the same concentration
of transported TCA-precipitable radioactivity as the homogenate (Fig. 1). There
is some enrichment of the label in the M fraction. However, the greatest proportion
of transported radioactivity is found in the fraction with the most protein, the P_2
fraction (Table 1).

The concentration of transported radioactivity in the soluble macromolecules
(S fraction) is very low, and represents only a few per cent of the total transported
radioactivity. On the other hand, the concentration of the transported TCA-

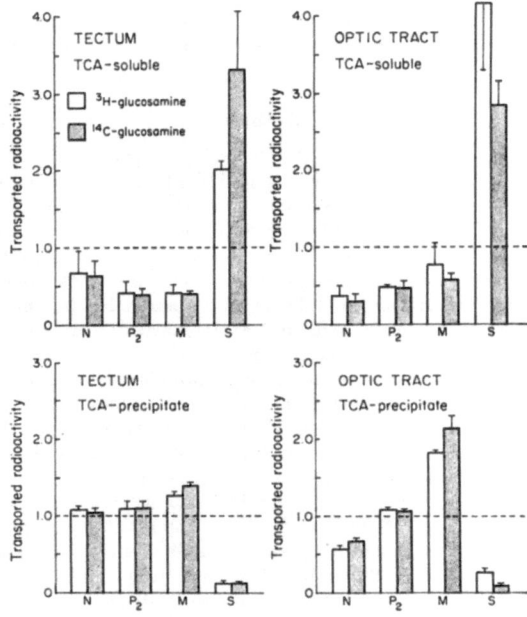

Fig. 1. Subcellular distribution of TCA-precipitable and TCA-soluble transported radioactivity in the optic tracts and tecta 24 h after the injection of radioactive glucosamine. D-Glucosamine-6-³H was injected into the right eye, and D-glucosamine-1-¹⁴C was injected into the left eye of the same fish. The concentration of transported radioactivity (dpm/mg protein) in each fraction has been divided by the concentration of transported radioactivity in the homogenate. N: "crude nuclear" fraction, P₂: "crude mitochondrial" fraction (mitochondria, synaptosomes, myelin fragments), M: microsomes, S: supernatant. Each value is the average of three experiments. Lines above the bars represent standard errors. Lipids were not extracted from the TCA precipitates

soluble radioactivity is high in the S fraction, and about two-thirds of the transported acid-soluble material is found in this fraction. The particulate fractions all have lower concentrations of transported TCA-soluble radioactivity than the homogenate.

A similar pattern is found in the tracts. TCA-soluble transported radioactivity in the tracts is found mainly in the S fraction, where this radioactivity has been considerably enriched. As in the tecta, the S fraction contains little TCA-precipitable transported radioactivity. However, in the tracts there is greater enrichment than in the tecta of transported incorporated radioactivity in the M fraction, which contains almost half of the transported TCA-precipitable radioactivity but less than a quarter of the total protein. The proportion of the total transported radioactivity which is TCA-soluble is higher in the tracts than in the tecta. This difference can also be seen in Table 2, which compares the TCA-soluble, chloroform-methanol extractable, and TCA-precipitable radioactivity found in tecta and optic tracts 24 h after glucosamine injections.

Table 1. *Distribution of recovered radioactivity and protein in subcellular fractions*

Per cent recovered in fraction	N (%)	P_2 (%)	M (%)	S (%)
Tecta				
Protein	17 ± 1	40 ± 0.4	20 ± 0.4	23 ± 1
Transported TCA-precipitable radioactivity	19 ± 1	50 ± 1	28 ± 2	3 ± 0.2
Background TCA-precipitable radioactivity	13 ± 1	42 ± 2	31 ± 1	13 ± 1
Transported TCA-soluble radioactivity	11 ± 2	17 ± 2	9 ± 2	64 ± 3
Background TCA-soluble radioactivity	9 ± 2	25 ± 2	15 ± 1	50 ± 3
Optic Tracts				
Protein	24 ± 2	30 ± 1	22 ± 1	24 ± 1
Transported TCA-precipitable radioactivity	15 ± 1	34 ± 2	47 ± 2	5 ± 1
Background TCA-precipitable radioactivity	14 ± 2	21 ± 3	26 ± 3	37 ± 3
Transported TCA-soluble radioactivity	7 ± 1	16 ± 1	11 ± 1	68 ± 1
Background TCA-soluble radioactivity	16 ± 3	17 ± 2	18 ± 2	54 ± 4

D-Glucosamine-6-^{3}H was injected into the right eye, and D-glucosamine-1-^{14}C was injected into the left eye 24 h before sacrifice. The values for ^{3}H and ^{14}C did not differ significantly, and they have been averaged together. "Background" radioactivity refers to radioactivity on the right side for ^{3}H and on the left side for [14]C. N: "crude nuclear" fraction, P_2: "crude mitochondrial" fraction (mitochondria, synaptosomes, myelin fragments), M: microsomes, S: supernatant. Values are the averages of three experiments $\pm$ standard errors. Average recoveries of protein and radioactivities range from $92-101\%$. The amount of protein in the 1.0 ml of tectum homogenate which was fractionated averaged 3.25 ± 0.06 mg, while in the case of the tracts the average was 0.38 ± 0.06 mg

Discussion

The cell fractionation experiments reported here confirm the particulate nature of the transported TCA-precipitable radioactivity, and the low level of labeling in soluble macromolecules (Forman *et al.*, 1971). It will be necessary to characterize the fractions biochemically and morphologically before any conclusions can be drawn about the subcellular location of this material. The enrichment of transported TCA-precipitable radioactivity in the M fraction of the optic tracts is reminiscent of the enrichment of rapidly transported amino acid-labeled proteins in microsomal fractions from nerves which has been observed by several authors (Ochs *et al.*, 1967; Kidwai and Ochs, 1969; Sjöstrand and Karlsson, 1969; D. Forman, unpublished results). However, the subcellular particles in which the label is concentrated have not yet been identified. Synaptic vesicles, smooth endoplasmic reticulum, and plasma membrane fragments are reasonable candidates. Preliminary experiments in which P_2 and M fractions from tecta or optic tract were subfractionated on continuous or discontinuous sucrose gradients have shown that very little of the transported radioactivity is associated with myelin (D. Forman, unpublished results). The enrichment of the transported TCA-soluble radioactivity in the S fraction might indicate that the TCA-soluble component is present in the cytoplasm rather than being packaged inside of membranous organelles.

D. S. Forman:

Table 2. *Distribution of radioactivity in optic tracts and tecta*

	^{3}H				^{14}C			
	Transported Radioactivity (L-R)		Background Radioactivity (R)		Transported Radioactivity (R-L)		Background Radioactivity (L)	
	dpm/mg	%	dpm/mg	%	dpm/mg	%	dpm/mg	%
Tecta—data from intact tecta								
P[a]	1638	59	722	44	489	64	334	44
L[b]	682	25	206	13	186	24	83	11
S[c]	446	16	694	43	89	12	338	45
Tecta—data from homogenized tecta								
P + L[d]	—	83	—	62	—	87	—	61
S	—	17	—	38	—	13	—	39
Optic Tracts—data from intact tracts								
P	1782	33	467	21	594	27	152	27
L	952	18	96	4	252	11	30	5
S	2592	49	1628	74	1364	62	392	68
Optic Tracts—data from homogenized tracts								
P + L	—	50	—	31	—	41	—	42
S	—	50	—	69	—	59	—	58

[a] = TCA precipitate after lipid extraction
[b] = Lipid (chloroform-methanol extract)
[c] = TCA-soluble
[d] = TCA precipitate, lipids not extracted

Distribution of radioactivity in optic tracts and tecta. Six large pond fish received 5 µl injections of 1 µCi D-glucosamine-6-^{3}H in the right eye and 0.4 µCi D-glucosamine-1-^{14}C in the left eye. They were sacrificed 24 h later, and the tissues processed as described under Methods. Values for homogenized tracts and tecta are from the homogenates of the cell fractionation experiments. Since different amounts of isotope were injected in each fractionation experiment, only the average per cent distribution of radioactivity is presented.

These experiments demonstrate that symmetrical double-labelling is a feasible approach for measuring axonally transported radioactivity in the presence of significant background labelling. The agreement between the results obtained with ^{3}H-glucosamine and ^{14}C-glucosamine in these experiments provides an internal control against the possibility that differences between the left and right samples arising during the fractionation have produced invalid calculations of transported radioactivity. In most of the data presented here the numerical values obtained with ^{3}H- and ^{14}C-glucosamine are very close. In the cases where the numbers diverge (e.g. the TCA-soluble radioactivity of the optic tracts), the two isotopes still illustrate similar quantitative relationships between the various chemical and subcellular fractions. It is important to note that where ^{3}H and ^{14}C label the same molecule in different positions, as is the case here, one may expect similar results with both isotopes when the precursor molecule is incorporated into macromolecules with little alteration, but the results could be quite different if the precursor is extensively metabolized. The agreement between the results for D-glucosamine-1-^{14}C and D-glucosamine-6-^{3}H are consistent with the hypothesis that the label has been incorporated into macromolecules (and possibly glycolipids) as N-acetylhexosamine or sialic acid. If a large fraction of the injected glucosamine has been converted to glucose and then to its metabolites, more divergent results would be expected.

Symmetrical double-labelling has the obvious advantage of producing twice as much data per experiment as experiments with one isotope. This benefit is somewhat offset by the additional difficulties in counting and calculation of radioactivity. Symmetrical double-labelling can also be used to compare transported and background labelling in the same tissue in cases where calculation of the amount of transported radioactivity is either unnecessary or impossible. For instance, one can use this technique with density gradients, chromatography, etc., to determine whether the patterns of transported and background labelling are similar or distinctly different without quantifying the amount of transported radioactivity. While the methods described here are useful for dealing with background labelling, it would clearly be preferable, if possible, to work with a background so low that it could be ignored. For instance, Elam and Agranoff (1971) have demonstrated that ^{3}H-proline labels transported proteins with background labelling so low as to be negligible. However, in the absence of such unusually favorable precursors or other means of suppressing background incorporation, symmetrical double-labelling provides a powerful method for studying axonally transported radioactivity in the presence of significant background labelling. Using this method, it will now be possible to study the chemical nature of the radioactivity which is axonally transported in the goldfish visual system after the injection of labelled D-glucosamine.

Bibliography

Barondes, S. H.: Incorporation of radioactive glucosamine into macromolecules at nerve endings. J. Neurochem. 15, 699—706 (1968).
— Dutton, G. R.: Acetoxycycloheximide effect on synthesis and metabolism of glucosamine-containing macromolecules in brain and in nerve endings. J. Neurobiol. 1, 99—110 (1969).
Bray, G. A.: A simple efficient liquid scintillator for counting aqueous solutions in a liquid scintillation counter. Analyt. Chem. 1, 279—285 (1960).
Burton, R. M., Garcia-Bunuel, L., Golden, M., Balfour, Y. McB.: Incorporation of radioactivity of D-glucosamine-1-C^{14}, D-glucose-1-C^{14}, D-galactose-1-C^{14}, and DL-serine-3-C^{14} into rat brain glycolipids. Biochemistry 2, 580—585 (1963).
Elam, J., Agranoff, B. W.: Rapid transport of protein in the optic system of the goldfish. J. Neurochem. 18, 375—387 (1971).
— Goldberg, J. M., Radin, N. S., Agranoff, B. W.: Rapid axonal transport of sulfated mucopolysaccharide proteins. Science 170, 458—460 (1970).
Davidson, E. A.: Metabolism of amino sugars. In: The Amino Sugars, Vol. II B, pp. 1—44. E. A. Jeanloz and R. W. Balazs, Eds. New York: Academic Press 1966.
Forman, D. S., McEwen, B. S., Grafstein, B.: Rapid transport of radioactivity in goldfish optic nerve following injections of labeled glucosamine. Brain Res. 28, 119—130 (1971).
Ginsburg, V., Neufeld, E. F.: Complex heterosaccharides of animals. Ann. Rev. Biochem. 38, 371—388 (1969).

Grafstein, B.: Transport of protein by goldfish optic nerve fibers. Science **157**, 196—198 (1967).
— Axonal transport: Communication between soma and synapse. Advances in Biochemical Psychopharmacology, Vol. I, pp. 11—25. E. Costa and P. Greengard, Eds. New York: Raven Press 1969.
Kidwai, A. M., Ochs, S.: Components of fast and slow phases of axoplasmic flow. J. Neurochem. **16**, 1105—1112 (1969).
Lowry, O. H., Rosebrough, N. J., Farr, A. L., Randall, R. J.: Protein measurement with the Folin phenol reagent. J. Biol. Chem. **193**, 265—275 (1951).
McEwen, B. S., Grafstein, B.: Fast and slow components in axonal transport of protein. J. Cell Biol. **38**, 494—508 (1968).
Ochs, S., Johnson, J., Ng, M.-H.: Protein incorporation and axoplasmic flow in motoneuron fibres following intra-cord injection of labelled leucine. J. Neurochem. **14**, 317—331 (1967).
Roseman, S.: Biosynthesis of glycoproteins, gangliosides, and related substances. Biochemistry of Glycoproteins and Related Substances, pp. 244—269. E. Rossi and E. Stoll, Eds. New York: S. Karger 1968.
Sjöstrand, J., and Karlsson, J.-O.: Axoplasmic transport in the optic nerve and tract of the rabbit: A biochemical and radioautographic study. J. Neurochem. **16**, 833—844 (1969).
Zatz, M., Barondes, S. H.: Rapid transport of fucosyl glycoproteins to nerve endings in mouse. J. Neurochem. (in press) (1971).

David S. Forman
The Rockefeller University
New York, N. Y. 10021
U.S.A.

Acta neuropath. (Berl.) Suppl. V, 179—186 (1971)
© by Springer-Verlag 1971

Single Cell Isotope Injection Technique, a Tool for Studying Axonal and Dendritic Transport

Peter Schubert, Hans D. Lux, and Georg W. Kreutzberg

Max-Planck-Institut für Psychiatrie, München, BRD

Summary. Radioactive precursors (amino acids and choline) were applied to cat spinal motoneurons by means of micro pipette electrophoresis. The amount injected was determined by the iontophoresis current used. Simultaneous recording of the electrical properties of the nerve cells allowed their identification and the control of the site and effect of injection. At different times after injection (4 min to 3 days) the cats were sacrified by formalin perfusion and autoradiographs were prepared from serial sections of the paraplast embedded spinal cord. This technique provides a high concentration of strictly intracellular radioactivity which is advantageous for the study of intracellular transport. The results indicate that proteins most probably synthetized within the nerve cell soma are transported within the dendrites nearly up to their terminals at a rate of at least 3 mm/h and within the axon at different rates of 0.5 and 1.7 mm/h. Following antidromic stimulation the synthesis of proteins within the nerve cell soma and their export into the axon was increased. Choline derivatives thought to be mainly phospholipids were also transported into dendrites and axon.

Key-Words: Axonal Flow — Dendritic Transport — Intracellular Iontophoresis — Autoradiography — Cat Spinal Motoneurons.

The use of radiochemicals for the demonstration of fluid convection in nerves introduced by P. Weiss *et al.* (1945) and H. Waelsch (1958) has turned out to be the most valuable tool for studying axonal flow (Weiss and Hiscoe, 1948). Since the pioneer experiments the techniques for demonstration of radioactive material have improved considerably (e.g., Droz and Leblond, 1963; Miani, 1963; Taylor and Weiss, 1965; Ochs *et al.*, 1967; Weiss and Holland, 1967; Barondes, 1968; Young and Droz, 1968). Autoradiography and liquid scintillation spectrography were instrumental in producing an impressive collection of data on axonal transport.

To learn more about intracellular transport in the neuron a new technique has been developed in our laboratories by combining single cell injection with simultaneous electrophysiological recording and subsequent demonstration of the radioactive material by autoradiography (Globus *et al.*, 1968). This technique was found useful for the investigation of the transport of proteins from the nerve cell soma to dendrites (1) and down the axon (2), to investigate this transport under various conditions (3), and to obtain some information about the distribution of other substances significant for neuronal function (4).

Methods

Three barreled glass electrodes with a tip of about 1μ were used. Two of the barrels contained the radioactive material within two glass capillaries (see Fig. 1). The substances used were: ^{3}H-glycine (spec. act. 2.3 C/mM), ^{3}H-histidine, (19 C/mM), ^{3}H-proline (1.2 C/mM) and ^{3}H-choline (15 C/mM). Commercial stock solutions (5 mC/5 ml, Radiochemical Centre

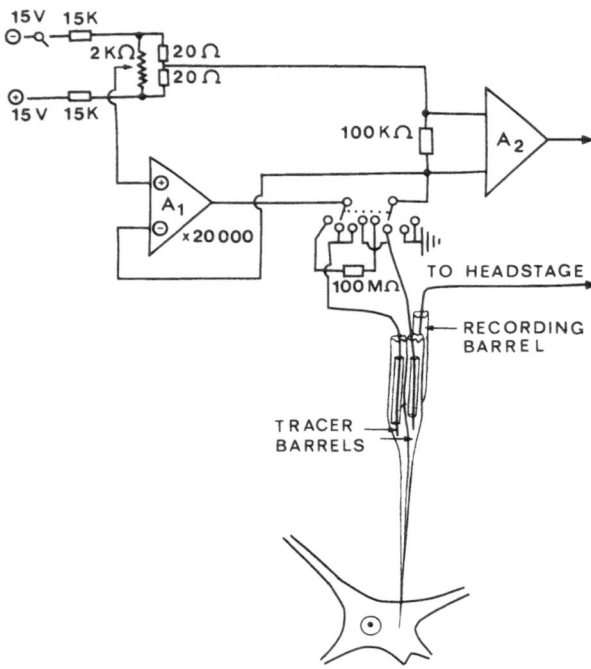

Fig. 1. Block diagram of the single cell injection technique. The three barreled electrode is inserted into the soma of a motoneuron. The recording electrode barrel is connected over an electrometer stage to an oscilloscope. Iontophoresis current in the range of 10^{-7} to 10^{-8} A is generated by a battery operating floating amplifier configuration providing a controlled current source. The current proportional feed back signal across the 100 kΩ resistor was amplified by a FET-differential amplifier which provided the necessary power for a panel meter or an oscilloscope display. The device permitted direct current measuring with an accuracy of about 5%. Current adjustment was linear for electrode resistances less than 200 MΩ. The current could be switched as cross barrel current or from either barrel to ground (across the membrane)

Amersham) were dried by means of a nitrogen stream and dissolved in 15 µl of equimolar acetic acid or potassium hydroxide. These solutions guaranteed a high concentration of charged radiochemicals necessary for the iontophoretic application as demonstrated in Fig. 1.

Cat spinal motoneurons were studied. Under Nembutal anaesthesia, flaxedil, and unilateral pneumothorax the spinal cord of the cat and the peripheral nerves were prepared for orthodromic and antidromic stimulation. The recording electrode served for registration of nerve cell responses. This permitted electrophysiological identification of the neurons and control of site and effect of the injection. Relocation of the cells in the autoradiographs was made possible by recording the exact stereotactic coordinates of every injected neuron (Globus et al., 1968; Lux et al., 1970a, b).

The cats were sacrificed by perfusion with buffered formalin, usually within 8 hours after intracellular injection. The surgery was done under sterile conditions in 4 cats, which were allowed to survive the injection unrestrained for 3 days with a prosthetic device replacing the spinal arcs. Three cats remained in rather satisfactory condition during this time. The spinal cord was embedded in paraplast and autoradiographs were prepared from 6 µ serial sections, after dipping into liquid emulsion (Kodak NTB 3). After an exposure time of 4 to 5 weeks the slides were developed, fixed, stained with toluidine blue, and mounted.

Results

The intracellular application of the radiochemicals was confirmed by the registration of antidromic spike potentials elicited by electrical stimulation of the ventral roots. Under stable recording conditions the site of injection was most probably the nerve cell soma. The application of ^{3}H-glycine was endured well by most of the neurons. This was indicated by the maintenance of neuronal potentials and excitability. Under these favorable conditions the autoradiographically demonstrable activity was well confined to the injected neuron (Fig. 2). It represented mainly (96%) synthetized proteins since most of the free amino acids were washed out during the autoradiographic procedure (Droz and Warshawsky, 1963; Peters and Ashley, 1967). Thus, the absence of labelling outside the nerve cells indicates that none of the unsoluble newly synthetized protein did leave the neuron. Moreover, it seems unlikely that significant amounts of the applied free glycine left the nerve cell. If free amino acid had been available outside the injected cell one should expect a labelling at least over the metabolically highly active nerve cells in the neighborhood. Therefore, if transfer of labelled material is observed this should be due to intracellular transport.

It was easy to trace the pathways of transport since the specific activity of the newly synthetized proteins was particularly high after direct intracellular injection and since the signal to noise ratio was further improved by the absence of extracellular labelling.

The results reported are derived from the study of 105 cat spinal motoneurons injected with ^{3}H-glycine. Glycine was prefered to proline (11 cells) and histidine (10 cells) since the latter substances demonstrated a tendency to leak out of the injected neurons. This caused various degrees of labelling in the surrounding neuropil and neighboring nerve- and glial cells. Otherwise, the results were similar to those of the glycine injection experiments.

Transport of Proteins from Soma to Dendrites

After the intrasomal injection of ^{3}H-glycine the dendritic tree was found to be labelled and the individual dendrites could be traced up to 1100 μ from the soma i.e. nearly up to the terminal branches (Globus et al., 1968; Lux et al., 1970 b). The radioactivity was clearly demonstrated in the dendrites (Fig. 2, 3). This provides direct evidence for the existance of somatodendritic material transport.

The possibility of labelled free amino acid being conveyed from the soma to be utilized in the peripheral dendrites has to be considered, but the capacity to synthetize proteins seems to be rather low in the dendritic periphery (Droz and Leblond, 1963; Rahmann, 1965; Droz and Koenig, 1970). More likely the dendritic labelling represents transported proteins, previously synthetized in the nerve cell soma.

A transfer of proteins from soma to dendrites was also concluded from the experiments of Droz and Leblond (1963); Rahmann (1965); Young and Droz (1968); Droz and Koenig (1970); Kramer and Sprenger (1970). After intraperitoneal injection of labelled amino acids radioactivity appeared in the neuropil with some delay compared with the early strong labelling of the nerve cell somas (Droz and Koenig, 1970).

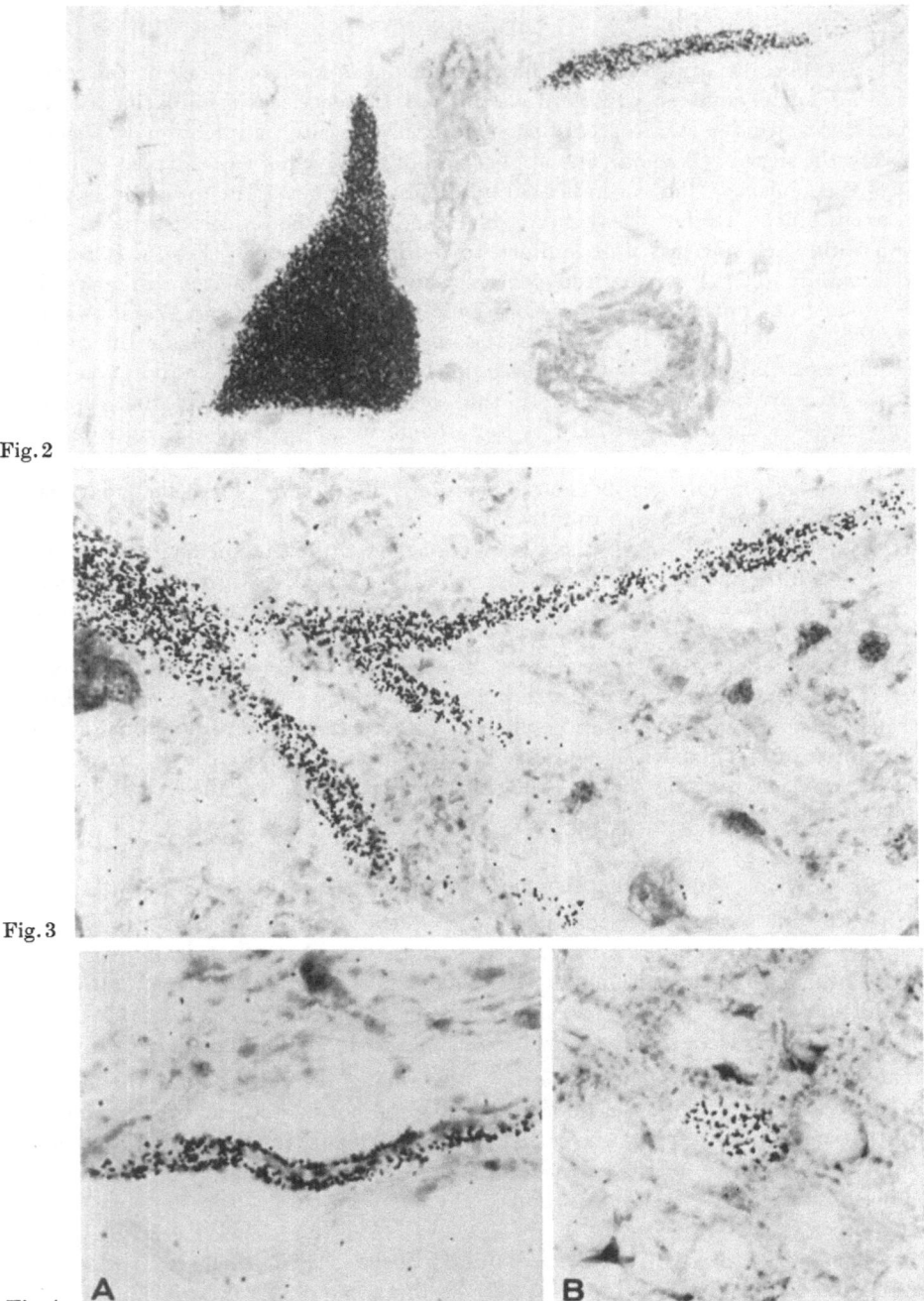

Fig. 2

Fig. 3

Fig. 4

Fig. 2. Autoradiograph of a cat spinal motoneuron injected iontophoretically with ³H-glycine 3 hours before sacrifice. The activity is confined to the soma and dendrites, no silver grains exceeding background level over the glial cells and neighboring nerve cells. Stained by tolui-dine blue, 530×

The time course of dendritic labelling suggests that a high percentage of proteins is transported at a fast rate. For an exact evaluation of the transport rates the intracellular injection technique seems to be more suitable than the intraperitoneal injection. The applied precursor is immediately available for synthesis; the time elapsed, until a sufficient amount of the precursor enters the blood stream, passes the blood brain barrier, and is taken up by the nerve cell, needs not to be taken into account.

Our calculations are based on a detailed analysis of 25 neurons of which the labelled dendritic tree was reconstructed from serial sections. Radioactivity in the dendrites could be traced up to 600 to 800 μ from the soma, if the formalin perfusion was started 15 to 20 min after intracellular injection, thus terminating the metabolism of the cells. In 3 experiments with shorter sacrifice times—i.e. when the perfusion was started 8 min after the beginning, 4 min after the end of the single cell injection, respectively—the radioactivity was demonstrated in dendrites as far as 400 μ from the soma. On the basis of these experiments the transportation rate for proteins in dendrites must be at least 3 mm/h. This is the order of magnitude of the fast transport found in axons (Ochs *et al.*, 1967; McEwen and Grafstein, 1968; Lasek, 1968; Karlsson and Sjöstrand, 1968).

In the short survival experiments a gradient of activity was evident within the labelled dendrites. The grain density decreased considerably with the distance from the soma. With time the grain density over soma and dendrites became more and more uniform which corresponds to the findings of Droz and Koenig (1970). This observation was confirmed by 3 experiments with longer survival times up to three days (Fig. 3). At this time the peripheral branches revealed nearly the same activity as the soma. This may indicate that the export of proteins previously synthetized in the soma continues for some time.

Protein Transport into Axons

Axons within the spinal cord were readily identified, in most instances, by a characteristic labelling pattern. In longitudinal sections the axons were outlined by a dense line of silver grains whereas the activity over their center was lower (Fig. 4A). This pattern distinguished axons from the dendrites in which the distribution of silver grains over their surface was more irregular (compare Fig. 3 and 4A). The individual labelled axon could be traced into the periphery in serial sections. Within the ventral roots the activity was uniformly distributed over the

Fig. 3. Radioactivity within dendrites, 3 days after intrasomal injection of ³H-glycine. At this stage, the peripheral branches reveal nearly the same grain density as the dendritic trunc. Autoradiography, stained with toluidine blue, 675×

Fig. 4A and B. Labelling of axons at different distances from the nerve cell soma. A Longitudinal section at the level of root formation within the spinal cord. The silver grains are densely packed over the surface, and more scattered over the central part. B Cross section of an axon within the ventral root, about 2.5 mm distant from the injected soma. The silver grains are uniformly distributed; no activity occurs within the myelin sheaths. The injection of ³H-glycine was performed 5 h (A) and 4 h (B) before sacrifice. Autoradiograph, stained with toluidine blue, 650×

entire axonal cross section (Fig. 4 B). The activity was confined to the axon at all levels confirming intraaxonal transport. A delivery of labelled material to the myelin sheats was not apparent.

The distribution of activity along the axon was determined by counting the number of silver grains per axonal cross section at different levels of the ventral roots (Lux et al., 1970a). Two waves of migrating proteins were found. The greater portion moved down the axon with a speed of 0.5 mm/h (S.D. 0.15 mm/h) which corresponds to the rate found by Koenig (1958) in sciatic nerves of cats. A smaller portion of the labelled proteins moved with a speed of 1.7 mm/h (S.D. 0.61 mm/h) corresponding to the data by Ochs (1966) and McEwen and Grafstein (1968).

Transport under Various Conditions

A study on the influence of efferent stimulation on synthesis and transport of proteins is presented as an example; it was reported in more detail by Lux et al. (1970a). The technique used provided an appropriate electrophysiological control of the effectiveness of stimulation and of the functional state of the neuron. The control of the intracellular iontophoresis current made it possible to apply predetermined amounts of precursor. Cells injected with the same iontophoresis current for the same time had received comparable amounts of labelled amino acids which were available for protein synthesis. A difference in the autoradiographic labelling of these cells is indicative of a different protein metabolism. It was found that effectively stimulated neurons showed increased protein synthesis compared to non stimulated control neurons. Also, the export of proteins into the axon was increased. The stimulated axons revealed a significantly higher activity over the whole length up to the distal front. No change in the speed of transport was observed.

Distribution of Choline Derivatives

Since choline is known as a precursor of the transmitter acetylcholine (Korey et al., 1951) we were interested in the distribution of the ^{3}H-choline derivatives. The intracellular injection of choline impaires the function of the neuron (Ito and Oshima, 1964). All of the 15 motoneurons studied showed a depolarization of some 10—30 mV, a reduction of spike high, or even loss of excitability during the post injection observation period of 5—15 min. The radioactivity was high in the injected pericaryon and dendrites, but not in the cell nucleus. This indicates a rather specific metabolism of the injected ^{3}H-choline of which a high percentage is probably synthetized to phospholipids (Kennedy, 1957). In contrast to the incorporated glycine, choline or its derivatives evidently left the nerve cell in greater amounts. Such leakage was found near the site of injection; also, a considerable amount of radioactive material that had been transported far into the dendrites apeared to have permeated into the neuropil. However, no obvious uptake was found by nerve cells located in the area of leakage.

The choline derivatives are also transported down the axon. Again, the radioactivity was accentuated over the axonal surface, even more pronounced than after glycine injection. Since phospholipids and proteins are important constituents of membranes this finding may reflect a substitution of structural components of the axolemma by material transported by the axonal flow. Such an exchange along the axon between transported and stationary material was also postulated by Miani (1964) and Grafstein and Murray (1969).

References

Barondes, S. H.: Further studies on the transport of protein to nerve endings. J. Neurochem. **15**, 343—350 (1968).

Droz, B., Koenig, H. L.: Localization of protein metabolism in neurons, pp. 93—106. In: A. Lajtha (ed.): Protein metabolism the of nervous system. New York-London: Plenum Press 1970.

— Leblond, C. P.: Axonal migration of proteins in the central nervous system and peripheral nerves as shown by autoradiography. J. comp. Neurol. **121**, 325—345 (1963).

— Warschawsky, H.: Reliability of the autoradiographic technique for the detection of newly synthetized protein. J. Histochem. Cytochem. **11**, 426—435 (1963).

Globus, A., Lux, H. D., Schubert, P.: Somadendritic spread of intracellularly injected glycine in cat spinal motoneurons. Brain Res. **11**, 440—445 (1968).

Grafstein, B., Murray, M.: Transport of protein in goldfish optic nerve during regeneration. Exp. Neurol. **25**, 494—508 (1969).

Ito, M., Oshima, T.: The electrogenic action of cations on cat spinal motoneurons. Proc. roy. Soc. B **161**, 92—108 (1964).

Karlsson, J. O., Sjöstrand, J.: Transport of labelled proteins in the optic nerve and tract of the rabbit. Brain Res. **11**, 431—439 (1968).

Kennedy, E. P.: Biological synthesis of phospholipids. Fed. Proc. **16**, 847 (1957).

Koenig, H.: The synthesis and peripheral flow of axoplasm. Trans. Amer. Neurol. Ass. **83**, 162—164 (1958).

Korey, S. R., De Braganza, B., Nachmansohn, D.: Choline acetylase V. Esterification and transacetylations. J. biol. Chem. **189**, 705 (1951).

Kramer, H., Sprenger, H.: Regionale Inkorporation von ^{3}H-markiertem Phenylalanin in Proteine des ZNS der Katze. Veröffentl. morph. Path. **82**, 1—55 (1970).

Lasek, R. J.: Axoplasmic transport in cat dorsal root ganglion cells as studied with ^{3}H-l-leucine. Brain Res. **7**, 360—377 (1968).

Lux, H. D., Schubert, P., Kreutzberg, G. W.: Direct matching of morphological and electrophysiological data in cat spinal motoneurones, pp. 189—198. In: P. Anderson and J. K. S. Jansen (eds.), Excitatory synaptic mechanisms. Oslo: Universitetsforlaget 1970b.

— — — Globus, A.: Excitation and axonal flow: Autoradiographic study on motoneurons intracellularly injected with ^{3}H-amino acid. Exp. Brain Res. **10**, 197—204 (1970a).

McEwen, B. S., Grafstein, B.: Fast and slow components in axonal transport of protein. J. Cell Biol. **38**, 494—508 (1968).

Miani, N.: Analysis of the somato-axonal movement of phospholipids in the vagus and hypoglossal nerves. J. Neurochem. **10**, 859—874 (1963).

— Proximo-distal movement of phospholipids in the axoplasm of the intact and regenerating neurons. In: M. Singer and J. P. Schadé (eds.): Mechanisms of neural regeneration. (Progr. Brain Res., vol. 13, pp. 115—126). Amsterdam: Elsevier 1964.

Ochs, S.: Axoplasmic flow in neurons, pp. 20—39. In: J. Gaito (ed.): Macromolecules and behavior. Amsterdam: North-Holland Publishing Comp. 1966.

— Johnson, J., Ng, M. H.: Protein incorporation and axoplasmic flow in motoneuron fibres following intra-cord injection of labelled leucine. J. Neurochem. **14**, 317—331 (1967).

Peters, T., Ashley, C. A.: An artefact in autoradiography due to binding of free amino acids to tissues by fixations. J. Cell Biol. **33**, 53—60 (1967).

Rahmann, H.: Zum Stofftransport im ZNS der Vertebraten. Z. Zellforsch. **66**, 878—890 (1965).

Taylor, A. C., Weiss, P.: Demonstration of axonal flow by the movement of tritium labelled protein in mature optic nerve fibers. Proc. nat. Acad. Sci. (Wash.) **54**, 1521—1527 (1965).

Waelsch, H.: Some aspects of amino acid and protein metabolism of the nervous system. J. nerv. ment. Dis. **126**, 33—39 (1958).

Weiss, P., Wang, H., Taylor, A. C., Edds, M. V., Jr.: Proximal-distal fluid convection in the endoneurial spaces of peripheral nerves, demonstrated by colored and radioactive (isotope) tracers. Amer. J. Physiol. **143**, 521—540 (1945).

Weiss, P., Hiscoe, H. B.: Experiments on the mechanism of nerve growth. J. exp. Zool. **107**, 315—395 (1948).

— Holland, Y.: Neuronal dynamics and axonal flow. II. The olfactory nerve as model test object. Proc. nat. Acad. Sci. (Wash.) **57**, 258—264 (1967).

Young, R. W., Droz, P.: The renewal of protein in retinal rods and cones. J. Cell Biol. **39**, 169—184 (1968).

Dr. Peter Schubert
Max-Planck-Institut für Psychiatrie
D-8000 München 23
Kraepelinstraße 2
Deutschland

Acta neuropath. (Berl.) Suppl. V, 187—197 (1971)
© by Springer-Verlag 1971

Neuronal Organelles in Neuroplasmic ("Axonal") Flow*

I. Mitochondria

Paul A. Weiss

Rockefeller University, New York

Robert Mayr

Department of Anatomy, University of Vienna

Summary. 1. Axonal mitochondria, carried cellulifugally by the axonal flow at its average rate of daily advance of 1 mm, accumulate not only at artificial nerve blocks (e.g., constrictions and transections) but at the normal distal ends of the axon as well (e.g., neuro-muscular junctions).

2. Mitochondria thus clustered, whether at normal endings or at artificial blocks break up within days. Their DNA→RNA→Protein production mechanism, thus spilled into the matrix of the axonal ending, might account for the reported neosynthesis of protein at peripheral nerve terminals.

3. Isolated nerve fragments left in the body for 5 to 31 days after transection show a large increase of protein synthesis (incorporation of ^{3}H-Leucine) near the levels of transection over the intermediate nerve stretch. This increase, averaging 77% for 314 specimens, expresses strong local wound effects evoked by the operation, presumably entailing, aside from cell debris, local accumulations and breakdown of cells.

4. The excess of protein synthesis in terminal over intermediate nerve samples disappears if the respective fragments have been exposed to chloramphenicol, a rather specific inhibitor of protein neosynthesis in mitochondria. It thus seems reasonable to attribute the local rise of protein production mainly to a clustering of either cells rich in mitochondria, such as Schwann cells, or even free mitochondria from disintegrated cells.

5. The fact that these accumulations of mitochondria in severed nerves occur on both sides of a cut (though on the distal side only fleetingly) even in fully degenerated nerves devoid of axons disposes, of course, definitively of their use as evidence for the possibility of retrograde (cellulipetally ascending) axonal flow.

6. In general, the results favor the hypothesis that protein neosynthesis observed at nerve endings is of mitochondrial origin.

Key-Words: Mitochondria, Axonal — Protein Synthesis — Axonal Transport — Nerve Endings.

The current status of the rapidly growing knowledge about "neuroplasmic flow" has been critically reviewed in several recent publications by the senior author (Weiss, 1967b, 1969, 1970). The term signifies that neuroplasm is being reproduced continuously throughout life in the nucleated soma (perikaryon) of the neuron, whence it is then conveyed cellulifugally into all cellular processes as a cohesive columnar mass.

At this point, a few supplementary remarks seem necessary. The rate (v) of the proximo-distal advance of the axonal mass has been established (and amply

* Work supported in part by grants from the National Institutes of Health (U.S.A. Public Health Service) and the Faith Foundation of Houston.

reconfirmed) to be of the order of one millimeter per day. However, the expression of this rate in terms of *linear* displacement, which has been generally adopted since the original description of the phenomenon by the author (1948), would be rigorously valid only if the longitudinal progression of the column were independent of the width of the flow channel ($r^2\pi$). This being unlikely, it would seem more appropriate, pending evidence to the contrary, to express the true rate in terms of displacement of unit *volume*, i.e., as $v = \frac{r^2\pi \times l}{t}$; assuming equal rates of substance convection in fibers of different calibers, the longitudinal advance would then be *inversely* proportional to the square of the respective diameters. The average mass of neuroplasm propelled linearly in the millimeter range calculates to about 10 cubic micra per minute; if this were constant for a wide spectrum of fiber sizes, the linear progress in millimeters would be almost ten times faster in an axon of 2 μm diameter than in a 6 μm one. On the other hand, considering that axon diameter is related to size of perikaryon and the latter may be an expression of production rate of neuroplasm, the interrelations may be less simple. At any rate, in making comparative statements about axonal flow, such geometric relations must be born in mind.

Since the newly produced neuroplasm feeds not only into the axon, but into the dendrites as well, even though in more diffuse form, the more general term "neuroplasmic flow" should be substituted for the more restrictive term of "axonal flow". The nature of the flow might best be characterized as being similar to the flow of lava or of glaciers, that is, as the non-Newtonian movement of a plastic semi-solid body. Moreover, just as there is rapid Newtonian flow of water in the crevices of glaciers at speeds far in excess of the sluggish advance of the ice itself, so the observation that there is also substance transport within axons at rates up to a hundred times faster than the movement of the axon itself, makes us postulate the existence of either intra-axonal microchannels for express liquid traffic or of pathways for rapid electric transfer from center to periphery. In contrast to the slow neuroplasmic flow as such, the nature, site, and mechanism of the fast transport have thus far received little elucidation. Our discussions in the following will not concern themselves with this *intra*-axonal flow, but bear solely on the cohesive neuroplasmic flow of the slow type.

The original suggestion (Weiss and Hiscoe, 1948, pp. 371—374) that axonal protein could serve as a diagnostic marker of neuroplasmic flow has been widely confirmed, and the method has come into universal use. It should be stressed, however, that it is grossly misleading to refer to the longitudinal displacement of the proteinaceous markres as "protein migration", as is frequently done in current literature, because certainly the vast mass of the axonal proteins marked by radioactive amino acid incorporated in them is not in solution and freely diffusible, but is part of larger macromolecular arrays or structured assemblies. (The identification of proteins extracted from axons as "soluble" proteins, of course, does not imply that they have been in solution in the living system.)

The mitochondrial population within the moving axon is very sparse. Extensive electronmicroscopic observations of normal myelinated fibers of peripheral nerves in mature rodents show on the average only about 2 mitochondria per 500 Å thick section. As was reported in an earlier paper (Weiss and Pillai, 1965), when

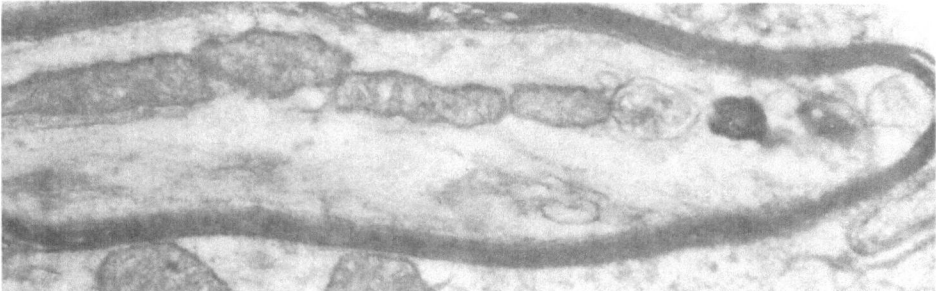

Fig. 1. Chain of mitochondria, trapped in blind pocket of constricted axon. Explanation in text. ×33,500

the axonal flow is throttled down by a local narrowing of the axon diameter, as in the standard constriction experiments, or is completely stopped by occlusion through a crush or severance of the nerve (Zelena, 1969), masses of mitochondria pile up at the proximal side of the obstruction within a few days. This has been shown to be due to the fact that the mitochondria are carried downward from their reproductive center in the cell body by the axonal flow as carrier system. In addition to the electronmicroscopic evidence, the piling up of mitochondria at sites where the axonal flow is blocked has also been demonstrated by statistical studies of mitochondrial distribution (Scharf and Blume, 1964) and by the accumulation in such places of mitochondrial enzymes (Friede, 1969,; Kreutzberg and Wechsler, 1963).

The electronmicroscopic studies revealed a massive and rapid breakdown of the stalled mitochondria. For details, the reader is referred to the earlier report by Weiss and Pillai. Merely as one example, Fig. 1 shows a tandem chain of mitochondria which have arrived from the left and been trapped with the axonal stream in a pocket of a constricted axon. The most recent (farthest left) arrivals have still their normal fine structure, but progressing to the right, one notes in sequence the increasingly severe signs of degeneration; from simple vacuolization, through swelling, to strong osmiophilia and eventually, fragmentation and dissolution. This mitochondrial "death history" repeats itself continually in front of any axonal constriction, the picture being the same regardless of whether the block has lasted for a few days or for a full year; that is to say, at the level of the block, the daily number of new arrivals (averaging 100 mitochondria per day per axon) is balanced by the disintegration of a corresponding number, with the piled-up surplus furnishing a measure of the breakdown time (by rough estimate, 5 to 7 days).

The reason why mitochondria in stalled flow disintegrate is unknown. Since motion pictures of living cells, taken in our laboratory (Taylor, 1961), have shown that mitochondria lose motility and break up when the pH of the medium sinks below 6, one might speculate that axoplasm subject to damming becomes locally acidified, which could explain the destruction of the accumulated mass of mitochondria, thereby engendering even further acidification. Yet, this being wholly conjectural, the question will have to remain open pending further exploration.

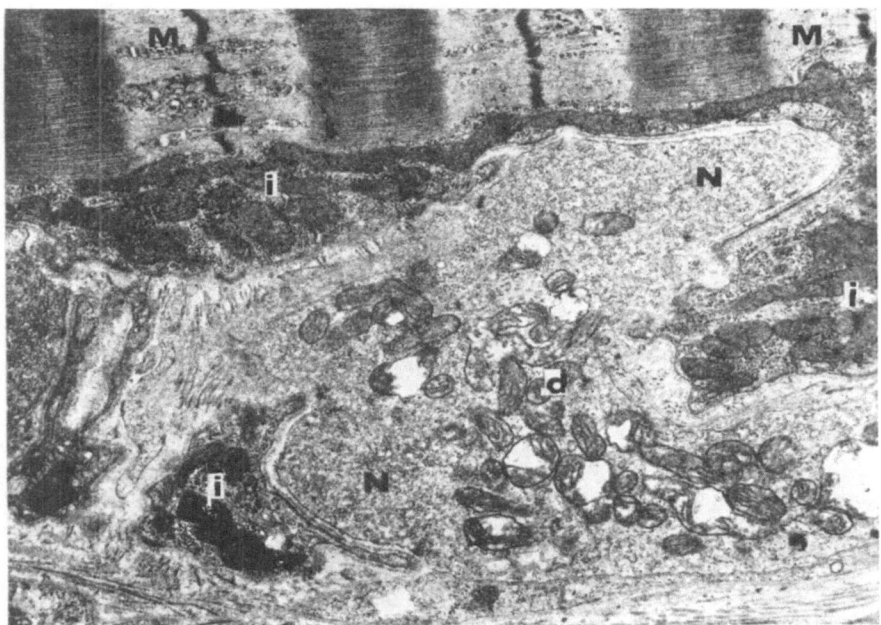

Fig. 2. Motor nerve ending (*N-N*) on extraocular muscle fiber (*M-M*) with fully intact mitochondria (*i*) on the muscular side and degenerating ones (*d*) in the neural part. × 11,500

At any rate, given the constancy of the phenomenon at artificial blocks, it was obvious to expect its occurrence at all blind ends of axons, hence at the normal peripheral endings; for instance, the neuro-muscular junctions at the motor endplate. Yet, although the accumulation there of mitochondria had been observed, breakdown had not. The observations summarized in the following prove that the postulated mitochondrial degeneration at axonal terminations is a fact.

Fig. 2 shows the junction between a motor nerve fiber and an extraocular muscle fiber of a rat. The section contains, besides an abundance of vesicles (most of them presumably synaptic), a pile of 40 mitochondria, thirteen of which are in the process of dissolution. By contrast, all 38 mitochondria of the muscular endplate portion contained in the picture are normal in shape and structure and show no signs of disruption. The fact that both kinds are seen side by side in the same section, but sharply confined each to its respective tissue compartment, proves that the abnormal configuration of the axonal mitochondria reflects the true state of the organelles in the living specimen and not an artificial distortion due to faulty technique of fixation and preparation for electronmicroscopy, of which one might have suspected it if the control forms were not present for comparison. Moreover, to clinch the argument, it should be added that although the jamming and breakdown of the mitochondria extends some distance backwards from the ending into the myelinated part of the axon, the axonal mitochondria at still farther proximal levels are quite intact and normal. Fig. 3, of a near-terminal section of a fiber, shows again side-by-side the degenerating mitochondria in the axon and the fully

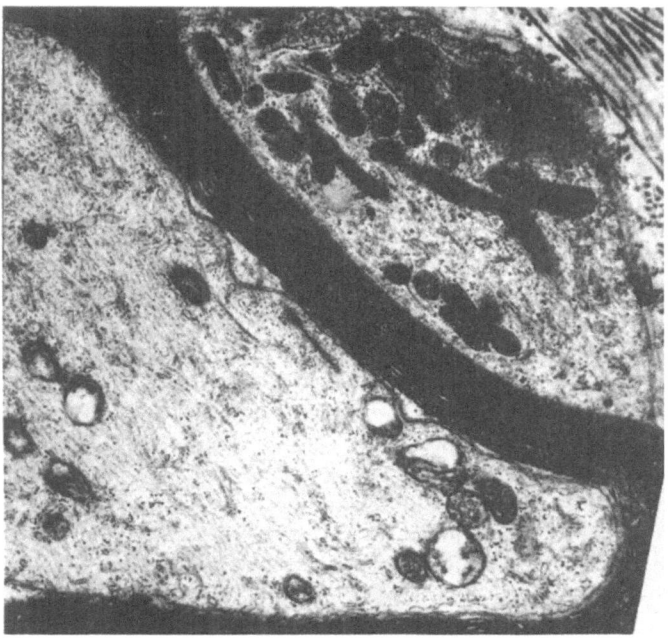

Fig.3. Section of axon near its termination, with its mitochondria already in dissolution, in contrast to the normal mitochondria of the enveloping sheath cell. ×21,500

intact mitochondria outside the axon — in this case, in the enveloping sheath cell of Schwann.

The examples here reproduced are representative of all specimens studied, including the nerve endings on intrafusal fibers of muscle spindles. Thus, the fact that axonal endings are mitochondrial grave yards seems rather conclusively established. In speculating about a possible functional significance of the pheno-menon, it had occurred to one of us (Weiss, 1970) to relate it hypothetically to miscellaneous reports of protein synthesis at nerve endings which at first seemed at variance with a strictly perikaryal monopoly for protein production. However, in view of the discovery of the presence in mitochondria of an autonomous DNA → RNA → Protein system (Chévremont, 1963; see, for instance, Lehninger, 1967), the possibility of linking the mitochondrial breakdown at endings to the local appearance of new protein seemed to merit consideration (see also Morgan and Austin, 1968).

In order to test this possibility, we resorted to a technique developed in our laboratory earlier (Weiss, 1967a) and standardized since. It consists of immersing segments of fresh sciatic nerve of a few millimeters length for 2 hours in a solution of ^{3}H-Leucine (1 mc/ml), at which time about $90^0/_0$ of the maximum attainable uptake of the label (after 5-hours' immersion) has been reached. It then takes a "chase" immersion of up to at least 4 hours to rid the tissue completely of its residual pool of unincorporated amino acid (surprisingly, this time was about the

same whether the balanced salt solution used for this chase did or did not contain
non-radioactive leucine), but since most of the residual pool was found to be
washed out after 2 hours, this value has been chosen as standard; at that time,
at least 50% of the radioactive label taken up by the live tissue during its 2-hour
bath in the solution has become incorporated in (chemically determined)
tissue protein. After thorough washing and blotting, the nerve pieces are subdivided into small segments of less than 1 cu mm; each segment is then dried on
aluminium foil, weighed, incinerated according to Gupta, and measured for radioactivity in a Packard liquid scintillation counter.

The applicability of this method to the mitochondrial tests seemed indicated
by the observations reported above of the local piling up of mitochondria at nerve
constrictions and total nerve interruptions. One ambiguity in the interpretation
of those observations, however, had to be cleared up first. It had been noted that
after drastic interventions, involving necessarily appreciable nerve damage, such
as after tight ligatures, crushing or transection, mitochondrial and mitochondrial-
enzyme accumulations occurred not only on the cell-near (upstream) side of the
lesion, where they would be readily accounted for by the damming of the axonal
flow, but also fleetingly for a few days, on the cell-far side near the break (Kreutzberg and Wechsler, 1963; Lubińska, 1964; Zelená, 1969). This centripetally oriented crowding had been cited as evidence of axonal flow in the reverse direction.
Such reversal being at variance with all direct observations of axonal flow in
mature nerve fibers, one of us (Weiss, 1967 b, 1969) had proposed that the bipolar
convergence of mitochondria and macromolecules upon the lesion might be merely
a local galvanotactic or electrophoretic displacement toward tissue debris of low
pH. The probability of this interpretation has greatly gained in credibility by the
following experiments, which revealed that the bipolar (or bidirectional) reaction
to a wound occurs just as well in degenerated nerve, in which, there being no
axon present, axonal flow reversal cannot be invoked as mechanism.

In preliminary studies, the rates of protein synthesis in live nerve fragments
of rats were compared by the described method between nerve stumps that were
in advanced stages of Wallerian degeneration, four weeks after proximal transection, and the contralateral intact nerves of the same animals. Radioactivity of
protein freshly synthesized in the 2-hour labelling period, expressed in counts per
minute per microgram, i.e. for equal weight fractions of degenerated and normal
control nerves, averaged 80% higher in the former than in the latter (10 pairs of
samples from 5 different animals). The result finds its obvious explanation in the
fact that the axoplasmic content of the intact control nerves takes no part in
protein synthesis, hence, is "dead weight", while in the degenerated ("aneuritic")
nerves its place has been filled by the hypertrophic and hyperplastic, actively
synthesizing Schwann cells (Büngner's cords). Considering that nerves contain,
besides nerve fibers, also endoneurial cells and blood vessels, about equal in their
contributions to radioactivity and weight measurements in both test and control
nerves, the Schwann cell share in the difference is, of course, even higher than the
80% determined for the bulk.

In passing, it is worth recording that the rate of incorporation into Schwann
cells was significantly higher (on a weight basis) than that into other tissues
(e.g., muscle; liver) tested by the same method, including also spinal ganglia and

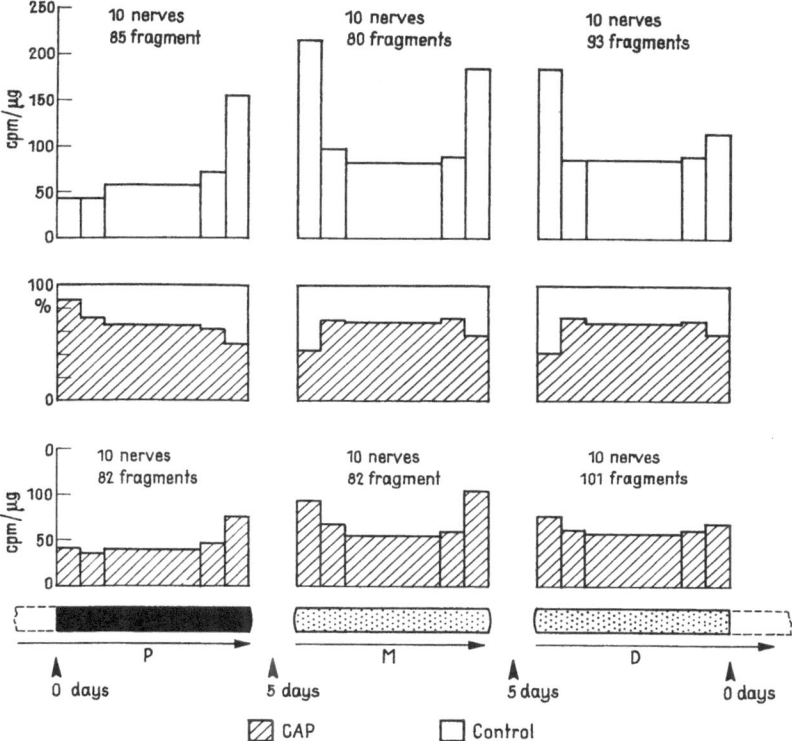

Fig. 4. Protein synthesis in untreated (top row, "T") and chloramphenicol treated (bottom row, "B", shaded) parts of proximal nerve stumps (P) and distal fragments (M, D), 5 days after transection. Middle row shows the inhibition by chloramphenicol in percentages of T

spinal cord with their large contingent of neuronal cell bodies besides glia cells. This might be a hint at a profound functional distinction between the peripheral (Schwann) and the central glia in line with Hyden's report (1967) that metabolic activity in isolated central glia cells is lower than it is in the adjoining neuronal cell bodies.

Given these background data of the rate of protein synthesis in degenerated ("aneuritic") nerve stumps, it was easy then to demonstrate the superimposed local effect of lesions[1]. To this end, sciatic nerves were severed by two transections about 10—15 millimeters apart (Fig. 4, bottom diagram), thus leaving in the animal a preparation that consisted of the still intact proximal stump (P), a middle piece (M) with cuts at both ends, and the remainder of the distal stump (D). After allowing 5 days for axonal breakdown to proceed in the two distal fragments, the middle piece, M, and pieces of equal length from the stumps P and D were removed from the animal and subdivided into 1 mm sections, each of which was then treated according to the standard procedure detailed above.

1 The valuable collaboration in these experiments by Yvonne Holland and Catherine Mytilineou is gratefully acknowledged.

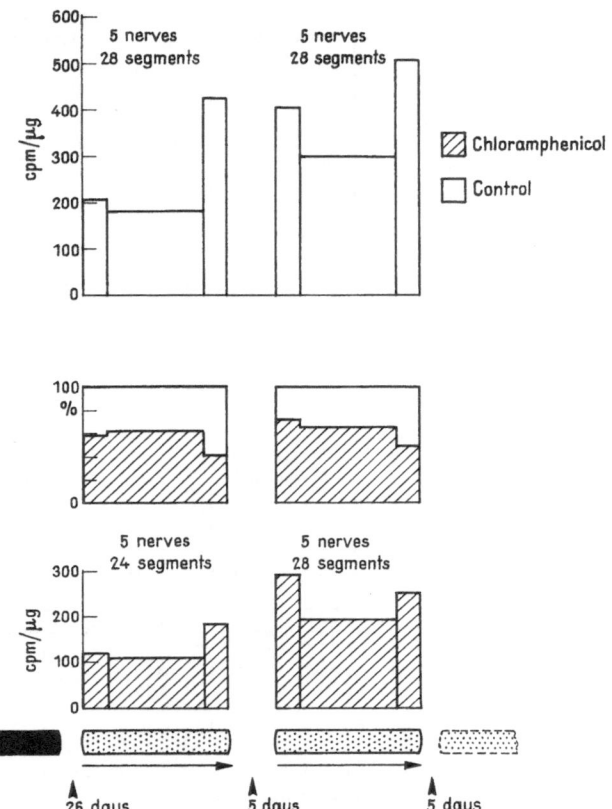

Fig. 5. Procedure as in Fig. 4, with 26 + 5 days of predegeneration after transection

The top record of figure 4 summarizes the 2-hour protein synthesis in 10 of the tandem triplets of pieces subdivided into 1 mm fragments, in proximal-distal sequence from left to right. Plainly, the four samples nearest to the two 5-day old transections showed, on an average, protein incorporation at about 3 times the rate of the intermediate samples of the same size; no similar rise is noted at the fresh cuts (farthest to the left and to the right) made just before the removal of the nerves from the animals.

This result proves conclusively that a nerve lesion engenders local processes which entail within days a dramatic rise of protein synthesis in the immediate neighborhood of the cut to either side. The fact that the effect extends in both directions over a distance of about one millimeter, which is roughly the length of one internode, hence, of a Schwann cell, points to a major involvement in the local reaction by these cells, but endoneurial cells and blood elements penetrating into the breach and possibly even into the open nerve ends must also be taken into account. On the other hand, these results cannot decide whether, as would seem plausible, the metabolic rise at the lesions can be ascribed to the observed concentration of mitochondria at those levels.

In order to decide the latter point, the experiments were actually carried out in two parallel series, using symmetrical nerves from both sides of the animal. Those of one side furnished the data presented in the preceding paragraphs, that is, total protein synthesis in normal and degenerated fragments, near to and distant from wounds. The contralateral nerves were treated in exactly the same way with the exception that a potent inhibitor specific for mitochondrial, as against cytoplasmic, protein synthesis, *chloramphenicol*, was added (1 mg/ml) to the ^{3}H-Leucine solution and the subsequent chase. The results, given in the lowest bar graph of Fig. 4, show a conspicuous reduction of protein synthesis in the 265 pieces that had been exposed to chloramphenicol, as compared to the 258 untreated pieces in the top graph. The graphs in the middle horizontal row give the differences between the top and bottom values in percentages of the rates of uninhibited synthesis. One recognizes that there is a markedly sharper decline of synthesis in the amphenicol-treated segments adjoining the lesions than in the uninjured segments of both the neuritic proximal piece, *P*, and the aneuritic distal pieces, *M* and *D*. One must conclude, therefore, that the high rate of protein synthesis at the lesion (top graph) is chiefly a feature of the amphenicol-susceptible mitochondria, crowded toward the old cuts. The slight additional surplus near the cuts even after amphenicol application in the bottom graph is presumably to be accounted for by the rapid infiltration into the lesion of masses of nonneural cells from the surroundings.

However, by themselves these experiments could not invalidate the contention that the mitochondrial accumulations at both cut ends of a fragment might simply be residual deposits of some bidirectional axonal flow during the days prior to the completion of axonal disintegration. In order to meet this objection, another set of experiments was carried out in which a much longer period was allowed for axonal degeneration (Fig. 5). Sciatic nerves were transected in both thighs; 26 days later, when Wallerian degeneration of the distal stumps had run its course, two new sections were made across those aneuritic stumps, and after a further interval of 5 days, the two isolated distal pieces of each limb were removed and treated as in the earlier experiments, comparing rates of amino acid incorporation with and without mitochondrial protein inhibitor. The graphs in Fig. 5 show essentially the same results as those of the former series, save for the lack of any sign of mitochondrial concentration near the 26-days old section; evidently the effect of wounding is a transitory one.

The conclusions to be drawn from these two concordant series of experiments, comprising 431 independent determinations of protein synthesis on nerve samples of sizes of 0.2—0.3 cu mm, are unequivocally as follows: (1) The observed accumulation of mitochondria at points of severe nerve lesions is correlated with a conspicuous rise of local protein synthesis per unit weight at those levels, the upstream one (in terms of axonal flow direction) enduring, the downstream one transitory (present at 5-day old cuts, absent at 26-day old ones). (2) Since the temporary concentration of mitochondria at the "upstream" end of a distal nerve stump occurs in completely axon-free (degenerated "aneuritic") nerve, it can be definitely ruled out as evidence for axonal stream reversal.

Whether mitochondria, whose motility has been amply illustrated cinemicrographically by Chévremont and Fréderic (1952); Pomerat (1961); and the extensive cell biological studies of this laboratory (e.g., Taylor, 1961), are converging on the wound galvanotactically or chemotactically, as suggested earlier (Weiss, 1970), or are rapidly multiplying in the cells of the woundbed and the wound-near nerve ends, or by any other means, will have to be determined by future studies. It even remains undecided whether the peaks of mitochondrial protein synthesis reflect a larger local density of *live* mitochondria or might not perhaps signify higher efficiency of the DNA → RNA → Protein process due to the release of the ingredients into the woundbed from their encasement in the live mitochondrion by the disintegration of the latter, as described in the first part of this paper. If the latter alternative could be confirmed, our hypothesis that the reported protein synthesis at nerve endings likewise originates from the demonstrated incessant breakdown of mitochondria at the blind ends of axons would greatly gain in convincingness. This view would be in good accordance with the demonstration of protein synthesis in the mitochondrial fraction of isolated synaptosomes by Morgan and Austin (1968).

A more comprehensive account of the data and conclusions of this paper with a fuller treatment of the relevant literature is planned for a later occasion in the broader context of neuronal dynamics and axonal flow in general.

References

Chévremont, M.: Cytoplasmic deoxyribonucleic acids: their mitochondrial localization and synthesis in somatic cells, under experimental conditions and during the normal cell cycle in relation to the preparation for mitosis. Symp. Internat. Soc. Cell Biol., 1963, vol. II, pp. 323—333.
— Fréderic, J.: Evolution des chondriosomes lors de la mitose somatique étudiée dans des cellules vivantes cultivées *in vitro* par microscopie et microcinématographie en contraste de phase. Arch. Biol. (Liège) **63**, 259—277 (1952).
Fréderic, J., Chévremont, M.: Recherches sur les chondriosomes de cellules vivantes par la microscopie et la microcinématographie en contraste de phase. Arch. Biol. (Liège) **63**, 109—132 (1952).
Friede, R. L.: Transport of oxidative enzymes in nerve fibers; A histochemical investigation of the regenerative cycle in neurons. Exp. Neurol. 1, 441—466 (1959).
Hydén, H.: In: The Neuron. Amsterdam-London-New York: Elsevier Publ. Comp. 1967.
Kreutzberg, G. W., Wechsler, W.: Histochemische Untersuchungen oxydativer Enzyme am regenerierenden Nervus ischiadicus der Ratte. Acta neuropath. (Berl.) **2**, 349—361 (1963).
Lehninger, A. L.: Cell organelles: The mitochondrion. In: The Neurosciences, pp. 91—100. Eds:. G. C. Quarton, T. Melnechuk, and F. O. Schmitt. New York: The Rockefeller University Press 1967.
Lubińska, L.: In: Mechanisms of neural regeneration. Vol. 13, p. 1—71. Eds.: M. Singer and J. P. Schadé. Amsterdam: Elsevier Publ. Comp. 1964.
Morgan, I. G., Austin, L.: Synaptosomal protein synthesis in a cell-free system. J. Neurochem. **15**, 41—51 (1968).
Pomerat, C. M.: Cinematography, indispensable tool for cytology. Internat. Rev. Cytol. **11**, 307—334 (1961).
Scharf, J.-H., Blume, R.: Über die Abhängigkeit der axonalen Mitochondrienzahl vom Kaliber der segmentierten Nervenfaser auf Grund einer Regressionsanalyse. J. Hirnforsch. **6**, 361—376 (1964).
Taylor, A. C.: Immediate response of cells to change of ion concentration in the medium. (Motion Picture). First Annual Meeting of the Society for Cell Biology, Nov. 2—4 (1961).

Weiss, P. A.: Neuronal dynamics and axonal flow III. Cellulifugal transport of labelled neuroplasm in isolated nerve preparations. Proc. nat. Acad. Sci. (Wash.) 57, 1239—1245 (1967a).
— Neuronal dynamics and axonal flow. Neurosci. Res. Progr. Bull. 5, 371—400 (1967b).
— Neuronal dynamics and neuroplasmic ("axonal") flow. In: Cellular dynamics of the neuron, pp. 3—34. Ed.: S. H. Barondes. Symposium of International Society for Cell Biology, Vol. 8. New York: Academic Press 1969.
— Neuronal dynamics and neuroplasmic flow. In: The Neuroscienes: Second study program, pp. 840—850. Ed.: F. O. Schmitt. New York: The Rockefeller University Press 1970.
— Hiscoe, H. B.: Experiments on the mechanism of nerve growth. J. exp. Zool. 107, 315—395 (1948).
— Pillai, Aiyappan: Convection and fate of mitochondria in nerve fibers: Axonal flow as vehicle. Proc. nat. Acad. Sci. (Wash.) 54, 48—56 (1965).
Zelená, J.: Bidirectional shift of mitochondria in axons after injury. In: Cellular dynamics of the neuron, pp. 73—94. Ed.: S. H. Barondes. Symposium of the International Society for Cell Biology, Vol. 8. New York: Academic Press 1969.

Prof. Dr. Paul A. Weiss
The Rockefeller University
New York, N. Y. 10021
U.S.A.

Dr. R. Mayr
II. Anatomisches Institut der Universität
A-1090 Wien, Währingerstraße 13
Österreich

Acta neuropath. (Berl.) Suppl. V, 198—206 (1971)
© by Springer-Verlag 1971

Neuronal Organelles in Neuroplasmic ("Axonal") Flow

II. Neurotubules *

Paul A. Weiss and Robert Mayr **

Rockefeller University, New York

Summary. Neurotubules are revealed to be firm structures which extend as single, continuous and undivided cylindrical bodies from their roots in the neuronal soma through the length of the axon to its peripheral ending. Counts of neurotubules in single branched axons have shown that the combined total of the numbers of tubules found in the distal branches equals the number present in the proximal undivided stem (Fig. 1). A theory is proposed according to which a tubule in a mature axon undergoes continuous growth in the following manner (Fig. 2): (1) it grows forth exclusively from its base by accretion of protein subunits at or beneath the surface of the nucleus (Fig. 2, E), the subunits arraying themselves in a linear string, which then keeps coiling itself helically on to the preceding coils (Fig. 2, T) whose radius thereby defines the lumen of the tubule; (2) the established stem of the tubule, which is firmly embedded in the advancing axonal column, is dragged along by the latter (Fig. 2, F) at the axonal flow rate of 1 mm per day; and (3) its distal end keeps disintegrating as it arrives at the axonal terminal. Quantitative and cytological (Fig. 3) evidence for an actual spinning off of the building material for the tubules by the rotation (Fig. 2, R) of the cell nucleus has added substantial support to the hypothesis.

Key-Words: Neurotubules — Protein Synthesis — Axonal Transport.

The presence in neuroplasm of microtubules ("neurotubules"), practically unrecognizable electronmicroscopically prior to the introduction of glutaraldehyde fixation, has since been firmly established (see recent review by Davison, 1970). They are cylindrical threads, judged to be hollow tubes with outer diameters variously given as between 220 and 260 Ångström and an inner lumen of about 150 Å. Their number varies, presumably according to the type of neuron. They are reported to conform to the pattern of microtubules in other types of cells, that is, to have walls consisting of 12—13 slightly twisted rows of globular protein subunits of a molecular weight of roughly 60.000 (see Schmitt, F. O., and F. E. Samson, 1968; Davison, P. F., and F. C. Huneeus, 1970). A distinctive property of this protein is its selective binding with colchicine (Borisy and Taylor, 1967; Shelanski and Taylor, 1968). In addition to other distinctions (e.g., amino acid composition), this colchicine affinity differentiates the tubular protein ("tubulin") sharply from the protein constituents of the "neurofilaments" (Schmitt and Samson, 1968). Taken together with electronmicroscopic evidence to be presented in a subsequent paper (P. A. Weiss and Mayr, 1971), these facts prove incontestably that tubules and filaments are intrinsically disparate in nature and that earlier suppositions to the effect that they are merely different states of aggrega-

* Work supported in part by grants from the National Institute of Neurological Diseases and Stroke (U.S. Public Health Service) and the Faith Foundation of Houston.

** Guest Investigator. Permanent address: Anatomisches Institut der Universität, Wien IX.

tion of the same units (Peters and Vaughn, 1967) can, therefore, be discounted. The colchicine-binding property has also furnished clues to a probable involvement of neurotubules in rapid intraaxonal substance traffic (Dahlström, 1968; Kreutzberg, 1969). At the same time, the facts (1) that the neurotubules seem to be firmly incorporated in the axis cylinder, (2) that the proximo-distal advance of the latter (the so-called "slow" phase of axonal flow) proceeds in a structurally consistent semisolid state, and (3) that the axonal mitochondria, not uncommonly seen associated with neurotubules in electronmicrographs, are also conveyed distally as inclusions of the axonal column, have led to the presumption that the neurotubules likewise are carried along by the advancing axonal column, in which they would lie firmly embedded. This would presuppose (a) that each neurotubule grows forth exclusively by continual accretion from a root-like base in the neuronal cell body, (b) that its stem then, during its proximo-distal shift, perseveres as a rigid structural entity, single and continuous from base to tip, and (c) that the tip dissolves with the rest of the intraaxonal structures when it arrives at the distal end.

Ordinary statistical data on neurotubular populations, assayed at different levels along a nerve trunk could not furnish a valid test of this concept of continuous neurotubular growth. Even if such a census were to reveal that the average *number* of tubules along a given nerve remains relatively constant, this would only indicate that the local population of tubules is under some density control, but it could not prove that the *individual* tubules counted at consecutive sampling levels are actually the same. The validation of the concept hinged on the feasibility of establishing the *lengthwise continuity* of individual tubules.

A practicable approach seemed to be offered by the study of *single branched* axons, for if tubules are unitary fixtures, their total number in the branches of a given axon should be equal to the number of tubules in the common stem proximal to the point of bifurcation. This actually proved to be the case, as will be documented in the following.

We shall deal here only with the *microtubular* contingent of axons, deferring the consideration of *neurofilaments* to a subsequent paper, because we found the two systems to be far too dissimilar to be treated profitably in conjunction. For the same reason, the results of purely statistical comparisons between the two fibrous constituents of neuroplasm, albeit valuable as census data (e.g., Friede and Samorajski, 1970), do not lend themselves to direct analytical interpretation.

The objects chosen for our present study were motor neurons (A alpha fibers) and a sensory neuron (Ia fiber), to the musculus lumbricalis of $150-250$ g albino rats, whose axons split into several branches in their terminal intramuscular course. After dissection from the Nembutal-anaesthetized, glutaraldehyde-perfused animals, the tissue was postfixed in 4% osmic acid solution, embedded in epon or araldite, and light microscopic serial sections alternating with ultrathin sections at proper intervals were cut perpendicular to the nerve fiber axis. It thus was possible to trace individual axons by ordinary light microscopy over their whole terminal length, follow them to their branching points and further down into the branches, and then submit selected cross sections from levels both through the undivided stem of a given axon and through its distal branches to electronmicroscopy for counts of the neurotubular profiles contained in them.

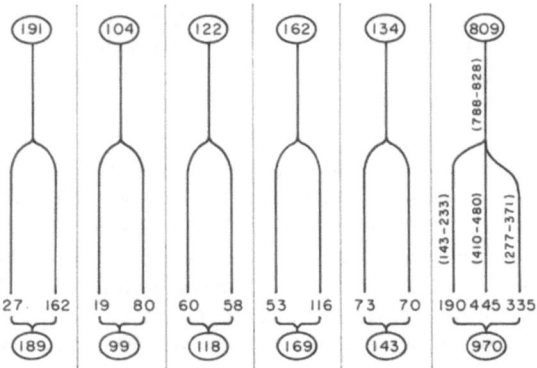

Fig. 1. Counts of numbers of neurotubules in the stem
and the branches of six divided single axons

Fig. 2. Schematic model of the formation and growth
of a neurotubule. — N Cell nucleus. — E Extrusion
of nuclear contribution to subunit protein across
nuclear pore. — R Direction of nuclear rotation. —
A Direction of movement of subunit string. — T Direction of apposition of subunit string to (dextral) coils;
the possibility of the tubule undergoing at the same
time a counterclockwise revolution around its axis in
the direction of T is left open. — F Direction of axonal
flow

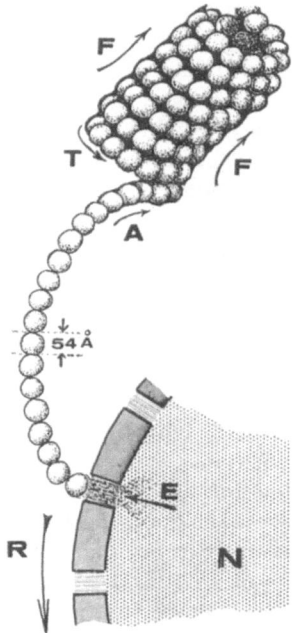

Fig. 2

The results of this laborious procedure in six single axons are summarized in
Fig. 1. The numbers give the average counts at different levels of single axons—on
top, of the axonal stem; at the bottom, of the derivative branches, both separately
and combined. The case at the far right with three branches (a Ia fiber at its
most proximal branching point and therefore still large in diameter with corre-
spondingly high numbers of tubules) was one of the very earliest counted and
reveals the relatively wide range (given in bracketed terms) of counting error
(about $\pm 13\%$) inherent in a preliminary investigation. Even so, the mere fact
that the distal for all three branches exceeded the stem count by only 20%
already signified that at least 80% of the individual tubules in the axonal stem
must have continued into the branches undivided. However, as one can readily
see, the remaining cases, exclusively preterminal motor axons with smaller numbers of tubules, yielded unequivocally consistent results; in each case, the total
number of tubules in the branches was nearly identical with the number present
in their common stem. It is safe, therefore, to conclude, in confirmation of our
initial premise, that each tubule is a single unitary entity, extending in uninterrupted and undivided continuity from its base in the cell body to its peripheral tip.

Moreover, the ratio between the number of neurotubules and the average
cross sectional area of a given axon continued to hold true for its branches with
the same proportionality factor, the smaller partner of a bifurcation receiving
proportionately fewer tubules than the larger one. This reveals the operation

of a true, but unknown, matrix-tubule control interaction, the exploration of which remains a task for future research.

The constancy and continuity of individual neurotubules all the way from the cell body to the nerve endings, proved by our measurements, cannot, however, of itself decide whether the tubule is a continuously *growing* unit, moving cellulifugally with the axonal stream, as we proposed, or is a skeletal fixture, past which the axonal flow would wash. The decision in favor of the former alternative, however, has come from recent experiments by Karlsson and Sjöstrand (1970). They followed the axonal flow in the optic nerve of rabbits by radioisotope labelling of the proteins at their retinal production site (see Taylor and Weiss, 1965) and found that the colchicine-binding protein species, diagnostic for microtubules, moved down the nerve from its source at the rate of 1.5—2 mm per day, which corresponds to the standard rate of the axonal flow (see also Grafstein et al., 1970; James and Austin, 1970).

There is thus gradually a fairly consistent picture emerging about the nature and origin of the axonal neurotubules, which in combination with some earlier observations and conjectures by one of us (P. W.) would lead to the following hypothesis (Fig. 2).

(1) The (colchicine-binding) protein subunits of a neurotubule originate in the immediate vicinity of the cell nucleus (Fig. 2, N) receiving essential intranuclear contributions extruded through nuclear pores (Fig. 2, E), which also may confer insolubility upon the product. The sites and steps of the synthesis and assembly of the subunits remain otherwise undefined.

(2) Due to the familiar phenomenon of the rotation of the nucleus relative to the cytoplasmic matrix (Fig. 2, R), new subunits are therefore continuously in the wake of the extrusions from the nuclear nozzles.

(3) A serial stacking of the anisotropic subunits by specific mutual bonding would then yield a continuously lengthening string of subunit beads connecting the most recent additions through their antecedents with the inner margin of the tubular wall. The tubule thus grows by recruitment of subunits to its basal edge.

(4) Assuming further that a coiled packing of the subunits, with 12 to 13 units per turn, has energetically an advantage over a mere linear array, the loose string of newly formed subunits would automatically keep adding fresh windings to the tubule (at A in Fig. 2).

(5) *Pari passu* with this continuous increment at its lower end, the finished shaft of the tubule, incorporated in the axonal matrix, is carried outward by the axonal flow (in direction of arrows F). Evidently, one must postulate that at its apical end the substance of the tubule is dissipated commensurate to its basal accretion; whether by dissolution or by fragmentation into vesicles (e.g., Pellegrino de Iraldi and de Robertis, 1968) remains problematical.

(6) Since, in accordance with (1) and (2), the rate of subunit generation would be a function of the velocity of the nuclear spin (R), the variable rate of the latter may represent a control mechanism to keep the basal growth of the tubule in balance with its elongation by the drag of axonal flow (F), the volume of the latter being, in turn, a function of the rate of perikaryal synthesis of all axonal proteins, including many other kinds besides the neurotubular one.

This concept of appositional growth, as here presented, has many counterparts in cellular and subcellular morphogenesis. On the cellular level, it corresponds to the general principle of "meristematic growth points" in plant development, or the formation of cellulose stalks in slime molds (Bonner, 1959) and on the sub-microscopic level, for example, to the outgrowth of cilia from their basal bodies in the cell or the basal stacking on of new lamellae in the visual cells (Young and Droz, 1968). But aside from such general similarities, more specific evidence for the applicability of the hypothesis to the neurotubules can be adduced from the following extensions of the six principal points made above.

ad (1). Nuclear pores and the extrusion of nuclear products are well attested (e.g., Swift *et al.*, 1956). The rotation of nuclei has been observed in many cell types (e.g., Hintzsche, 1956; Pomerat, 1953), although its mechanism is still obscure. (The nuclear extrusions, operating in an essentially incompressible environment, are perhaps generating the spinning motion in the manner of a jet turbine.)

ad (2). In his meticulous analysis of the fate of newly formed proteins in the neuronal cell body, Droz (1967) has distinguished two classes according to their residence times in the cell body of one day and up to two weeks, respectively. The former are evidently the ones that pass rather directly into the axon. The early appearance of labelled neurotubular (colchicine-binding) protein in the axon would favor its belonging to this class, which would strengthen our premise of there being a physical molecular connection between the nuclear surface and the base of each tubule.

ad (3). Our hypothesis construes the axial orientation of the linear array of units that is to build the tubular wall (arrow at A, Fig. 2) to be transversal (arrow T) with regard to the tubular axis, rather than longitudinal, as has been generally assumed (e.g., Porter, 1966). The tubule would be wound in a tight coil, like a solenoid, from a single continuous string, rather than be made up of $12-13$ separate component "protofibrils", oriented longitudinally parallel to each other and to what would thereby become the main axis of the assembled tubule. Our thesis would explain the statement by Davison (1970) that microtubules are very resistant to lateral dissociation, and when fragmenting, break transversally, sharply ended; this definitely indicates greater cohesion of the units in the transverse direction (arrow T) than in the direction of the tubular axis (arrows F).

ad (4). The amount by which the winding on of each new turn to the tubular base shortens the free feeder line of subunits can be roughly calculated as follows. An average tubule with outer and inner diameters of 250 and 200 Ångströms, respectively, can accommodate in its 700 Å circumference 13 globular subunits of approximately 54 Å transverse length each. [Since the girth of the tubule will not be an exact multiple (13) of the diameter of the units, neighboring coils will be out of mutual register by a constant fraction; this would explain the "twisted" shift in the alignment of subunits of consecutive coils that gives the visual illusion of longitudinal "protofibrils".] To lengthen the tube at its base by 1 mm, in compensation for its daily distal shift by the axonal flow, would require a daily production of at least 26×10^5 subunits, winding themselves into 2×10^5 coils of a minimum height of 50 Å each. This corresponds to a production rate per second of 30 subunits forming a row of 1500 Å length, which would wind into 2.3 coils

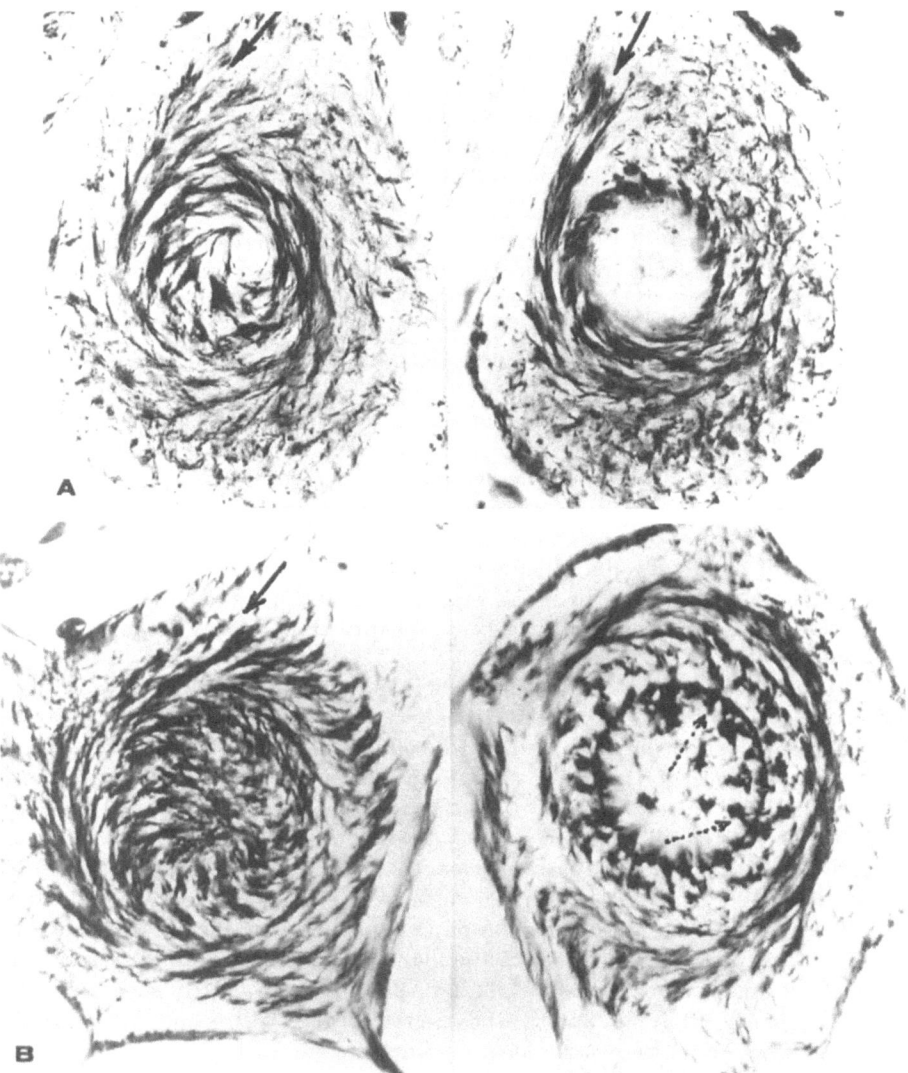

Fig. 3. Optical cross sections through cell bodies of motor neurons to electric organ of Torpedo (courtesy of Professor Hermann Hoepke, Heidelberg). Each horizontal pair represents the same cell at different levels

for a gain in tubular length of 115 Å. Correcting for the probable underestimation of the height of the subunits, and hence, of the coils, a closer approximation to reality would be an increment per second of 2300 Å uncoiled length of the string, or 180 Å addition to the length of the tubule after coiling. This then amounts to a longitudinal growth rate of the tubule of about $1\,\mu$ per minute, $60\,\mu$ per hour, hence, ca. 1.5 mm per day.

ad (6). The required rate of spinning off such a string of subunits at 2300 Å per second (see preceding paragraph) must be compared with the known spinning rates of nuclei to establish whether or not our suggestion of a *physical* connection between the two processes is at all reasonable. Quantitative data on nuclear spin rates (Pomerat, 1953; Hintzsche, 1965; P. Weiss, extensive unpublished recordings) give an average range, depending on cell type and conditions, between 1 and 6 min per revolution. Taking a mean value of 200 sec for a full revolution and a circumference of about 50 μ for a medium-sized neuronal nucleus of 16 μ diameter, the distance which an average nuclear pore would span in one second would be about 0.25 μ (= 2500 Å). This then is the length of the string of subunits left behind each second in the wake of the emissions from a single pore. And as this value coincides closely with the requisite generation rate calculated above (2300 Å per second), the confidence value of our hypothesis gains considerably in strength. Considering the many quantitative uncertainties in our assumptions, the closeness of this detailed correspondence may be coincidental, but the general agreement by order of magnitude is undoubtedly significant. The diagram of Fig.2 is, of course, greatly schematized, particularly in showing a single string of subunits issuing from a single pore. In reality, on the premise that there would be as many linear subunit strings produced in each neuron as there are tubules to be kept growing, there would have to be an equal number of intranuclear sites for the production of the respective discharges, each utilizing a fairly large number of neighboring outlets.

Tentative as our concept of tubular growth may be, it receives strong additional reinforcement from direct cytological observations. Fig.3 presents optical cross sections through silver-impregnated motor cells of the nerves to the electric organ of *Torpedo ocellata*, given generously to one of us (P. W.) by Prof. Hoepke of Heidelberg. They clearly show (a) an intimate association between the origins of "neurofibrils" in the microscopic sense and a set of essentially equidistant points along the nuclear surface; (b) a conspicuous spirality of the course of the fibrils; and (c) the convergence of the fibrils upon the exit of the axon from the cell body. There is as yet no systematic information available on how the gross microscopic picture of "neurofibrils" is related to the filamentous microstructures resolved by the electron microscope. But since neurofibrils have been clearly seen under the light microscope in living unperturbed nerve fibers (Weiss and Wang, 1936; Levi and Meyer, 1937), they must have a counterpart in the living state. Evidently they represent fascicles of submicroscopic fibrillar structures that have a different refractive index than that of the axonal matrix. Among the possible candidates for ultramicroscopic representatives of the microscopic fibrils are bundles of neurofilaments and neurotubules, coarsified in silver-impregnated preparations by their metallic coats.

Though it is uncertain whether the tubules are preserved by the light microscopic fixation technique applied, the pattern of neurofibrils in Fig.3 favours the assumption that it represents, maybe not exclusively, the distribution of neurotubules, as we recognize it as exactly the picture to be expected from our hypothesis: (a) the bundles emerge close to the surface of the nucleus (or perhaps even from the interior; see dotted arrows); (b) their spiral course in the nuclear vicinity is attributable to the fact that their older distal parts are embedded in the cytoplasm, while their proximal generative bases are spun around by the revolving nucleus; and (c) the straightening of their course as they approach the axon (solid arrows) indicates the cellulifugal drag of the axonal flow.

In conclusion, what we have attempted here has been to construct a tangible *model* of the origin and growth of neurotubules and their relation to neuroplasmic flow. One could hardly pretend that the data on which our conclusions have been based, although derived from quite a variety of unrelated observations and deductions, would have lend themselves to such a unified and consistent interpretation by sheer coincidence without some basic verisimilitude. Even so, the final validation remains still a task for the future. Regardless of how the details of the concept may change, we hope to have demonstrated the practicability of identifying not only, as is the usual procedure, biochemical bulk displacements of materials in the neuron (e.g., "neurotubular protein migrates" or "is transported"), but concrete physical operations and instrumentalities through which such translocations are effected. Being quite diverse (e.g., growth, flow in conduits, interfacial spreading, electric or osmotic gradients, pumping mechanisms, etc.), the dynamics involved and their structural foundations will not reveal themselves to any one single method of study and hence will escape resolution by purely chemical bulk determinations.

References

Bonner, J. T.: The cellular slime molds. Princeton: Princeton University Press 1959.
Borisy, G. G., Taylor, E. W.: The mechanism of action of colchicine. Binding of colchicine-^{3}H to cellular protein. J. Cell Biol. **34**, 525—548 (1967).
Dahlström, A.: Effect of colchicine on transport of amine storage granules in sympathetic nerves of rat. Europ. J. Pharmacol. **5**, 111—113 (1968).
Davison, P.: Microtubules and neurofilaments: possible implications in axoplasmic transport. In: Biochemistry of Simple Neuronal Models, pp. 289—302. Eds.: E. Costa and E. Giacobini. Advances in Biochemical Psychopharmacology, Vol. 2. New York: Raven Press 1970.
Davison, P. F., Huneeus, F. C.: Fibrillar proteins from squid axons. II. Microtubule protein. J. molec. Biol. **52**, 429—439 (1970).
Droz, B.: Synthèse et transfer des protéines cellulaires dans les neurones ganglionnaires; étude radioautographique quantitative en microscopie électronique. J. Microscopie **6**, 201—228 (1967).
Friede, R. L., Samorajski, T.: Axon caliber related to neurofilaments and microtubules in sciatic nerve fibers of rats and mice. Anat. Rec. **167**, 379—388 (1970).
Grafstein, B., McEwen, B. S., Shelanski, M. L.: Axonal transport of neurotubule protein. Nature (Lond.) **227**, 289—290 (1970).
Hintzsche, E.: Wachstum, Kernrotation und Kerngröße von Epithelkulturen aus Nierenpapillen junger Mäuse. Z. Zellforsch. **43**, 526—542 (1956).
James, K. A. C., Austin, L.: The binding in vitro of colchicine to axoplasmic proteins from chicken sciatic nerve. Biochem. J. **117**, 773—777 (1970).
Karlsson, J.-O., Sjöstrand, J.: Transport of neurotubular protein and the effect of colchicine on axonal transport. Acta physiol. scand. Suppl. **357**, 11—12 (1970).
Kreutzberg, G.: Neuronal dynamics and axonal flow IV. Blockage of intraaxonal enzyme transport by colchicine. Proc. nat. Acad. Sci. (Wash.) **62**, 722—728 (1969).
Levi, G., Meyer, H.: Die Struktur der lebenden Neuronen. Die Frage der Präexistenz der Neurofibrillen. Anat. Anz. **83**, 401—456 (1937).
Pellegrino de Iraldi, A., de Robertis, E.: The neurotubular system of the axon and the origin of granulated and non-granulated vesicles in regenerating nerves. Z. Zellforsch. **87**, 330 to 344 (1968).

Peters, A., Vaughn, J. E.: Microtubules and filaments in the axons and astrocytes of early postnatal rat optic nerves. J. Cell Biol. **32**, 113—119 (1967).
Pomerat, C. M.: Rotating nuclei in tissue cultures of adult human nasal mucosa. Exp. Cell Res. **5**, 191—196 (1953).
Porter, K. R.: Cytoplasmic microtubules and their function. In: Ciba Foundation Symposium on Principles of Biomolecular Organization, p. 308. Eds.: A. E. W. Wolstenholme and M. O'Connor. Boston: Little Brown 1966.
Schmitt, F. O., and Samson, F. E.: Neuronal fibrous proteins. Neurosci. Res. Progr. Bull. **6**, 113—219 (1968).
Shelanski, M. L., Taylor, E. W.: Properties of the protein subunit of central-pair and outer-doublet microtubules of sea urchin flagella. J. Cell Biol. **38**, 304—315 (1968).
Swift, H., Rebhun, L., Rasch, E., Woodard, J.: The cytology of nuclear RNA. In: Cellular Mechanisms in Differentiation and Growth, pp. 45—59. Ed.: Dorothea Rudnick. Princeton: Princeton University Press 1956.
Taylor, A. C., Weiss, P. A.: Demonstration of axonal flow by the movement of tritium-labelled protein in mature optic nerve fibers. Proc. nat. Acad. Sci. (Wash.) **54**, 1521—1527 (1965).
Weiss, P. A., Mayr, R.: Organelles in neuroplasmic ("axonal") flow: Neurofilaments. Proc. nat. Acad. Sci. (Wash.) **68**, 846—850 (1971).
— Wang, Hsi: Neurofibrils in living ganglion cells of the chick, cultivated in vitro. Anat. Rec. **67**, 105—117 (1936).
Young, R. W., Droz, B.: The renewal of protein in retinal rods and cones. J. Cell Biol. **39**, 169—184 (1968).

Prof. Dr. Paul A. Weiss   Dr. Robert Mayr
The Rockefeller University   II Anatomisches Institut der Universität
New York, N. Y. 10021   A-1090 Wien, Währingerstr. 13
U.S.A.   Österreich

Acta neuropath. (Berl.) Suppl. V, 207—215 (1971)
© by Springer-Verl. 1971

Axonal Transport of Proteins in the Optic Nerve and Tract of the Rabbit

J.-O. Karlsson and J. Sjöstrand

Institute of Neurobiology, University of Göteborg, Göteborg, Sweden

Summary. The intraaxonal transport of protein in the optic nerve and tract of the rabbit occurs at four different velocities; 150, 40, 6—12 and 2 mm/day respectively. The two most rapidly migrating phases of axonal transport were predominantly associated with light particulate fractions and had a relatively rapid turnover in the nerve terminals. The third phase of axonal transport, which moved down the axon at a rate of 6—12 mm/day, was possibly associated with the migration of mitochondria or lysosomes. The most slowly migrating proteins in the axon, which moved at an average rate of 2 mm/day, carried predominantly soluble proteins down to the nerve terminals. These proteins had a half-life of 9.6 days in the nerve terminals in the lateral geniculate body. The colchicine-binding microtubular protein was a constituent of this slowly migrating phase. The different phases of axonal transport were of different magnitudes. As measured from the maximal amount of radioactivity present in the nerve terminals, the relative amount of radioactivities of the four phases were: 1; 1.8; 1.5; 8.5.

Colchicine has profound effects on the axonal transport of protein in this system. Very low doses of colchicine cause a total inhibition of the three rapidly transported protein phases. In contrast to this it was impossible to inhibit the slow transport completely with colchicine.

Key-Words: Axonal Transport — Protein Synthesis — Radioactivity — Mitochondria — Lysosomes.

Introduction

The concept of a proximo-distal transport of axonal constituents, first demonstrated by Weiss and Hiscoe (1948), has been well established. It is now commonly believed that axonal transport occurs at a minimum of two velocities (Lasek, 1966, 1968; Grafstein, 1967; McEwen and Grafstein, 1968; Livett *et al.*, 1968; Karlsson and Sjöstrand, 1968; Ochs and Johnson, 1969), and that there is a different subcellular localization of the proteins belonging to these two phases (McEwen and Grafstein, 1968; Bray and Austin, 1969; Kidwai and Ochs, 1969; Sjöstrand and Karlsson, 1969).

However, little is known about the transport of specific proteins within the axon. The fate of the transported proteins in the axon and in the nerve terminals is not known either.

The mechanism responsible for the transport of proteins in the axon is not yet known, although several investigators have suggested that the neuronal microtubules or neurotubules play an important role in this process (Kreutzberg, 1969; Dahlström, 1968; Karlsson and Sjöstrand, 1969; James *et al.*, 1970; Sjöstrand *et al.*, 1970; Karlsson *et al.*, 1971).

The present communication is a review of our studies during the preceding year on axonal transport in the optic system of the rabbit. The presence of at least four different phases of axonal transport in the retinal cells is described, and the effects of colchicine on these transport phases are discussed. It is also shown that the colchicine-binding microtubular protein of Weisenberg *et al.* (1968) is a constituent of the slow phase of axonal transport.

Results and Discussion

Albino rabbits of both sexes, weighing between 2 and 3.5 kg, were used. The animals were injected with 50 μCi (^{3}H) leucine, or in some cases with 50 μCi (^{14}C) leucine in sterile aqueous solution into the vitreous body of one or both eyes. For further details see Karlsson and Sjöstrand (1971 b).

Following its injection into the eye, the isotope rapidly disappeared from the vitreous body. The retina rapidly incorporated the isotope into protein during the first three hours after injection. Three hours after injection the retina contained about 16×10^6 d.p.m., and this level of radioactivity was stable during the following 15 h. The protein-bound radioactivity of the retina rapidly decreased during the interval 16 h to 36 h after injection. The half-life of this rapidly declining component was approximately one day. After 1.5 days the labelled protein of the retina disappeared at a slower rate (half-life = 6.4 days).

Labelled proteins from the retina reached the optic nerve about one hour after injection and the amount of radioactivity in the nerve increased rapidly thereafter. A corresponding increase in radioactivity of the optic tract occurred between 2.8 h and 9 h after injection. The protein-bound label reached the lateral geniculate body at about 4.4 h and the labelled proteins increased rapidly up to about 10 h after injection (Fig. 1).

After about 10 h a decrease in the radioactivity of this rapidly transported phase in the lateral geniculate body was observed. As can be seen in Fig. 1, the half-life of the protein of this phase must be in the order of hours. As calculated from the time interval between arrival of labelled proteins to the optic tract and to the lateral geniculate body, respectively, the maximal transport rate in the optic tract for this phase was approximately 150 mm/day. At this velocity the phase should reach the lateral geniculate body 4 h after injection. When this is compared to the observed value of about 4.4 h, it is possible to estimate that the time needed for synthesis and elaboration of these proteins in the perikaryon is 0.4 h. Since the rate of increase of labelled material in the lateral geniculate body was most marked at about 5 h, it can be assumed that the major portion of transported material in phase I reached the nerve terminals at this time. By estimating the average intraocular length of the axons to be 4 mm, and the average time needed for synthesis of these proteins in the retinal ganglion cells to be approximately 25 min, an average transport rate of 150 mm/day can be calculated for phase I. Phase I corresponds to the rapid component of axonal flow, previously reported to move at a rate of 110—150 mm/day in the optic pathway (Karlsson and Sjöstrand, 1968).

A second increase of radioactivity occurred in the lateral geniculate body at about 14 h after injection (Fig. 1). The average transport rate of this phase (phase II), as calculated from the time interval between injection and arrival of a peak of radioactivity in the optic tract, and the time of rapid increase in the lateral geniculate body, was 35 and 43 mm/day, respectively. If we assume that the time needed for synthesis of proteins in this phase is of the same order as that for the proteins in phase I, the average transport rate for phase II is about 40 mm/day. From 24 to 36 h after injection a rapid decrease of radioactivity was observed, indicating a fast turnover rate for this phase.

After the decline in radioactivity of phase II the radioactivity in the lateral geniculate body reached an almost constant level. During the time interval 2 to 4 days after the injection a doubling of the amount of radioactivity was observed (Fig. 1), indicating the arrival of a third component of axonal transport (phase III) to the nerve terminals in the lateral geniculate body. The amount of radioactivity in this phase was of about the same magnitude as that of phase II.

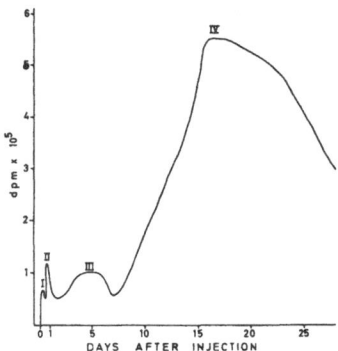

Fig. 1. Radioactivity in the lateral geniculate bodies at different intervals following intraocular injections of (^{3}H) leucine. I, II, III and IV show the different phases of axonal transport that arrived to the lateral geniculate body. (From Karlsson and Sjöstrand, 1971 b)

The maximal transport rate of this phase as calculated from the time of arrival to the lateral geniculate body was 6—12 mm/day.

The slow component of axonal transport previously described in this system (Karlsson and Sjöstrand, 1968) reached a maximum in the optic nerve at about 5.5 days in the optic tract about at 13 days and in the lateral geniculate body 16 days after injection (phase IV) as shown in Fig. 1. The average transport rate for this slow component as calculated from the time periods, at which the radioactivity was at a maximum in the optic nerve, and the optic tract was 2.1 and 1.9 mm/day respectively. The maximal transport rate for this phase as measured from the time of arrival to the lateral geniculate body was about 3 mm/day.

After about 22 days following injection, when no appreciable radioactivity entered the nerve terminals from the optic tract, the radioactivity in the lateral geniculate body decreased with a half-life of 9,6 days.

The four different phases of radioactivity that reached the lateral geniculate body were of different magnitudes. As calculated from the maximal amount of radioactivity present in the lateral geniculate body, the relative amount of radioactivity in phase I; II; III; IV was about 1; 1.8; 1.5; 8.5. These data concerning the quantitative relations between the phases are of course valid only if the proteins of the different phases contain the same relative amount of leucine, and if differences in turnover rates both in the axons and in the nerve terminals are neglected.

In addition to the classical fast and slow rates of protein transport in the axon we have found evidence for the presence of at least two phases with transport rates between the fast and the slow phase. These phases move at a rate of 40 mm/ day (phase II) and 6 to 12 mm/day) (phase III). An intermediate phase of axonal transport with a rate of 40 mm/day has recently also been found in the motor neurons of the cat (Lux *et al.*, 1970). These observations demonstrate that the transport mechanism in the axon is very complex. Even though the possibility of the existence of different populations of axons with different transport rates has not been excluded in the present study, it is probable that all the phases of transport can exist in the same axon. Radioautography has shown that both the rapid and the slow phases are present in the majority of the axons (Sjöstrand and Karlsson, 1969).

In previous studies we have shown that after an intra-ocular injection of ³H-leucine most of the radioactivity in the optic nerve, optic tract and lateral geniculate body is confined to the axon and their terminals (Karlsson and Sjöstrand, 1968; Sjöstrand and Karlsson, 1969). Therefore, after subcellular fractionation of the lateral geniculate body we would expect to find the radioactivity in the crude mitochondrial fraction where the detached nerve endings are usually found (Gray and Whittaker, 1962). However, we found a considerable amount of radioactivity in all the particulate fractions and in the soluble proteins. About 28 per cent of the radioactivity in the lateral geniculate body was always found in the 'nuclear' fraction, regardless of the phase which was present in the lateral geniculate body. This 'nuclear' fraction was obtained after a mild homogenization procedure and was very heterogenous. We consider that most of the radioactivity in the nuclear fraction is due to synaptosomes trapped by the cell debris and/or to the fact that a population of synaptosomes of retinal origin is so large and heavy that it ordinarily sediments in this 'nuclear' fraction.

When the slow phase of axonal transport (phase IV) is present in the lateral geniculate body about 41 per cent of the radioactivity is found in the soluble proteins. Most of this radioactivity must be derived from disrupted synaptosomes or axons. Data from a previous study (Sjöstrand and Karlsson, 1969) showed that about 51 per cent of the radioactivity of the slowly migrating phase in the optic nerve and tract consists of soluble proteins. With 51 per cent of the radioactivity in the axon and 41 per cent of the radioactivity in the lateral geniculate body being soluble, it can be calculated that about 80 per cent of the nerve terminals of retinal origin in the lateral geniculate body are disrupted during our fractionation procedure. This figure is based upon the assumption that the slowly migrating labelled soluble proteins in the axon still behave as soluble proteins in the nerve terminals.

With 80 per cent of the nerve terminals of retinal origin disrupted and 28 per cent of the radioactivity of the lateral geniculate body found in the nuclear fraction, one can assume that few nerve terminals of retinal origin are recovered in the crude mitochondrial fraction. It is therefore probable that the labelled material in this fraction consists mainly of free organelles derived from the terminals or the axons.

Subfractionation of the crude mitochondrial fraction on continuous or discontinuous sucrose gradients indicated that phases I and II were associated with the lighter particulate fractions, whereas phase III had a high relative specific radioactivity in fractions enriched with mitochondria and lysosomes. It is possible that a population of mitochondria or lysosomes reaches the nerve terminals with this phase. By measuring the rate of accumulation of cytochrome oxidase proximal to a ligation of the cat hypogastric nerve, Banks et al. (1969) found a rate of movement of mitochondria of about 14 mm/day. This value corresponds fairly well to our estimate of the transport rate for phase III in our system, which is about 6—12 mm/day.

The slow phase (phase IV) of axonal transport in our system contains a considerable amount of soluble proteins (Sjöstrand and Karlsson, 1969). However, there is also radioactivity among the soluble proteins in the other phases. In order to determine whether the same protein is transported at different rates in the axon, or whether the transport of a certain protein is restricted to one phase, we investigated the labelling pattern of the soluble proteins of phases I and IV. After labelling the proteins of phase I with ^{3}H-leucine and of phase IV with ^{14}C-leucine, the soluble proteins in the optic nerve and tract was subjected to gel electrophoresis (Karlsson and Sjöstrand, 1971a).

The results show that most of the soluble proteins from the optic nerve and tract separated by gel electrophoresis are ^{14}C-labelled. The radioactivity profile more or less corresponded with the densitometric tracing of these proteins. This result indicates a homogeneous labelling of the soluble proteins of the slow phase. As we have previously shown that the protein-bound radioactivity is confined to the axons in the optic pathway of the rabbit (Sjöstrand and Karlsson, 1969), it can be inferred that the axons contain a large number of soluble proteins which are transported with the slow phase. In the crayfish nerve cord gel electrophoresis has also shown a complex labelling pattern of the proteins transported at a slow rate in the axons (Fernandez et al., 1970). The absence of significant labelling of the three most rapidly migrating protein bands shows that these proteins are not constituents of the slow phase. In contrast to the slow phase radioactivity in the rapid phase is only confined to certain protein bands in the polyacrylamide gel. At least six labelled bands of the rapid phase are distinguished both in the optic nerve and tract.

In a previous study (Sjöstrand and Karlsson, 1969) it was shown that the proteins of the rapid phase in the optic nerve and tract were mainly associated with the microsomal fraction. Triton X-100 extraction of the microsomal fraction solubilized a relatively small amount of proteins with a very high specific radioactivity. Gel electrophoresis showed that the bulk of these proteins together with the majority of both the ^{3}H- and ^{14}C-label were associated with fractions having a low electrophoretic mobility.

To follow the axonal transport of a single protein we isolated a specific colchicine-binding protein from the optic nerve and tract at various intervals, following intraocular injection of ^{3}H-leucine (Karlsson and Sjöstrand, 1971c).

At various intervals following the injections the retina, optic nerves and optic tracts were dissected out, and the colchicine-binding protein was isolated by a batch DEAE Sephadex elution procedure, essentially as described by Weisenberg et al. (1968). After reduction and alkylation the isolated protein migrate as a single band on 7.5 per cent polyacrylamide gels. Incubation of the purified protein with ^{3}H-colchicine showed that it bound 0.24 moles colchicine per 120,000 g protein.

Determination of the specific radioactivity of the colchicine-binding protein at various intervals following injection showed that this protein was synthesized by the retinal ganglion cells and transported along their axons with the slow phase of the axonal transport (Fig. 2). Recently, James and Austin (1970) also found evidence for a slow transport of the colchicine-binding protein in the peri-

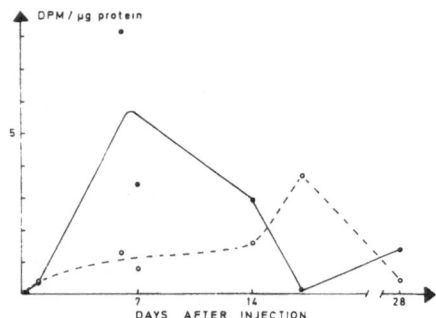

Fig. 2. Radioactivity in the colchicine-binding protein of the optic nerve (solid line) and the optic tract (dashed line) at various intervals following intraocular injection of tritiated leucine into both eyes. (Compiled from Karlsson and Sjöstrand, 1971 c)

pheral nerve. In experiments where we injected tritium labelled colchicine (which binds to the microtubular protein *in vitro*) into the eye, we could not trace any transport of this compound to the optic tract or to the lateral geniculate body. This is in contrast to the findings of Grafstein *et al.* (1970) on the goldfish optic system, where they found that ^{3}H-colchicine was associated with the slow phase of axonal transport.

The microtubules have been implicated in the mechanisms of axonal transport (Kreutzberg, 1969; Dahlström, 1968; Karlsson and Sjöstrand, 1969; James *et al.*, 1970; Sjöstrand *et al.*, 1970; Karlsson *et al.*, 1971), because colchicine, which causes a depolymerization of the microtubules, can block axonal transport.

After an intra-ocular injection of colchicine, there is no depression in the capacity for protein synthesis in the retina and choroid, if colchicine is injected 24 h before the isotope (Table 1). There are also no effects on protein synthesis at longer intervals following colchicine injection. Perhaps there is a slight depression of protein synthesis in the retina and choroid during the first hours following colchicine injection, as indicated by the somewhat lower specific radioactivity of the retina and choroid when the isotope was injected together with colchicine.

An almost complete inhibition of the rapid phase of axonal transport occurs if 2.5 µg or more colchicine is injected into the eye 24 h before the isotope is injected (Fig. 3). 2.5 µg of colchicine produces about 90 per cent inhibition and 10 µg about 95 per cent inhibition of the transport of the proteins of phase I. About 5 per cent of the radioactivity in the lateral geniculate body 7—8 h after the intraocular injection of isotope is due to blood carried background radioactivity (Karlsson and Sjöstrand, unpublished data). This means that we have a complete inhibition of the rapid transport when colchicine in a dose of 10 µg or more is injected into the eye 24 h before the isotope.

From Fig. 3 it is also clear that there is a certain lag period before the effects of colchicine are noticed, as indicated by the very low inhibition that occurs when colchicine is injected at the same time as the isotope. The actions of colchicine seems to be relatively long lasting as indicated by the clear effects on the rapid phase even after intervals as long as 8 and 47 days.

Axonal Transport of Proteins213

Table. *Effect of colchicine on the protein synthesis in the retina and choroid. All animals were sacrificed 7.5 h after the isotope injection, i.e. at a time when the radioactivity in the retina and choroid has reached its maximal level*

Dose of colchicine in μg	Interval between colchicine and isotope injection	Sp. act. of retinal and choroid proteins, dpm/μg protein	Number of animals
0	—	990	4
2.5	0 h	655	2
2.5	24 h	1030	2
10	24 h	930	3
25	24 h	930	1
10	8 days	900	1
10	47 days	1030	1

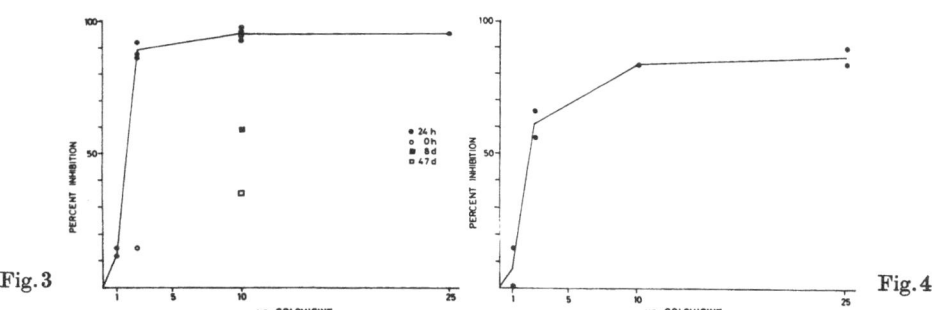

Fig. 3   Fig. 4

Figs. 3 and 4. The effect of colchicine on phase I (Fig. 3) and phase IV (Fig. 4) of the axonal transport in retinal ganglion cells. The animals were injected with different amounts of colchicine into the left eye and with ³H-leucine into the same eye after the indicated time period. Fig. 3: Animals sacrificed 7.5 h after isotope injection, when phase I of the axonal transport has reached the lateral geniculate body. Fig. 4. Animals sacrificed 16 days after isotope injection when phase IV of the axonal transport has reached the lateral geniculate body. Data are expressed as the percentage inhibition of the appearance of labelled protein in the lateral geniculate body when compared to animals not injected with colchicine. (From Karlsson *et al.*, 1971)

In contrast to the rapid phase of axonal transport the slow phase seems to be more resistant to colchicine treatment (Fig. 4). 2.5 μg produces about 50 per cent inhibition and 10—25 μg colchicine causes about 85 per cent inhibition of the slow phase of axonal transport. About 0.5 per cent of the radioactivity in the lateral geniculate body 16 days after isotope injection is due to blood carried background radioactivity (Karlsson and Sjöstrand, unpublished data). The same dose-dependent degree of inhibition was seen in the optic nerve and tract when the slow phase of axonal transport was present at these sites. No evidence was obtained for a change in rate of transport in the optic nerve and tract for the slow phase of axonal transport.

Acknowledgements. This investigation has been supported by grants from the Swedish Medical Research Council (No. B70-13X-2226-04B), Swedish National Cancer Society (No. 265-B69-01X), Svenska Sällskapet för Medicinsk Forskning, Magnus Bergvalls Stiftelse and Svenska Livförsäkringsbolags nämnd för medicinsk forskning. The skilful technical assistance of Mrs. Marie-Louise Eskilson and Miss Barbro Lilja is gratefully acknowledged.

References

Banks, P., Mangnall, D., Mayor, D.: The re-distribution of cytochrome oxidase, noradrenaline and adenosine triphosphate in adrenergic nerves constricted at two points. J. Physiol. (Lond.) **200**, 745—762 (1969).

Bray, J. J., Austin, L.: Axoplasmic transport of ^{14}C proteins at two rates in chicken sciatic nerve. Brain Res. **12**, 230—233 (1969).

Dahlström, A.: Effect of colchicine on transport of amine storage granules in sympathetic nerves of rat. Europ. J. Pharmacol. **5**, 111—113 (1968).

Fernandez, H. L., Huneeus, F. C., Davison, P. F.: Studies on the mechanism of axoplasmic transport in the crayfish cord. J. Neurobiol. **1**, 395—409 (1970).

Grafstein, B.: Transport of protein by goldfish optic nerve fibers. Science **157**, 196—198 (1967).

— McEwen, B. S., Shelanski, M. L.: Axonal transport of neurotubule protein. Nature (Lond.) **227**, 289—290 (1970).

Gray, E. G., Whittaker, V. P.: The Isolation of nerve endings from brain: An electron-microscopic study of cell fragments derived by homogenization and centrifugation. J. Anat. (Lond.) **96**, 79—88 (1962).

James, K. A. C., Austin, L.: The binding in vitro of colchicine to axoplasmic proteins from chicken sciatic nerve. Biochem. J. **117**, 773—777 (1970).

— Bray, J. J., Morgan, I. G., Austin, L.: The effect of colchicine on the transport of axonal protein in the chicken. Biochem. J. **117**, 767—771 (1970).

Karlsson, J.-O., Hansson, H.-A., Sjöstrand, J.: Effect of colchicine on axonal transport and morphology of retinal ganglion cells. Z. Zellforsch. **115**, 265—283 (1971).

— Sjöstrand, J.: Transport of labelled proteins in the optic nerve and tract of the rabbit. Brain Res. **11**, 431—439 (1968).

— — The effect of colchicine on the axonal transport of protein in the optic nerve and tract of the rabbit. Brain Res. **13**, 617—619 (1969).

— — Characterization of the fast and slow components of axonal transport in retinal ganglion cells. J. Neurobiol. **2**, 135—143 (1971a).

— — Synthesis, migration and turnover of protein in retinal ganglion cells. J. Neurochem. (in press) (1971b).

— — Transport of microtubular protein in axons of retinal ganglion cells. J. Neurochem. (in press) (1971c).

Kidwai, S. M., Ochs, S.: Components of fast and slow phases of axoplasmic flow J. Neurochem. **16**, 1105—1112 (1969).

Kreutzberg, G. W.: Neuronal dynamics and axonal flow, IV. Blockage of intra-axonal enzyme transport by colchicine. Proc. nat. Acad. Sci. (Wash.) **62**, 722—728 (1969).

Lasek, R. J.: Axoplasmic streaming in the cat dorsal root ganglion cell and the rat ventral motoneuron. Anat. Rec. **154**, 373—374 (1966).

— Axoplasmic transport in cat dorsal root ganglion cells as studied with (^{3}H)-leucine. Brain Res. **7**, 360—377 (1968).

Livett, B. G., Geffen, L. B., Austin, L.: Proximo-distal transport of (^{14}C) noradrenaline and protein in sympathetic nerves. J. Neurochem. **15**, 931—939 (1968).

Lux, H. D., Schubert, P., Kreutzberg, G. W., Globus, A.: Excitation and axonal flow: Autoradiographic study on motoneurons intracellulary injected with a ^{3}H-amino acid. Exp. Brain Res. **10**, 197—204 (1970).

McEwen, B. S., Grafstein, B.: Fast and slow components in axonal transport of protein. J.
    Cell Biol. 38, 494—508 (1968).
Ochs, S., Johnson, J.: Fast and slow phases of axoplasmic flow in ventral root nerve fibres. J.
    Neurochem. 16, 845—853 (1969).
Sjöstrand, J., Frizell, M., Hasselgren, P.-O.: Effects of colchicine on axonal transport in
    peripheral nerves. J. Neurochem. 17, 1563—1570 (1970).
— Karlsson, J.-O.: Axoplasmic transport in the optic nerve and tract of the rabbit: A bio-
    chemical and radioautographic study. J. Neurochem. 16, 833—844 (1969).
Weisenberg, R. C., Borisy, G. G., Taylor, E. W.: The colchicine-binding protein of mammalian
    brain and its relation to microtubules. Biochemistry 7, 4466—4479 (1968).
Weiss, P., Hiscoe, H. B.: Experiments on the mechanisms of nerve growth. J. exp. Zool. 107,
    315—396 (1948).

J.-O. Karlsson and J. Sjöstrand
Institute of Neurobiology
University of Göteborg
Göteborg, Sweden

Acta neuropath. (Berl.) Suppl. V, 216—225 (1971)
© by Springer-Verlag 1971

Changes in Microtubules and Neurofilaments in Constricted, Hypoplastic Nerve Fibers *

REINHARD L. FRIEDE

Institute of Pathology, Case Western Reserve University, Cleveland, Ohio

Summary. Hypoplastic nerve fibers were produced by applying a snug ligature around rat sciatic nerves by the 14th postnatal day, allowing the nerves to compress themselves with subsequent growth. This technique produced hypoplastic axons distal to the compression of caliber ranges consistent with arrested growth, or atrophy, respectively.

Hypoplastic axons showed increased microtubular density and increased density of axoplasmic organelles, including mitochondria, smooth endoplasmic reticulum and vesicles. The increased microtubular density in the hypoplastic fibers corresponded to a loss of 50% or more of the axonal neurofilaments at the level of compression, with a proportional decrease in axon caliber and an increase in the tubule/filament ratio. These changes restituted rapidly to normal fiber structure upon release of the compression. The tubule/filament ratio of restituted fiber was low, indicating massive "outgrowth" of neurofilaments.

The model described permits a highly selective experimental manipulation of axonal neurofilaments. The corresponding changes in the hypoplastic fibers are suggestive of the existence of a relation between the densities of microtubules and cytoplasmic organelles, including mitochondria. There was no indication, on the other hand, of a relationship existing between the axoplasmic organelles and the neurofilaments, although the latter appeared to be in quantitative relation to the volume of amorphous axoplasm as well as to axon caliber.

Key-Words: Axonal Neurofilaments — Axoplasmic Organelles — Microtubules — Electron Microscopy.

Introduction

The data reported here are a portion of an experimental program attempting to retard or accelerate axon growth; its ultimate goal is to determine how the rate of myelin formation by the sheath cells is affected by changes in axon caliber. Extremely slow compression was produced by applying a snug ligature around the sciatic nerve of rats by the 14th postnatal day, allowing the nerve to compress itself by its subsequent growth (Duncan, 1948). This technique produces "chronic" axon swellings proximal to the constriction and axonal hypoplasia distal to it, both changes being capable of rapid restitution upon removal of the ligature. The "chronic" axon swellings differ in axoplasmic composition from the "reactive" swellings found in the stumps of transected nerve fibers in that the swelling of the axon is due entirely to the accumulation of excessive amorphous axoplasm, with no significant increase in the density of axoplasmic organelles. A quantitative analysis of the fine structure of sheaths and axoplasmic composition of "chronic" axon swellings, including the changes upon restitution, was the subject of a separate investigation (Friede and Miyagishi, 1971). The present report concerns changes in axon caliber, number of neurofilaments and microtubules, and in

* This investigation is supported by U.S. Public Health Grant NS 06239 from the National Institute of Neurological Diseases and Stroke.

density of axoplasmic organelles in the hypoplastic portions of the fibers distal to the compression. A reduction in the axon caliber of these fibers was found to correspond to a loss of 50 per cent or more of the neurofilaments with little or no change in the number of microtubules.

Material and Methods

The left sciatic nerve of Sprague Dawley rats, 14 days-old, was exposed under pentothal anesthesia, and a black silk ligature was applied snugly around the nerve in the upper thigh, several mm above the point of branching. Extreme care was taken to tighten the knot slowly; there was usually no reaction in the limb; a slight twitching indicated maximum permissible compression. Selection of the proper age was critical for the sucess of the experiment as earlier ligation was likely to strangulate the fibers while later ligation may be ineffective in compressing the nerve. At the age at which the ligature was applied, practically all the fibers that are myelinated in adults have acquired their sheaths, but they are only about half way toward the normal adult caliber range (Friede and Samorajski, 1968). Following surgery the rats showed no signs of paresis, but some developed a slight weakness of the leg during the subsequent weeks, which was considered a symptom of effective compression. Rats were sacrificed 10, 20 and 30 days after application of the ligature. In another series of experiments the ligatures were removed surgically at the 40th day and their location was marked with a small deposit of india ink on the nerve. These animals survived another 10, 20 and 30 days. One animal for each period (2 for day 20) was studied with the electron microscope, but 1 μ thick sections from additional animals were available for comparison. Previously studied material on the progress of myelination in the sciatic nerves of normal rats (Friede and Samorajski, 1968) also was available for comparison.

All animals were sacrificed under deep pentothal anesthesia and the nerves were removed, postfixed for 24 hours in glutaraldehyde at 4° C and stored at the same temperature in 0.15 M cacodylate buffer, pH 7.2. Samples were immersed in 2⁰/₀ osmic acid for 1 to 2 hours, dehydrated and embedded in Maraglas. Sections were cut with an MT2 Porter Blum ultramicrotome, using glass knives. Sections approximately 1 μ thick were stained with a modified p-phenylenediamine method. Thin sections were mounted on 200 mesh copper grids, stained with uranyl acetate and lead citrate and studied with an RCA EMU-3 electron microscope. All specimens used for measurements were carefully oriented to provide sections cut precisely perpendicular to fiber axes.

Sections 1 μ thick were photographed with a Zeiss Ultraphot photomicroscope at a primary magnification of 1000× and enlarged 4.9 times on 16×20 inch prints. The inner circumferences of the myelin sheaths were measured with a Dietzgen plan meter. Fibers were selected at random by drawing a grid of equidistant, parallel lines across the prints, sampling every fiber touched by a line. This sampling method is biased in favor of the large fibers; however, it effectively eliminates subjective bias in sampling and does not affect the comparison of the fiber spectra obtained.

In electron micrographs, axon circumferences were measured with a Dietzgen plan meter at the axon membrane; myelin lamellae were counted with the aid of a binocular microscope. For the convenience of counting, a myelin lamella was defined as the electron dense, fused portion of two Schwann cell membranes (Friede and Samorajski, 1967). The cross-sectional area of axoplasm was determined with a precision Ott disc planimeter. The density of axoplasmic organelles was determined with a method of line sampling (Martinez and Friede, 1970), which consists of drawing a grid of equidistant, parallel lines across each print; the length of the lines crossing axoplasm is determined as well as the length crossing axoplasmic organelles; 3 to 8 such determinations were made for each fiber. Mitochondria, multivesicular bodies, smooth endoplasmic reticulum and vesicles were compounded, but neurofilaments and microtubules were excluded. The combined volume of the organelles was obtained in terms of per cents of axoplasmic volume, without correction for changes in organelle volume which may occur during processing or embedding of the tissue. Neurofilaments (approximately 100 Å high density dots in cross-sections) and microtubules (approximately 200 Å circular profiles) were counted.

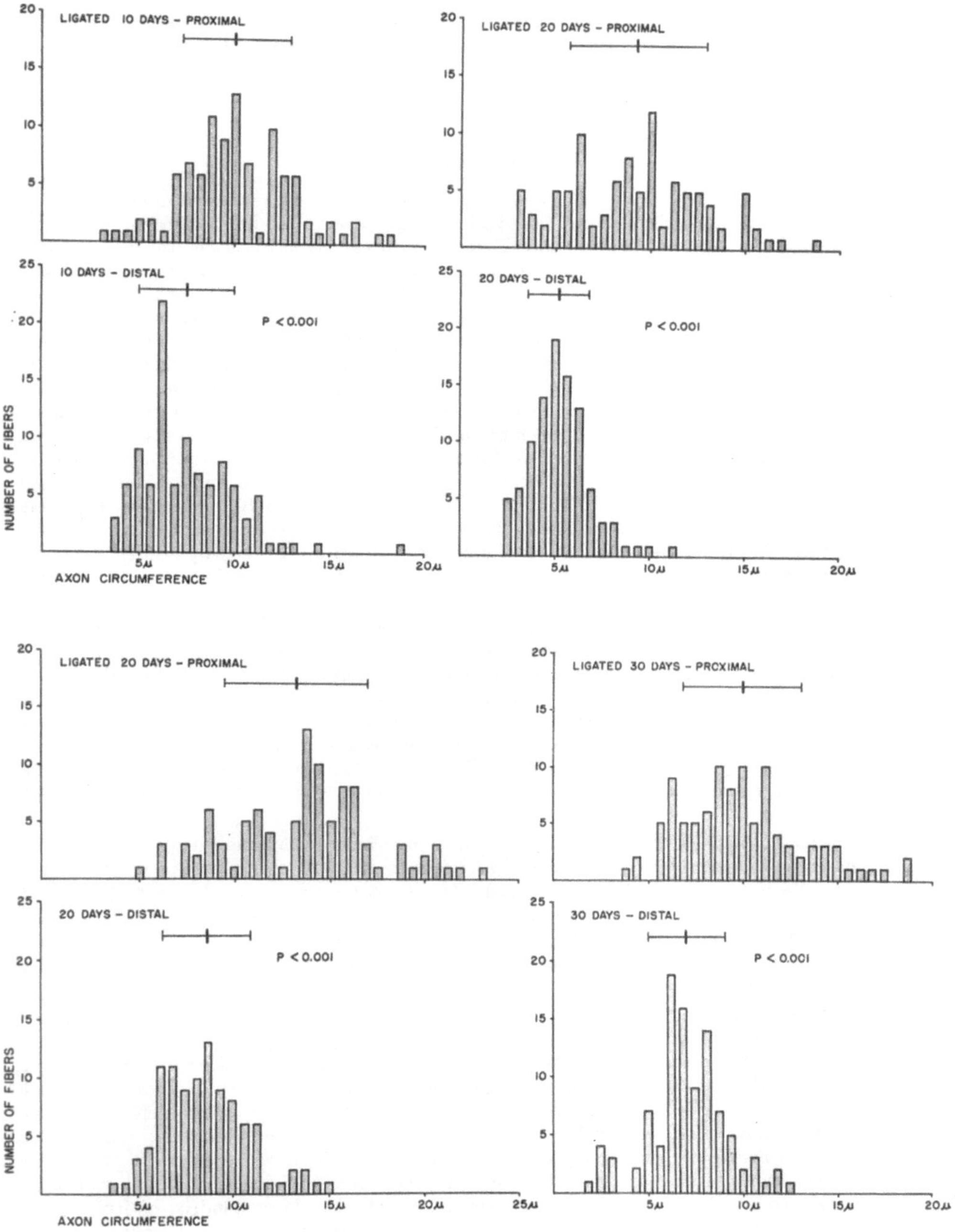

Fig. 1. Histograms of axon calibers in ligated nerves, sampled 5 mm proximal or distal, respectively, to the ligature

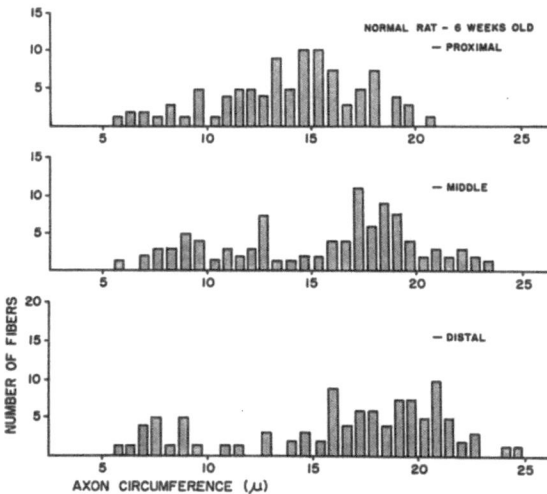

Fig. 2. Histograms of axon calibers in normal rat sciatic nerve, sampled at the same distance as the nerves shown in Fig. 1. Average fiber caliber in this control is slightly larger than the proximal samples in Fig. 1, as the control was older

Statistical analysis included calculation of means, standard deviations and *t*-tests. Regression analyses were done, where pertinent, by the least squares method, calculating correlation coefficients, their significance, and the slopes and intercepts of the regression curves.

Results

1. Hypoplasia of Nerve Fibers

Nerves were examined 10, 20 and 30 days after application of the ligatures. Plastic-embedded sections, approximately 1 μ thick, of the distal portion of the nerve showed myelinated fibers of markedly smaller calibers than is normal for nerves of that age. Histograms of axon calibers of nerves sampled 100 mm proximal and distal to the compression showed statistically highly significant changes in the fiber spectra (Fig. 1). These changes were not due to a normal tapering of the fibers, as verified in controls of normal nerves sampled at the same intervals (Fig. 2). The caliber spectra proximal to the ligature were alike those of normal nerves of the same age (Friede and Samorajski, 1968); the site of sampling was at two to three times the distance within which the "chronic" axon swellings formed.

Fig. 1 shows variation in the degree of hypoplasia, which evidently resulted from variance in the degree of compression rather than its duration. Nerves with moderate hypoplasia showed normal density of the myelinated fibers without indication of loss of fibers. Severe hypoplasia was associated with reduced density of myelinated fibers, probably due to atrophy of some of the myelinated fibers to the extent that they were not discernible with the light microscope; the presence of such fibers was confirmed in electron micrographs.

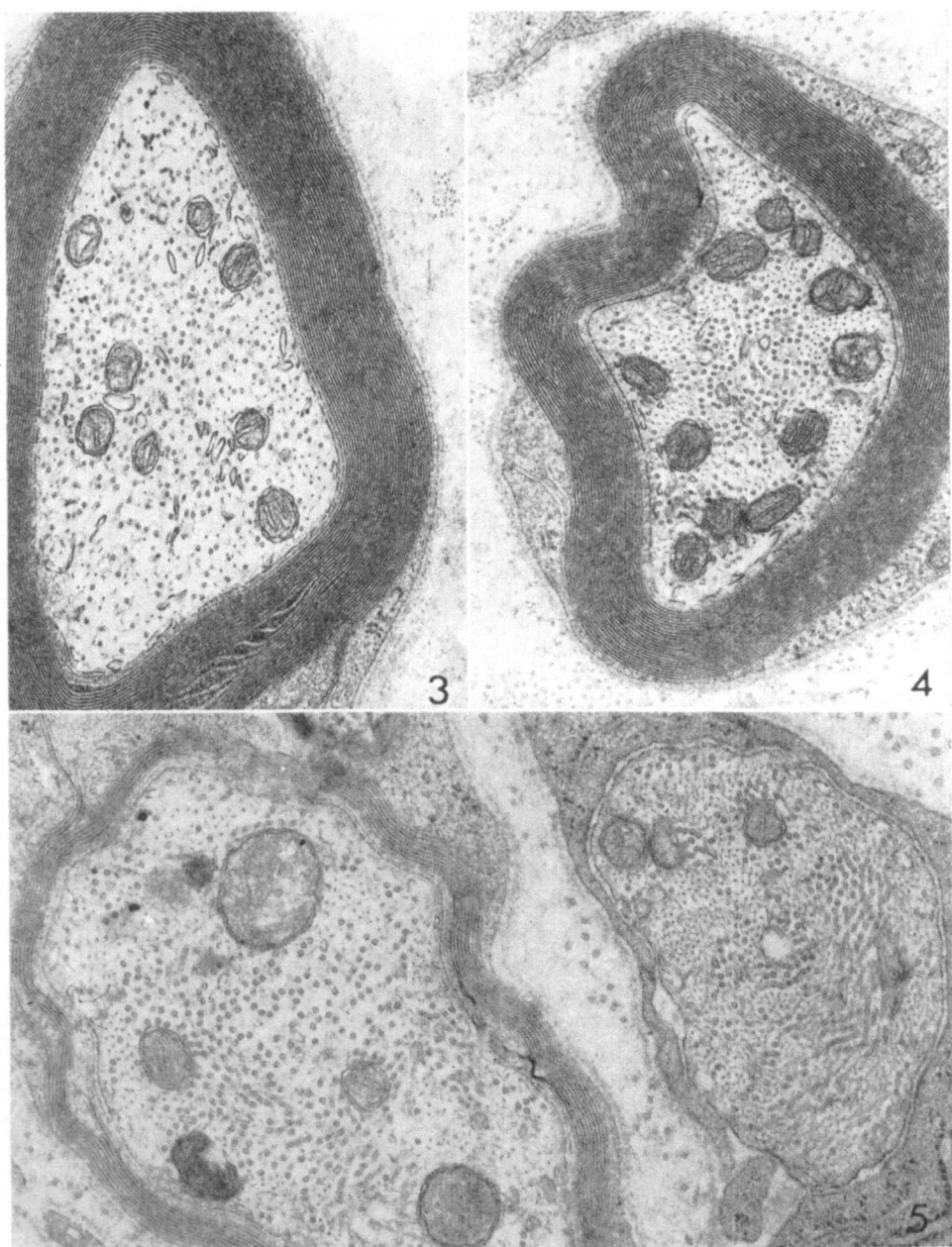

Figs. 3 and 4. Electron micrographs of hypoplastic fibers distal to the compression show essentially normal fine structure, with an increase in the number of microtubules and relatively few neurofilaments. Fig. 4 shows central bundling of the microtubules. The density of mitochondria and smooth endoplasmic reticulum is also increased, more in Fig. 4 than in Fig. 3.

31.900 ×

Fig. 5. Fine structure of fibers at the level of maximum compression underneath the ligature. The sheaths of these fibers are attenuated, and some relatively large axons lack sheaths (right). A marked increase in microtubular density is evident, with occasional clustering of tubules.

31.900 ×

2. Fine Structure of Hypoplastic Fibers

Electron micrographs of the nerve distal to the compression showed myelinated fibers having normal proportions of sheath thickness and axon caliber and a normal envelope of Schwann cell cytoplasm. The axoplasm showed somewhat increased spacing of the neurofilaments and microtubules; however, there were relatively more microtubules or fewer neurofilaments respectively than in normal fibers (Figs. 3, 4). Other axoplasmic organelles, including mitochondria, showed normal fine structure. Increased mitochondrial density was evident (Fig. 4), particularly for the very hypoplastic fibers which often were crowded with mitochondria.

Bundles of apparently normal nonmyelinated fibers were dispersed throughout the nerve; a possible increase in microtubule density was difficult to assess because nonmyelinated fibers normally have more microtubules than neurofilaments (Friede and Samorajski, 1970). In addition, there were abnormally large single nonmyelinated fibers, each having an individual Schwann cell envelope. There were also very thinly myelinated fibers with a few turns of lamellae, which are seen in normal rat sciatic nerve only during the first two weeks of life; such fibers with less than 10 lamellae become sparse thereafter (Friede and Samorajski, 1968). Fibers undergoing degenerative changes of axoplasm or sheath were not a characteristic feature but were observed in isolated instances.

The changes in axoplasmic composition were verified by determinations of neurofilament and microtubule densities. Myelinated fibers of normal rat sciatic nerves of various ages have a microtubule/neurofilament ratio ranging between 0.24 and 0.36 (Friede and Samorajski, 1970). The ratio in hypoplastic fibers ranged between 0.42 and 1.14 (Table) and was highest for the nerve with the greatest reduction in axon caliber (Fig. 1).

The tubule/filament ratios of myelinated fibers were analyzed further by plotting tubular or fibrillar densities as a function of the cross-sectional area of the axon. Plottings for normal sciatic fibers showed that both the number of tubules and filaments increased with axon caliber, although the tubules at a much slower rate than the filaments (Friede and Samorajski, 1970). The slopes of the regression curves for hypoplastic fibers were more alike for tubules and filaments, indicating increased microtubules and decreased neurofilaments (Fig. 6).

Determinations of the density of axoplasmic organelles, including mitochondria smooth endoplasmic reticulum and vesicles, by a method of line sampling showed statistically highly significant increases in organelle density for all specimens (Table), the increase being greatest for the nerve having maximum hypoplasia and maximum change in the tubule/filament ratio.

3. Changes Proximal to the Compression

The changes in the fine structure of the "chronic" axon swellings proximal to the compression (Friede and Miyagishi, 1971) are reviewed only in abstract. All myelinated fibers were swollen, with little difference in the extent of swelling, 10, 20 and 30 days after ligation. The myelin sheaths were markedly expanded and attenuated. The increase in axoplasmic volume was entirely due to the accumulation of pools of excessive, amorphous axoplasm at the periphery of the fiber and between the neurofilaments, separating the latter into individual bundles.

Table. *Axoplasmic composition of hypoplastic fibers*

Duration of compression	Number of fibres	Tubule/filament ratio (S.D.)		Organelle density (S.D.)	
10 days	20	0.42	(0.02)	16.9	(7.3)
20 days	22	1.14	(0.52)	31.0	(12.9)
20 days	22	0.51	(0.03)	21.0	(8.3)
30 days	41	0.56	(0.11)	15.5	(9.3)
Averages for normal fibers	—	0.24—0.37 (Friede and Samorajski, 1970)		6.3—8.7 (Friede and Martinez, 1970)	

The nerves are the same for which the caliber spectra are given in Fig. 1; maximum change in the tubule/filament ratio and in mitochondrial density correspond to nerve with maximum hypoplasia.

Microtubules traversed these pools separately. Determination of the density of axoplasmic organelles by the same method of line sampling as above showed normal or slightly below normal organelle densities (6.1 to 8.2).

Near and within the constricted portion of the nerve there was reduction in the volume of excess axoplasm. Increase in the density of microtubules was evident, especially for the maximally compressed fibers underneath the ligature (Fig. 5). Loss of neurofilaments, therefore, must have occurred proximal to the maximum constriction at about the same level where the pooling of the excess amorphous axoplasm occurred.

5. Changes after Releasing the Compression

Portions of nerves distal to the compression restituted rapidly—within 10 to 20 days—to a normal caliber range upon removal of the ligature. The effectiveness of the compression had been verified at the time of the removal of the ligature, when the distal portion of the nerve showed a markedly reduced caliber and, sometimes, a slightly more greyish color. The caliber range of restituted fibers showed no significant difference when compared with the proximal portion of the nerve. The thickness of the myelin sheaths also was in normal proportions with axon caliber. Determinations of the tubule/filament ratios for three restituted nerves gave the following ratios: 10 days after removal of ligature, 0.15 ± 0.05 (standard deviation); 20 days, 0.12 ± 0.03; and 30 days, 0.11 ± 0.04. These ratios were slightly below the averages for normal nerves; they indicated that the restitution corresponded to a massive "outgrowth" of neurofilaments into the hypoplastic portion of the fiber, with a corresponding increase in axon caliber.

Discussion

Our data indicate that there is a significant retardation of axon growth distal to a local compression of nerve fibers (Fig. 1). The caliber range of these hypoplastic axons remained the same as for normal axons at the age when the ligature was applied (3—15 µ; Friede and Samorajski, 1968). Hence, the hypoplasia was

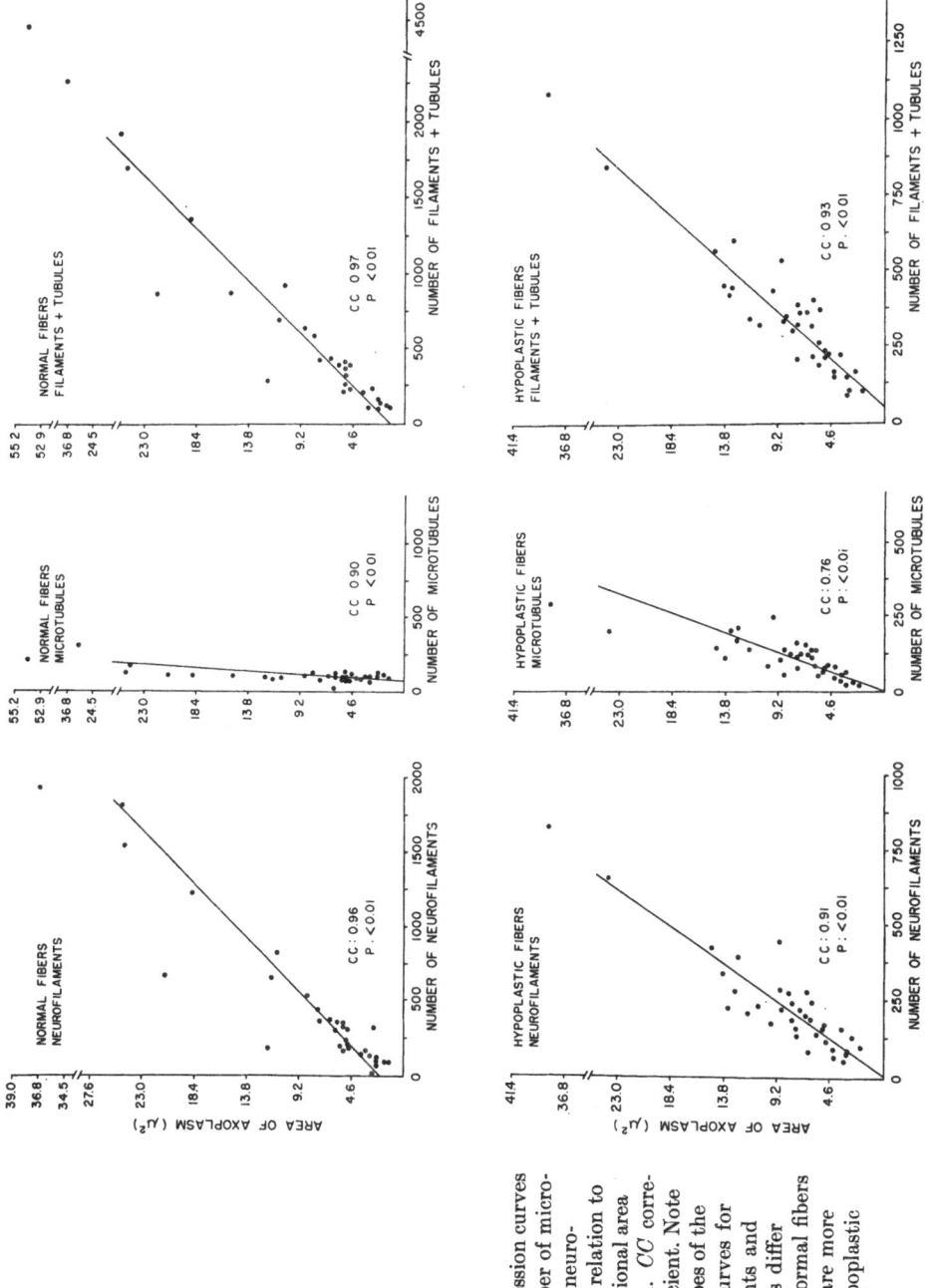

Fig. 6. Regression curves of the number of microtubules and neurofilaments in relation to te cross-sectional area of axoplasm. *CC* correlation coefficient. Note that the slopes of the regression curves for neurofilaments and microtubules differ greatly in normal fibers while they are more alike for hypoplastic fibers

mainly due to arrested growth, probably also including actual atrophy of severely compressed nerve fibers.

The most characteristic alteration in the fine structure of the hypoplastic fibers was an increase in the ratio of microtubules to neurofilaments (Figs. 3, 4) above the range for normal fibers of comparable calibers (Friede and Samorajski, 1970).

Reduction in the mean axon calibers for the four nerves shown in Fig. 1 was: 10 days, 0.75; 20 days, 0.57; 20 days, 0.63 and 30 days, 0.70. This corresponds to decreases in cross-sectional area by 0.56, 0.33, 0.40 and 0.49. If there were a corresponding, selective loss of neurofilaments, the average tubule/filament ratios would increase to: 0.53, 0.89, 0.75 and 0.63 (calculated from an average ratio of 0.3 for normal myelinated fibers). These calculated ratios corresponded rather well to those determined in the Table (0.42 to 1.14). One may assume, therefore, that the loss of neurofilaments at the compression was highly selective, the average myelinated nerve fiber in our nerves having lost approximately one half or more of its neurofilaments, with a proportionate decrease in axon caliber.

The data on axoplasmic organelles indicate that a fairly abrupt loss of approximately 50 per cent of the neurofilament population per fiber did not cause a decrease in the concentration of axoplasmic organelles including mitochondria, smooth endoplasmic reticulum and vesicles. Indeed, these organelles were normal proximal ot the constriction (Friede and Myagishi, 1971) and significantly increased distal to it (Table). Hence, there is no indication that a direct relation exists between the number of neurofilaments and the density of axoplasmic organelles. There may be a relation, on the other hand, between the microtubules and the organelles; both increased similarly in the hypoplastic fibers, the magnitude of the increases corresponding to the degree of hypoplasia. It may be more than a coincidence that the microtubular density (Friede and Samorajski, 1970) and the mitochondrial density (Samorajski and Friede, 1968) of normal nonmyelinated and myelinated fibers show similar, parallel trends, both densities being higher for the nonmyelinated fibers, and the differences being of corresponding magnitude. These observations lend support to the concept that microtubules are related in some way to the density and/or intracellular redistribution of cytoplasmic organelles (Tilney, 1965; Porter, 1966; Freed and Lebowitz, 1970).

The loss of approximately 50 per cent of the neurofilament population in the hypoplastic fibers was probably related to the accumulation of excess amorphous axoplasm in the swollen axons proximal to the constriction. The precise topographic relation between these two changes could not be defined since a search for alterations which would identify the stumps of the neurofilaments in longitudinal sections was unsuccessful. However, the available data indicate strongly that a relation exists between the loss of neurofilaments and the accumulation of excess amorphous axoplasm in the swollen fibers proximal to the constriction.

Our observations imply that both neurofilaments and microtubules extend over great distances along the axon, without having the facility of converting into each other. The number of neurofilaments appears to be related to the volume of amorphous axoplasm, and both these factors appear to be in turn related directly with axon caliber. The number of microtubules appears to be related to the density of axoplasmic organelles, including mitochondria.

Our technique offers a unique model for the experimental manipulation of neurofilaments in nerve fibers. The simplicity of the model and the selectivity of the axoplasmic changes invite further exploration toward possible correlations between changes in fine structure and changes in the rates of axonal flow.

References

Duncan, D.: Alteration in the structure of nerves caused by restricting their growth with ligatures. J. Neuropath. exp. Neurol. 7, 261—273 (1948).

Freed, J. J., Lebowitz, M. M.: The association of a class of saltory movements with microtubules in cultred cells. J. Cell Biol. 45, 334—354 (1970).

Friede, R. L., Miyagishi, T.: Adjustment of the myelin sheath to changes in axon caliber. (In preparation.)

— Samorajski, T.: Relation between the number of myelin lamellae and axon circumference in fibers of vagus and sciatic nerve of mice. J. comp. Neurol. 130, 223—232 (1967).

— — Myelin formation in the sciatic nerve of rat. A quantitative electron microscopic, histochemical and radioautographic study. J. Neuropath. exp. Neurol. 27, 546—571 (1968).

— — Axon caliber related to neurofilaments and microtubules in sciatic nerve fibers of rats and mice. Anat. Rec. 167, 319—378 (1970).

Martinez, A. J., Friede, R. L.: Accumulation of axoplasmic organelles in swellen nerve fibers. Brain Res. 19, 183—198 (1970).

Porter, K. R.: Cytoplasmic microtubules and their function. I. Ciba Foundation Symposium on Principles of Biomolecular Organization, p. 308. M. O'Connor and G. E. W. Wolstenholme, Eds. London: J. and A. Churchill, Ltd 1966.

Samorajski, T., Friede, R. L.: Size dependent distribution of axoplasm, Schwann cell cytoplasm and mitochondria in the peripheral nerve fibers of mouse. Anat. Rec. 161, 281—292 (1968).

Tilney, L. G.: Microtubules in the asymmetric arms of actinosphaerium and their response to cold, colchicine and hydrostatic pressure. Anat. Rec. 151, 426 (1965).

Reinhard L. Friede
Institute of Pathology
Case Western Reserve University
Cleveland, Ohio (U.S.A), 44106

Acta neuropath. (Berl.) Suppl. V, 226—237 (1971)

Effects of Vinblastine and Colchicine on Monoamine Containing Neurons of the Rat, with Special Regard to the Axoplasmic Transport of Amine Granules

Annica Dahlström

Institute of Neurobiology, Department of Histology, University of Göteborg, Sweden

Summary. The effects of vinblastine and colchicine on monoamine neurons has been studied by a histochemical fluorescence method. The results obtained indicate that both substances, when applied locally to adrenergic nerves, cause an inhibition in the proximo-distal transport of amine granules. These effects are discussed in relation to the destroying effects of the substances on the axonal microtubules. The effective concentrations were lower for vinblastine (10^{-3}—10^{-4} M) than for colchicine (0.05 M) and it is suggested that this effect of the drugs to inhibit granule transport may be due to their microtubule disrupting effect. The low pH of vinblastine solutions is probably not involved in this effect, since isotonic-citrate-buffer solutions of the same pH had no observable effect on granule transport.

Application of vinblastine to ganglia in concentrations high enough to cause a marked inhibition of amine granule transport, resulted in degeneration of the nerve terminals.

Also the bulbo-spinal NA and 5-HT neurons were effected by the mitosis inhibitors. This may indicate that also in the CNS the transport of amine granules in NA and 5-HT systems, may be related to microtubules.

Key-Words: Amine Granules — Axoplasmic Transport Inhibition — Vinblastine — Colchicine — Microtubules.

Introduction

In sympathetic adrenergic neurons the noradrenaline (NA) storing amine granules appear to be transported distally in the axons at fast rates (several mm/h, Dahlström and Häggendal, 1966). The rate in rat sciatic nerves appear to be about 5 mm/h, i.e. about 120 mm/day. The transport of amine granules thus belongs to the category of fast axoplasmic transport, in contrast to the slow flow of 1—2 mm/day, first described by Weiss and Hiscoe (1948).

The mechanism for the slow flow has been suggested to be the continuous outgrowth of axoplasm from the perikarya (cf. Weiss, 1961), whereas the mechanism for the fast transport is so far essentially unknown. In 1967 it was proposed that the fibrous proteins of the axons, particularly the microtubules, could act as a structural basis for fast transport systems (e.g. Taylor, 1967; Schmitt, 1968).

Certain mitosis inhibitors, e.g. colchicine and vinblastine have been found to selectively destroy the organization of microtubules (Borisy and Taylor, 1967; Weisenberg, 1968; Weisenberg and Timasheff, 1969). These substances have been applied locally to adrenergic neurons to test the possibility that the fast transport of amine granules may be dependent on the microtubules in the adrenergic axons. In a preliminary report the effect of colchicine on adrenergic nerves has been described (Dahlström, 1968). The results obtained indicated that colchicine interrupted the transport of the granules. This effect was discussed as possibly being due to the ability of colchicine to disrupt the microtubules in the neurons, furnishing some support for the hypothesis that the microtubules were involved in transport of granules.

Also vinblastine has now been tested on adrenergic neurons[1], and the present article will describe and discuss the results obtained with both vinblastine and colchicine, locally applicated to monoamine containing neurons in the rat.

Material and Methods

Male albino rats of the Sprague-Dawley strain were used. Colchicine (Sandoz) or vinblastine (Velbe®, Lilly) were dissolved in saline at concentrations of 20% (corresponding to 0.5 M), 2%, 0.2%, and 1% (corresponding to about 0.01 M), 0.1%, 0.01% and 0.001%, respectively. Three to five rats were used for each group. All operations were performed under ether anaesthesia. After dissection of the tissues, the specimens were frozen in liquid propane, cooled by liquid nitrogene, freeze-dried at $-50°$C to $-35°$C for $1-3$ days. Thereafter they were treated with paraformaldehyde and handled according to the histochemical fluorescence method of Hillarp and Falck for the visualization of catecholamines and 5-hydroxytryptamine (5-HT) (for references and description see e.g. Falck and Owman, 1965; Corrodi and Jonsson, 1967; Eränkö, 1967).

Four different monoaminergic systems were studied:

a) The lumbar sympathetic chain, giving adrenergic axons to i.a. the sciatic nerve, was exposed by laparatomy, and small cotton pellets which were soaked with the test-solutions, were carefully placed over the ganglia. Ten min later the pellets were removed, and the treated area was carefully cleaned with pellets, soaked in saline. The abdomen was closed by silk ligatures and external clips. Twentyfour hours after this operation the sciatic nerves were ligated (crushed) bilaterally according to Lubińska (1959) (Fig. 1a). The animals were killed 2 h after the ligations, and the lumbar ganglia and the sciatic nerves were dissected out. Animals treated with saline on the ganglia served as controls for the mechanical handling. In some cases the ganglia were dissected out 3 h after the initial operation.

Some animals were treated with an isotonic citrate-buffer (McIlvaines, pH 4.5) to serve as controls for the low pH of the vinblastine solutions (the pH of 0.1% vinblastine in saline $\approx$ 4.5). Some rats, the ganglia of which had been treated with 0.1% solution of vinblastine, were given reserpine (10 mg/kg i.p.) 7 h before death.

b) With a thin cannula (gauge 27) small amounts of the solutions $(3-5 \mu l)$ were injected unilaterally under the perineurium of the sciatic nerve, at a high level (about 1 cm below the for. infrapiriformis). The contralateral nerve was injected with saline. Twentyfour hours later ligations were performed bilaterally at a level about 2 cm below the level of the injections (Fig. 1b). The animals were killed 2 h later and the sciatic nerves, from the for. infrapir. and distally just beyond the site of ligation, were dissected out in one piece.

c) The cervical superior ganglion unilaterally was carefully soaked for 15 min with the test-solutions, applied to small cotton pellets. In this group only vinblastine was used. The contralateral ganglion was treated with saline (control for the mechanical handling). At different time intervals after this operation (18, 24, 48 h and 5 days) the ganglia and the irides were dissected out. The irides were spread on glass-slides, air-dried, and treated for fluorescence microscopy according to Falck et al. (1962) and Malmfors (1965).

Some rats, the ganglia of which had been treated with 0.1% vinblastine 24 h prior to death, were given α-methyl-NA (Corbasil®, Hoechst) (0.1 mg/kg i.v.) 30 min before death.

d) For studying the effect of the mitosis inhibitors on central monoamine neurons, the spinal cord was exposed at a mid-thoracic level by removal of one vertebral lamina. A small cotton pellet, soaked with the test-solution, was carefully spread over the exposed area, with particular care taken that the lateral edges of the pellet reached the dorsal part of the lateral funiculi. Ten min after the application of the pellets, these were removed. Animals treated with saline served as controls for the mechanical manipulations.

---

1 Results with vinblastine have briefly been presented at Bayer Symposium II, October, 1969 (Dahlström, 1970).

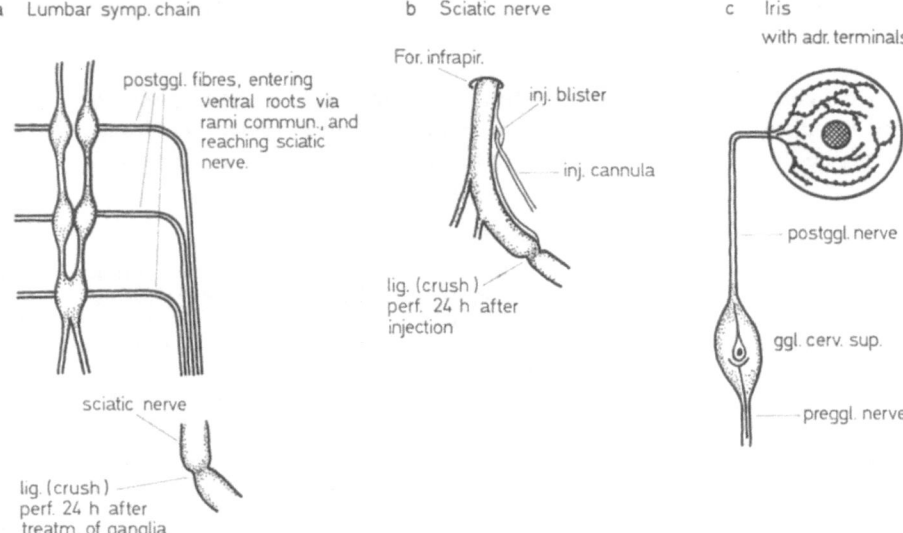

a Lumbar symp. chain

postggl. fibres, entering
ventral roots via
rami commun., and
reaching sciatic
nerve.

sciatic nerve

lig. (crush)
perf. 24 h after
treatm. of ganglia

b Sciatic nerve

For. infrapir.

inj. blister

inj. cannula

lig. (crush)
perf. 24 h after
injection

c Iris
with adr. terminals

postggl. nerve

ggl. cerv. sup.

preggl. nerve

Fig. 1a—c. Schematic illustrations of the peripheral neuron-systems studied

Results and Discussion

The green fluorescence observed under the microscope in perikarya, axons and nerve terminals of peripheral adrenergic neurons is due to the presence of NA (for discussion see e.g. Norberg and Hamberger, 1965; Corrodi and Jonsson, 1967). Therefore, the changes observed in amount and intensity of green fluorescent material will in the following be referred to as changes in NA content or concentration. Likewise, the green fluorescence observed in the spinal cord is most probably due to the presence of NA, while the yellow fluorescence is due to 5-HT (see discussion in e.g. Dahlström and Fuxe, 1965).

a) Lumbar sympathetic ganglia. In normal or saline treated ganglia the cytoplasm of the cell bodies shows low to medium fluorescence intensities. Some cells are non-fluorescent, and probably represent cholinergic nerve cell bodies (see discussion in Norberg and Hamberger, 1965). The intraganglionic axons are thin and smooth, and of low fluorescence intensities (Fig. 2a).

In ganglia treated with vinblastine or colchicine a marked increase in the NA content of both perikarya and axons was observed. Already 3 h after soaking the ganglia with the test solutions some cell bodies had developed strong fluorescence intensities, and so had some of the intraganglionic axons. Twentyfour hours after the treatment almost all cell bodies had a markedly increased NA content, and this increase was often most marked in the periphery of the cells (Fig. 2b). The intraganglionic axons were enlarged in diameter, and strongly fluorescent. Such effects were observed with 20 % and 2 % (0.05 M) colchicine, while 0.2 % solutions had very little or no effects. Vinblastine was effective in concentrations of 1 %, 0.1 % and 0.01 % (10^{-4} M), while the 0.001 % concentrations caused weak to

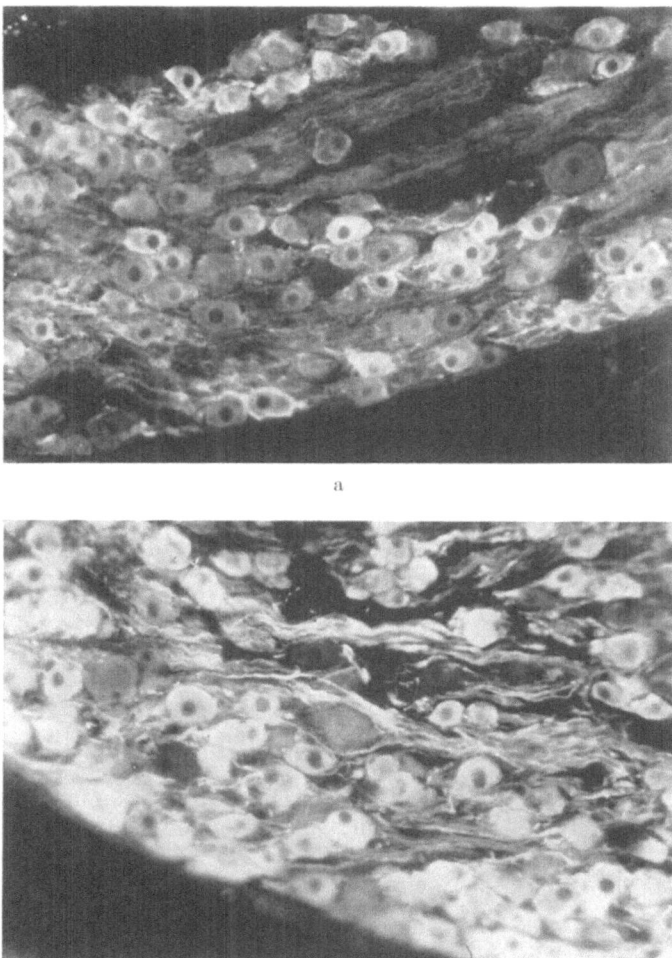

Fig. 2. a Lumbar sympathetic ganglion, treated locally with saline 24 h before sacrifice. The green fluorescence observed is due to the presence of noradrenaline (NA). The cell bodies have weak or medium fluorescence intensities, while the intraganglionic axons are thin, smooth and of weak fluorescence intensity.   b Lumbar sympathetic ganglion treated with 20% colchicine in saline 24 h before death. Most cell bodies have strong fluorescence intensities, often specially marked in the periphery of the perikarya. The intraganglionic axons are dilated, and of strong fluorescence intensity, indicating a marked increase in NA content after the colchicine treatment. Fluorescence microphotographs, ×220

moderate changes in half of the animals, and no observable change in the rest of the group.

This increase in NA in perikarya and axons was probably due to an increase in NA, bound to a specific storage protein, since reserpine administration could completely abolish all NA fluorescence in the ganglia. It is thus possible that the

NA increase was due to an increased number of amine storage granules in perikarya and axons. Electronmicroscopical studies together with Hökfelt (Hökfelt
and Dahlström, 1970, 1971) have shown an increased number of dense cored
vesicles in perikarya of colchicine or vinblastine treated ganglia.

In the sciatic nerves of rats, the ganglia of which showed a marked increase in
NA, no or little NA accumulated above the ligations. In saline treated rats normal
amounts of NA were accumulated (see Fig. 7 in Dahlström, 1970).

These results seem to indicate that both vinblastine and colchicine, applied
to the lumbar ganglia, inhibit the transport of amine granules from the cell
bodies and intraganglionic axons to the axons in the sciatic nerve. The increased
NA content observed in the cell bodies may be due to a continued production of
amine granules (or precursors of amine granules) in the cell bodies together with
the inhibition of the export from the cell bodies of the formed granules.

At present, this explanation seems to be reasonable. It is possible that this
effect of the two substances is related to their capacity to destroy microtubules.
Colchicine had to be applied in rather high concentrations (c:a $0.05-0.5$ M),
while vinblastine was effective in $10^{-3}-10^{-4}$ M concentrations. Therefore, one
may speculate as to wheather the vinblastine effect is more specific than the
effect of colchicine. However, since the substances were sokaed on the ganglia
and not injected into them, and since the cotton pellets with the solution were
removed 10 min after the application, differences in rates of diffusion between
the two substances may play a role.

The vinblastine substance has a buffer capacity, and e.g. a 0.1% solution in
saline has a pH of about 4.5. In order to see if the low pH of the solutions had
any part in the vinblastine effects observed, an isotonic citrate-buffer of pH 4.5
(McIlvaines buffer) was tested. The picture obtained after buffer treatment was
very similar to the picture obtained in saline controls, and normal amounts of
NA were found accumulated in the sciatic nerves. Therefore, it seems unlikely
that the effects of vinblastine should be due to the low pH of the solutions.

b) Sciatic nerves. Also when the test solutions were applied to axons, marked
effects were noticed. The saline injected area of the sciatic showed in most cases
a normal appearance, but occasionally a few axons with swollen appearance and
strong fluorescence were observed. These NA accumulations were probably due
to the trauma caused occasionally by the injection. In such nerves the amount
of NA accumulating above the low ligation, was normal. In vinblastine or colchicine
injected nerves dilated, strongly fluorescent fibres were seen all through the nerve
diameter (see Fig. 8a in Dahlström, 1970). Such accumulated fibres were observed
within and above the area of the injection blister. Since the perineurium
is a rather elastic sheath, it was difficult to decide how far in both directions the
injected solutions had penetrated along the nerve. In those nerves with pronounced
NA accumulations at the level of the injection no, or occasionally a few, weakly
fluorescent fibres were observed above the low ligation (see Fig. 8 b in Dahlström,
1970).

The effective concentrations of the respective substances were similar to those
mentioned in a). Thus, 0.2% colchicine or 0.001% vinblastine caused no or minor
changes.

The results obtained indicate that both substances, when injected perineurally in the sciatic nerve, cause an arrest in the proximodistal transport of amine granules in the adrenergic axons of this nerve. The granules which were being transported down from higher levels of the nerve could obviously not pass through the area of the injection, hence the pronounced accumulations of NA in dilated adrenergic fibres in this region. The lack of NA accumulations above a low ligation, performed 22 h after injection, supports this interpretation.

Depolymerization of the axonal microtubules may be the reason of this interruption in transport of NA granules. After local treatment with vinblastine of the interganglionic nerves of the lumbar sympathetic chain, which induces accumulations of NA in the fibres, a large number of dense cored vesicles have been observed at the ultrastructural level (Hökfelt and Dahlström, 1970, 1971). Glutaraldehyde-osmium fixation of such nerves revealed a picture where microtubules were not observed. Thus, the data obtained so far seem to support the hypothesis that microtubules are involved in transport of amine granules.

Kreutzberg in 1968 performed similar experiments with injections of colchicine under the perineurium of the rat sciatic nerve. He found that acetylcholine-esterase (AChE) accumulated above and within the injection area, and furthermore, no AChE accumulated above a low ligation of the same nerve, performed several hours later (Kreutzberg, personal communication 1968, 1969). This may indicate that also AChE, intraaxonally probably bound to the membrane of the smooth endoplasmic reticulum, travels distally in axons by some mechanism related to the microtubules.

c) Cervical Superior Ganglion with its Adrenergic Nerve Terminals. This neuron system was studied since the nerve terminals of the treated ganglion cells were easily accessible, and could be observed in the irides by a simple technique. The question had arisen during the progress of the forementioned experiments: What happens to the nerve terminals after treatment of the cell bodies with vinblastine ?

Since vinblastine had been found to be effective in smaller concentrations than colchicine and since this substance was less toxic than colchicine, only vinblastine was used in these experiments.

The ggl. cerv. sup. are larger than the lumbar ganglia and the cotton pellets were therefore left *in situ* for 15 min instead of 10 min, to allow more time for diffusion of the substance into the ganglion. Essentially the same observations were made in this ganglion as in the lumbar ganglia after vinblastine treatment. However, since the efferent fibres are more aggregated in bundles in the neck ganglia, a common feature was the presence of huge amounts of NA, accumulated in these efferent fibres (Fig. 3).

The effective concentrations of vinblastine were 1% and 0.1%. With 0.01% varying results were obtained, and with 0.001% clear accumulations of NA were observed only in one animal. It must be pointed out that the route of administration does not allow a quantitation of the amount of substance which reaches the cells. The cotton pellets were of similar size, but variation in e.g. the thickness of the capsule and of the ganglion may well influence the results.

In the irides of the saline treated sides the adrenergic nerve terminals formed a dense plexus, with distinct and strongly fluorescent varicosities (Fig. 4a). After vinblastine treatment the number of terminals decreased. At 18 h the intensity

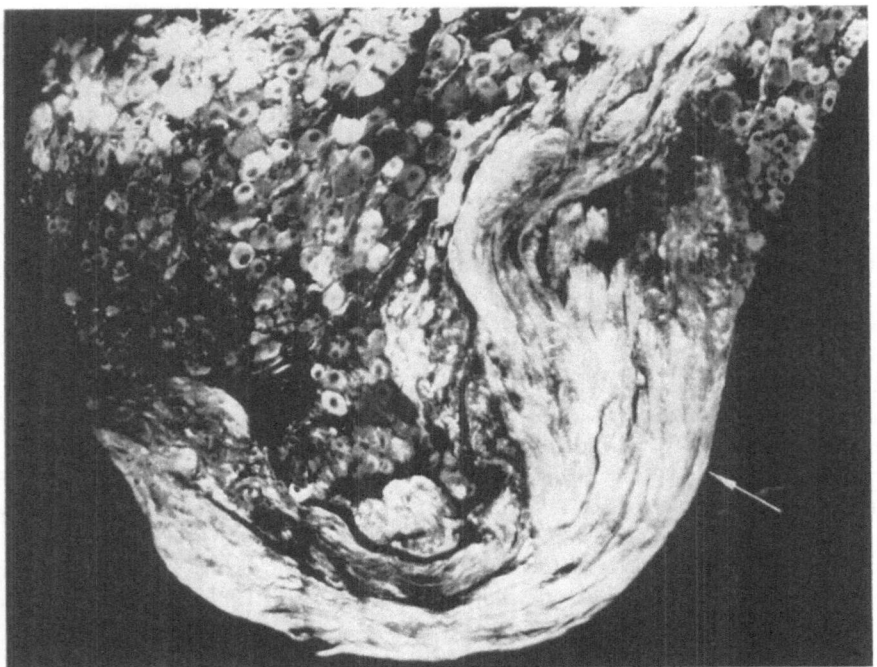

Fig. 3. Cervical sympathetic ganglion from a rat, treated with 0.1°/₀ vinblastine 24 h before death. A high number of fluorescent cells of supranormal intensity can be observed. The axons, normally of weak fluorescence intensity, are strongly fluorescent, which is particularly striking in the efferent bundle (→). The fluorescence is due to the presence of NA. Fluorescence microphotographs, ×100

of many terminal fibres was decreased, but the number still appeared to be unchanged. Six hours later most terminals had disappeared, a few had a very weak fluorescence intensity and had lost the characteristic varicose appearance, while some terminals looked quite normal (Fig. 4b)[1]. The amount of remaining terminals with normal appearance was related to the concentration of vinblastine used.

---

[1] At this time ptosis was present on the vinblastine treated side (Dahlström, Häggendal and Linder, in preparation).

Fig. 4a—c. Set of photographs illustrating the effects on adrenergic nerve terminals of vinblastine treatment of the cervical superior ganglion. a Whole mount preparation of an iris of a rat treated locally with saline on the ipsilateral cervical ganglion 24 h before sacrifice. The adrenergic nerve terminal plexus is dense, and shows the characteristic appearance of strongly fluorescent varicosities along the fibres. b Iris-preparation from the contralateral side of the same rat as in a). The cervical ganglion of this side was treated with 0.1°/₀ vinblastine 24 h before death. The density of terminals is clearly reduced, one terminal fibre of normal fluorescence with its arborizations is seen, together with some fibres with very low fluorescence (→). c Iris from a rat with 1°/₀ vinblastine treatment on the ipsilateral cervical ganglion. The iris is almost devoid of fluorescent nerve terminals. One single, faintly fluorescent fibre is observed, running diagonally in the picture. Fluorescence microphotographs, ×400

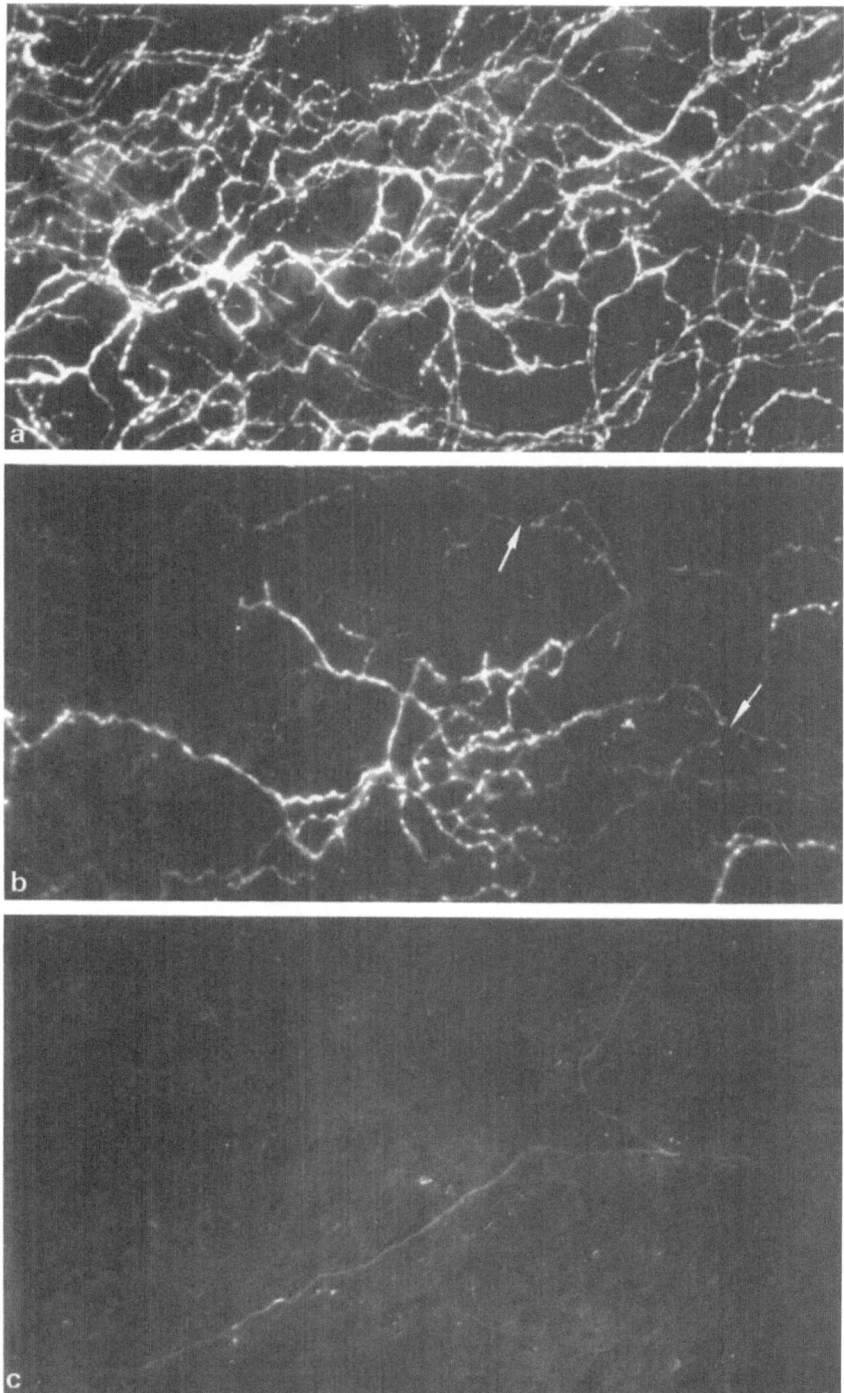

Fig. 4 a—c

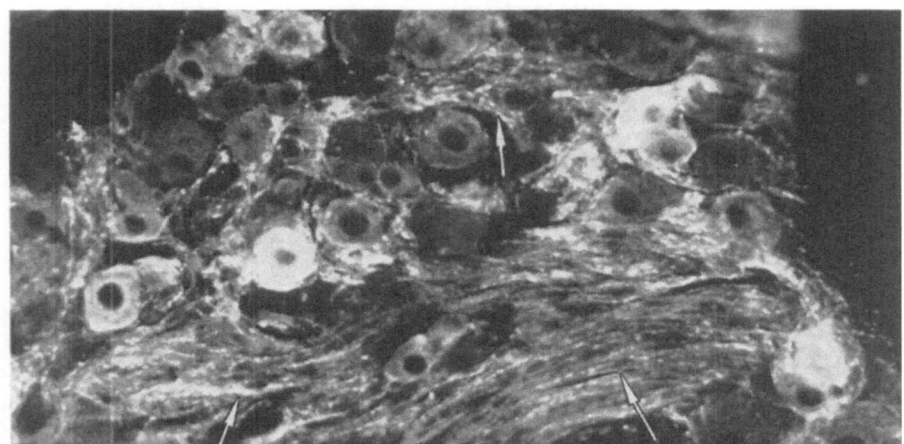

Fig. 5. Cervical superior ganglion, treated with 0.1% vinblastine 5 days before sacrifice. Many weakly fluorescent and a few strongly fluorescent cell bodies are seen. A large number of thin fibres of moderate fluorescence intensity and with irregular varicosities are indicated (→). These fibres may represent regenerating axons. Fluorescence microphotograph, ×400

Thus, in irides, the ganglia of which were treated with a 1% solution no (Fig. 4c) or only very few normal fibres were remaining 24 and 48 h after treatment. After treatment with 0.1% some more normal fibres were observed, while treatment with 0.01% in some iride caused only a moderate decrease in nerve terminals.

In order to find out if the invisible nerve terminals were degenerated or only lacked the NA content, α-methyl-NA was given to 3 rats, unilaterally treated with 0.1% vinblastine. The amounts of fluorescent nerve terminals was essentially similar to the number observed without α-methyl-NA. Since α-methyl-NA is taken up through the nerve membrane, but not deaminated by MAO, it is accumulating in intact nerve terminals, and gives rise to a fluorescence like that of NA. The appearent inability of the α-methyl-NA treatment to increase the number of fluorescent nerve terminals was indicative of a true degeneration of the nerve terminals.

Five days after treatment, the few remaining normal nerve terminals showed signs of outgrowth into the areas which lacked nerve terminals. Growth cones were frequently observed. According to Olson and Malmfors (1970) the growth of "adult" adrenergic terminals can only be induced by a truly denervated tissue. Thus, this also indicates that the invisible nerve terminals were really degenerated.

In the ganglia at 5 days the marked accumulations of fluorescent material in cell bodies and axons had almost disappeared. Some cells were still of strong intensity, but most cells had a weak fluorescence intensity (Fig. 5). A common feature in these ganglia was the over all presence of thin, varicose fibres, with a medium fluorescence intensity (Fig. 5). These fibres, not observed in the control ganglion, may possibly be regenerating axons.

d) Spinal Cords. The application of vinblastine or colchicine to the spinal cords caused marked accumulations of NA and 5-HT in the descending axons of bulbo-

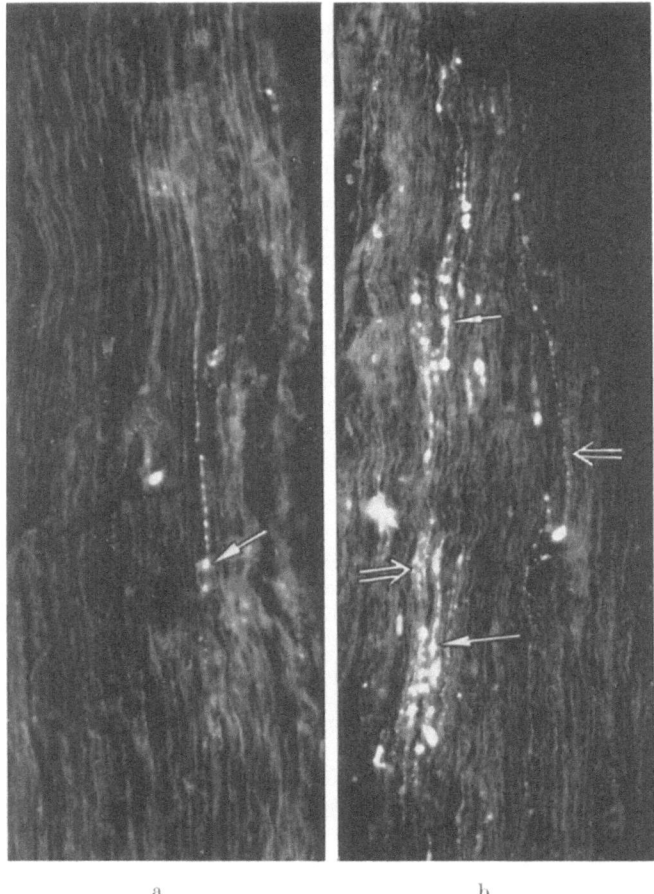

a   b

Fig. 6. From the spinal cord (lateral funiculus) of rat 3 h (a) and 24 h (b) after local treatment with 0.1% vinblastine. Accumulations of green NA induced fluorescence ($\rightarrow$) and of yellow 5-HT induced fluorescence ($\Rightarrow$) are observed in bulgy, dilated fibres. The fibres with 5-HT accumulations are generally thinner than the fibres with NA accumulations. Fluorescence microphotographs, $\times 260$

spinal NA and 5-HT containing neurons, respectively. (For disc. on monoamine systems in the spinal cord see Dahlström and Fuxe, 1965.) Three hours after treatment accumulated fibres were observed (Fig. 6a), and the number of accumulated material within the fibres was clearly increased at 24 h (Fig. 6b).

The colchicine applications had a very toxic effect on the animals, and 5 out of 6 treated rats died in convulsions within 24 h. Two of the rats developed convulsions very soon after arousal from the anaesthesia. The concentrations used were 20% and 2%. In addition to the accumulated NA and 5-HT fibres, the rest of the fibres of the cord showed degenerative changes.

The vinblastine treatment appeared much less toxic. The animals appeared normal, as compared to the saline treated controls, during the 24 h-period, and no paresis was apparent. The sensory system, as tested by pinching the tails, seemed to function.

The results may indicate that also in central monoamine neurons, the two mitosis inhibitors arrest the proximo-distal transport of amine granules. This transport, as regards the NA neurons is probably slower than in the peripheral adrenergic neuron (only some 20 mm/day, Häggendal and Dahlström, 1969), and may be referred to as of intermediate speed and may, thus, possibly be connected to the microtubules, as suggested by the inhibition caused by vinblastine and colchicine.

The results of this study may indicate that proximo-distal flow of amine granules in central and peripheral monoamine neurons is connected to the microtubules, The interpretation of effects obtained with mitosis inhibitors must, however, be made with caution, particularly since Wilson et al. (1970) have demonstrated that vinblastine also has effects on other proteins than microtubule protein in cells. An interesting observation which should be mentioned in this connection has been made by Järlfors and Smith (1969) in cholinergic neurons of the lamprey. They found synaptic vesicles, aggregated along microtubules in a very regular pattern. In cross sections it was observed up to 5 vesicles, surrounding each microtubule, sometimes connected with the tubular wall by thin side arms. In the synaptic region the vesicles were not connected with tubules, but "naked" tubules were observed. This picture may possibly indicate that the microtubules in this neuron system are the "highways" for a tentative distally directed transport of transmitter vesicles in the axons.

Acknowledgement. The studies reported in this article have been supported by grants from the Swedish Medical Research Council (grants no. B70-14X-2207-04, K70-40P-3045-01A, B71-14X-2207-05A), by a grant from Magnus Bergwalls Foundation, from Gustav and Majen Lindgrens Foundation, and from Wilhelm and Martina Lundgrens Foundation.

For generous supply of drugs I thank Swedish CIBA, Stockholm (reserpine, Serpasil®), Swedish Hoechst, Stockholm (α-methyl-noradrenaline, Corbasil®) and Eli Lilly Co. (vinblastine, Velbe®).

The skilful technical assistance of Mrs. Kirsten Collin and Mr. Pär-Anders Larsson is gratefully acknowledged.

References

Borisy, G. G., Taylor, E. W.: The mechanism of action of colchicine. Binding of colchicine-³H to cellular protein. J. Cell Biol. **34**, 525—533 (1967).

Corrodi, H., Jonsson, G.: The formaldehyde fluorescence method for the histochemical demonstration of biogenic amines. A review on the methodology. J. Histochem. Cytochem. **15**, 65—78 (1967).

Dahlström, A.: Effect of colchicine on transport of amine storage granules in sympathetic nerves of rat. Europ. J. Pharmacol. **5**, 111—113 (1968).

— The effect of drugs on axonal transport of amine storage granules. In: New Aspects of Storage and Release of Catecholamines. Bayer Symposium II, pp. 20—36. Berlin-Heidelberg-New York: Springer 1970.

— Fuxe, K.: Evidence for the existence of monoamine containing neurons in the central nervous system. II. Experimentally induced changes in the intraneuronal amine levels of bulbo-spinal neuron systems. Acta physiol. scand. **64**, Suppl. 247, 1—36 (1965).

— Häggendal, J.: Studies on the transport and life-span of amine storage granules in a peripheral adrenergic neuron system. Acta physiol. scand. **67**, 278—288 (1966).

Eränkö, O.: The practical histochemical demonstration of catecholamines by formaldehyde induced fluorescence. J. roy. Micr. Soc. 87, 259—276 (1967).

Falck, B., Hillarp, N. Å., Thieme, G., Torp, A.: Fluorescence of catecholamines and related compounds condensed with formaldehyde. J. Histochem. Cytochem. 10, 348—354 (1962).

— Owman, Ch.: A detailed methodological description of the fluorescence method for the cellular demonstration of biogenic monoamines. Acta Univ. lund., sect. II. 7, 1—23 (1965).

Häggendal, J., Dahlström, A.: The transport and life-span of amine storage granules in bulbospinal noradrenaline neurons of the rat. J. Pharm. Pharmacol. 21, 55—57 (1969).

Hökfelt, T., Dahlström, A.: Electronmicroscopical observations on the distribution and transport of noradrenaline storage particles after local treatment with mitosis inhibitors. Acta physiol. scand. Suppl. 357, 10—11 (1970).

— — Effects of colchicine and vinblastine on the distribution and transport of noradrenaline storage particles, studied by electron and fluorescence microscopy. Z. Zellforsch. (in press) (1971).

Järlfors, U., Smith, D. S.: Association between synaptic vesicles and neurotubules. Nature (Lond.) 224, 710—711 (1969).

Kreutzberg, G.: Neuronal dynamics and axonal flow. IV. Blockage of intra-axonal enzyme transport by colchicine. Proc. nat. Acad. Sci. (Wash.) 62, 722—728 (1969).

Lubińska, L.: Region of transition between preserved and regenerating parts of myelinated nerve fibres. J. comp. Neurol. 113, 315—335 (1959).

Malmfors, T.: Studies on adrenergic nerves. The use of rat and mouse iris for direct observations on their physiology and pharmacology at cellular and subcellular levels. Acta physiol. scand. 64, Suppl. 248, 1—93 (1965).

Norberg, K.-A., Hamberger, B.: The sympathetic adrenergic neuron. Some characteristics revealed by histochemical studies on the intraneuronal distribution of the transmitter. Acta physiol. scand. 63, Suppl. 238, 1—42 (1964).

Olson, L., Malmfors, T.: Growth characteristics of adrenergic nerves in the adult rat. Acta physiol. scand. Suppl. 348 (1970).

Schmitt, F. O.: The molecular biology of neural fibrous proteisn. Neurosci. Res. Progr. Bull. 6, 119—144 (1968).

Taylor, E. W.: Contractile proteins and cytoplasmic movement. Neurosci. Res. Progr. Bull. 5, 333—337 (1967).

Weisenberg, R. W.: Studies on the chemistry of microtubule protein. Ph. D. Thesis, University of Chicago 1968.

— Timasheff, S. N.: Aggregation of microtubule protein induced by vinblastine. Biophys. J. 9, A 174 (1969).

Weiss, P.: The concept of perpetual neuronal growth and proximodistal substance convection. In: Regional Neurochemistry (S. S. Kety and J. Elkes, eds.) p. 220. New York: Pergamon Press 1961.

— Hiscoe, H.: Experimentals on the mechanism of nerve growth. J. exp. Zool. 107, 315—396 (1948).

Wilson, L., Bryan, J., Ruby, A., Mazia, D.: Precipitation of proteins by vinblastine and calcium ions. Proc. nat. Acad. Sci. (Wash.) 66, 807—814 (1970).

Annica Dahlström
Institute of Neurobiology
Department of Histology
University of Göteborg
Göteborg, Sweden

Acta neuropath. (Berl.) Suppl. V, 238—248 (1971)
© by Springer-Verlag 1971

The Importance of Axoplasmic Transport of Amine Granules for the Functions of Adrenergic Neurons *

JAN HÄGGENDAL and ANNICA DAHLSTRÖM

Department of Pharmacology and Department of Histology
(Institute of Neurobiology), University of Göteborg, Göteborg, Sweden

Summary. In the adrenergic neurons, the amine granules which are formed in the cell bodies and transported to the nerve terminals at a rate of several mm/h, probably play an important role for the functions of the nerve terminals. Results obtained with and without reserpine pre-treatment indicate that the average life-span of the granules with regard to their capacity to store endogenous noradrenaline (NA) is about 4 weeks. The capacity of the granules to store ^{3}H-NA, on the other hand, appears to be rather short-lasting, in the order of a few days. This indicates that the new amine granules may be more active in storing ^{3}H-NA than the older granules. Hypothetically, also the release of the transmitter may occur predominatly from the new granules.

Experiments with axotomy at different levels in non-reserpinized animals indicate that some factor, needed for the maintenance of the nerve terminals, is transported distally in adrenergic axons at a rate of about 10 mm/h. It is discussed if this factor may be the amine granules.

Key-Words: Adrenergic Neuron — Amine Granules — Axoplasmic Transport — Nerve Function.

Amine storage granules from adrenergic nerves were demonstrated in 1956, when Euler and Hillarp (1956) could isolate a noradrenaline (NA) storing particle from homogenates of bovine splenic nerves. These particles were found to have many characteristics in common with amine granules from the adrenals, but some differences have also been pointed out (see review in e.g. Iversen, 1967).

I. Properties of Amine Granules

Isolated nerve granules contain a specific NA storage protein, named chromogranin, and large amounts of ATP, which are essential for the intragranular storage of NA. They also contain the protein dopamine (DA)-β-hydroxylase, which converts DA to NA. The granules thus participate in the synthesis of NA, which occurs in all parts of the neuron, but predominantly in the nerve terminals. The nerve terminals contain the majority of the amine granules in the neuron (for references see review by Iversen, 1967).

* The studies were supported by grants from the Swedish Medical Research Council (grants nr. B71-14X-166-07C, B71-14X-2207-05A), from the Medical Faculty at the University of Göteborg (Gustav and Majen Lindgrens Foundation), from Wilhelm and Martina Lundbergs Science Foundation, and from Magnus Bergwall Foundation (A. Dahlström).

We are grateful for the generous supply of drugs from the Swedish CIBA, Stockholm (reserpine, Serpasil®).

The isolated granules have certain characteristic physiological and pharmacological properties. They take up and store amines. The NA storage mechanism is reserpine-sensitive, i.e. addition of reserpine to the incubation medium causes a leakage of the amines from the granules, and an inability of the particle to store NA (cf. Stjärne, 1964).

The adrenergic neurons of normal animals react to pharmacological treatments in such a way that it may be assumed that the major part of the intraneuronal NA is bound to "amine granules". The term "amine granules" is thus used for a particle with certain physiological and pharmacological properties.

Electronmicroscopists have tried to correlate this physiologico-pharmacological concept with a morphological structure. The dense cored vesicles, probably both the small *and* the large types, have been identified in $KMnO_4$ fixed tissues to represent the amine granules (cf. Hökfelt, 1968). These vesicles have a typical triple-layered membrane, and have been found in high numbers in adrenergic nerve terminals, but in small numbers in axons and adrenergic perikarya (Hökfelt, 1969). It has been claimed that the amount of dense cored vesicles observed in perikarya and axons is too low to account for the amount of reserpine-depletable NA. It is possible that aggregations of storage proteins with NA but without e.g. the external "envelope" may in the perikarya react to pharmacological treatment like fully developed amine granules. In this connection it must be observed that much knowledge about the properties of granules have been obtained from granules isolated from the axons of the splenic nerve; "mature" granules are thus present in the non-terminal axons of adrenergic neurons.

The amine storage granules are, after having been formed in the perikarya of adrenergic neurons, transported proximo-distally in the axons to the nerve terminals. The rate of this proximo-distal axonal transport seems to be several mm/h, as observed by different methods (Dahlström and Häggendal, 1966a; Laduron and Belpaire, 1968; Livett et al., 1968; Banks et al., 1969). Electronmicroscopically, rapidly occurring accumulations of dense cored vesicles have been observed in ligated nerves, suggesting a transport in the axon of morphologically "mature" amine granules (Geffen and Ostberg, 1969).

Thus, the nerve terminals continuously seem to be supplied with a certain amount of new amine granules per unit of time. The average life-span of the granules in the nerve terminals, with respect to their capacity to store endogenous NA, has been calculated to about 4 weeks (see e.g. Dahlström and Häggendal, 1970; Häggendal and Dahlström, 1971b).

II. Amine Granules and Functional Parameters of the Neuron

The levels of *endogenous NA* are mainly depended on NA stored in the amine granules. The granules protect the NA from deamination by MAO, which rapidly metabolites free NA in the cytoplasm (e.g. Iversen, 1967).

The life-span of the granules must be clearly distinguished from the turn-over of NA in the nerve terminals. Since the granules themselves participate in the synthesis of NA, and since the turn-over of NA in nerve terminals appears to be very fast (in the order of some hours or several times per day, for reference see Iversen, 1967), the granules probably turn over their own NA content several times during their life-span. The amount of NA reaching the nerve terminals via the down-transport of granules contribute only with a few $^0/_0$ per day to the NA stores in the nerve terminals (cf. Dahlström and Häggendal, 1966a).

The *retention of tracer amounts of* ^3H-NA in the tissue appears to be dependent on functioning amine granules. The ^3H-NA is taken up into the nerve terminals by the "membrane pump", but is not (if MAO is not inhibited) stored and retained in the terminals unless this occurs in functioning amine granules (cf. Andén *et al.*, 1969; Jonsson *et al.*, 1969).

Some observations indicate that functioning amine granules are necessary for the *release of transmitter* at nerve-activity. In reserpinized animals transmission is impaired during a certain period, due to the lack of transmitter in the terminals. However, even if the intraneuronal NA levels are increased by MAO inhibition and subsequent administration of exogenous NA, no or very little of this NA, located to the major part in the cytoplasm, appears to be released during nerve stimulation. This indicates that the intraneuronal presence of the transmitter is not sufficient for normal transmission, but that the transmitter must be stored in functioning amine granules (cf. Häggendal and Malmfors, 1969).

III. Studies in Reserpine Treated Animals

A. Endogenous NA and Transport of Granules

Reserpine (10 mg/kg i.p. to rats) depletes the tissue stores of NA by causing a long-lasting (cf. Carlsson, 1965) or practically irreversible (Dahlström and Häggendal, 1966b, 1970; Häggendal and Dahlström, 1971a) block of the amine storage mechanism of the granules. The amines leak out from the granules and become deaminated by MAO (see e.g. Carlsson, 1965).

The recovery of the levels of endogenous NA in the nerve terminals after reserpine appears to be dependent on the axonal down-transport of new amine granules. After reserpine, the earlist signs of recovery of NA in the neurons have been found in the *perikarya*, where a perinuclear ring of NA-induced fluorescence appears about $12-15$ h after reserpine. This indicates that the new NA-forming and -storing granules are synthesized in the cell bodies. At $15-18$ h the axonal down-transport of such new granules has been detected in adrenergic *axons* (Dahlström, 1967; Dahlström and Häggendal, 1969). At the beginning, the amount of NA-storing granules passing down the axons appears to be low, but it rapidly increases, and during the second to fifth day after reserpine the amount appears to be clearly supranormal (Fig. 1). Thus, the cell bodies seem to produce and send down supra-normal amounts of amine granules during a certain period after reserpine treatment (Dahlström and Häggendal, 1969). After this period the amounts of down-transported granules appears to decrease, being subnormal during the 9th to 13th day (see Fig. 1).

In the *nerve terminals* the levels of endogenous NA start to increase between 24 and 36 h, whereafter the levels steadily rise (Häggendal and Dahlström, 1970, 1971a). This rise in NA in the nerve terminals can be delayed by axotomy or by removal of their cell bodies. Table 1 shows the results obtained from two series of reserpine-pretreated rats with unilateral removal of the cervical superior ganglion and contralateral preganglionic denervation of this ganglion

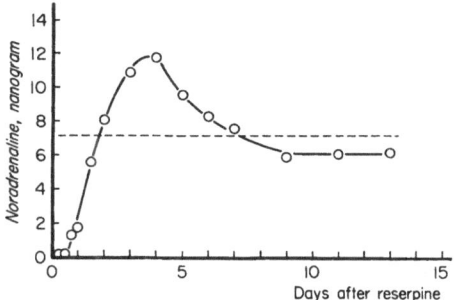

Fig. 1. The amount of NA transported down and accumulated above a 6 h ligation of rat sciatic nerves at different times after reserpine treatment (10 mg/kg i.p.). The values are taken from Fig. 1 in Dahlström and Häggendal (1969) and are obtained by the subtraction of the NA amount in unligated nerves from the amount in the 6 h ligated nerves. The NA values probably reflect the number of NA storing granules which accumulate above the ligation. (From Häggendal and Dahlström, 1971 a)

(to reduce the influence of nerve activity). The operations were performed 12 h before killing in all cases. The NA content in the salivary glands was estimated (for method see Häggendal, 1963). Between 24 and 36 h the NA levels started to increase in the glands with intact ganglia. The NA levels in the glands on the ganglionectomized side were clearly lower than those on the intact side 36, 48, and 72 h after reserpine. The difference in NA content is greatest at 72 h. This may be considered in relation to the amounts of amine granules, transported down the axons to the terminals, which is larger at this time period than earlier (Fig. 1).

The NA recovery in the nerve terminals then proceeds fairly rapidly up to the second week, when the rate of the recovery slows down (Häggendal and Dahlström, 1971 a). In the axons at this time there seems to be a decrease in the number of granules that are transported down. Thus, the NA recovery in the nerve terminals

Table 1. *Content of endogenous noradrenaline (NA) in rat salivary glands after reserpine (10 mg/kg i.p.). Twelve hours before death unilateral ganglionectomy was performed, and the contralateral ganglion was preganglionically denervated (decentralized). The NA values are given in per cent of the NA content in normal salivary glands (239 ± 16.9 ng, n = 7). Roman figures indicate corresponding pairs of glands*

Time after reserpine in hours		18	24	36	48	72
Decentralized side	I	2.5	1.6	3.3	9.3	15.7
	II	1.7	2.1	3.9	13.6	29.3
	I	1.9	1.2	— [a]	3.3	5.0
Ganglionectomized side	II	1.7	1.3	0.9	7.7	13.4
Mean values for the difference between decentralized and ganglionectomized pair of glands		0.3	0.6	2.7	6.0	13.3

[a] Omitted due to technical error.

Table 2. *Concentrations of endogenous noradrenaline (NA) in cranial and caudal parts of rat spinal cord 24 h after midthoracic transection. Reserpine (10 mg/kg i.p.) was given at different times before death. Spinal cords from 4 to 7 rats were pooled. The results are expressed in per cent of the concentrations found in corresponding parts of the spinal cord of non-reserpinized rats with 24 h transections. Roman figures indicate estimation series. Figures within brackets indicate the NA concentrations in ng/g found 24 h after the transection in non-reserpinized animals. The 0.5 cm part just cranial to the lesion was omitted in all rats, since the accumulations of NA in the transected axons (cf. Dahlström and Fuxe, 1965) would disturb the comparison between the cranial and caudal parts of NA recovery in the nerve terminals of the spinal cord*

Time after reserpine		0 h	1 d.		2 d.		3 d.	4 d.	
Cranial part	I	100 (195)	2.9		28			64	
				4.3[a]		26[a]			57.5[a]
	II	100 (249)	5.6		24		42	51	
Caudal part	I	100 (245)	1.8		4.2			48	
				4.2[a]		4.6[a]			41[a]
	II	100 (302)	6.6		5.0		22	34	
Mean values for the difference between cranial and caudal parts			0.1		21		20	16.5	

[a] Mean value of the 2 Figs.

appears to be a reflection of the amount of granules which are transported distally in the axons per unit of time. This relation, together with the delay in NA recovery caused by axotomy indicate that the proximo-distal transport of new amine granules is of great importance for the recovery of endogenous NA in adrenergic nerve terminals after reserpine. Also in the CNS the NA recovery after reserpine follows a multiphasic course (Häggendal and Dahlström, unpublished). For further discussion of the multiphasic recovery curve, see Häggendal and Dahlström, 1971a. It should be pointed out that the amount of NA in the down-transported granules is an indication of the relative number of granules which are transported. This NA is probably exchanged several times in the nerve terminals like in the normal animal.

Also in the CNS the NA recovery in nerve terminals after reserpine is most probably depending upon the supply of new granules from the cell bodies. If the spinal cord of a rat is sectioned at a mid-thoracic level 24 h before the sacrifice at different times after reserpine, the NA recovery in the caudal half of the cord is delayed as compared to the cranial half. Table 2 shows the results from two series of experiments (I and II), where cords from 4—7 rats were pooled for every estimation. The values are expressed in % of the NA levels in non-reserpinized animals, transected 24 h before death, estimated at every series. The figures, although few in number, seem to indicate that transection of the spinal cord, i.e. interruption of the axoplasmic flow of e.g. amine granules from the NA cell bodies in the brain stem to the NA terminals in the caudal half of the cord, causes a delay in the NA recovery after reserpine. The transection time used may appear long, but in the CNS the NA nerve terminals degenerate slower than in the PNS upon axotomy (e.g. Dahlström and Fuxe, 1965). It is interesting to observe that the delay in recovery appears to correspond to 24 h.

Thus, the NA recovery in both peripheral and central NA nerve terminals after reserpine appears to be dependent on the axonal transport of some factor, probably the amine granules.

B. Retention of ^{3}H-NA and Transport of Amine Granules

It is well known that the uptake-retention capacity of the nerve terminal granules is lost after reserpine treatment (cf. Carlsson, 1965). The recovery of this capacity appears to start about 36 h after a large dose of reserpine (10 mg/kg i.p. to rats) and is normalized within a few days (for references see Andén, Carlsson and Häggendal, 1969). The recovery of this function has often been discussed to be due to the recovery of the old, reserpine-blocked granules in the nerve terminals. However, an alternative explanation has been proposed. The recovery of ^{3}H-NA retention was suggested to depend upon the arrival in the nerve terminals of new granules, formed in the perikarya after the reserpine injection, and having a particularly high ability for storing ^{3}H-NA (Dahlström and Häggendal, 1966 b). This hypothesis has been tested in peripheral tissues of the rat (Häggendal and Dahlström, 1970, 1971 b, c).

^{3}H-NA (2.5 µg/kg, spec. act. 2.33 Ci/mmole, Amersham) was given i.v. 30 min before death to rats, pretreated with reserpine (10 mg/kg i.p.) at different times before death, in which the cervical superior ganglion was removed unilaterally (ganglionectomized or axotomized side) 12 h before death. At the same time the contralateral ganglion was preganglionically denervated (decentralized side, side with intact adrenergic neurons or "intact side").

In the glands on the "intact side" the ^{3}H-NA retention started to recover 24—36 h after reserpine (Häggendal and Dahlström, 1970). Normal levels of

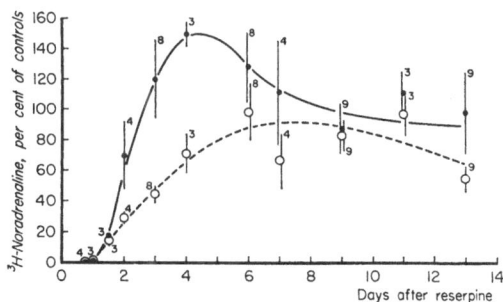

Fig. 2. The uptake-retention of ^{3}H-NA in rat salivary glands (30 min after an i.v. injection of l-^{3}H-NA, 2.5 µg/kg) at different times after reserpine treatment. Unilateral removal of the cervical superior ganglion and contralateral preganglionic denervation of this ganglion were performed 12 h before death. The values are expressed in $^0/_0$ of the uptake-retention of ^{3}H-NA in operated controls (preganglionically denervated glands 12 h beforehand) without reserpine treatment. Mean values ± S.E.M. (vertical bars) are given. Small figures indicate number of estimations. •———• indicates the values in glands of the denervated side (with intact adrenergic neurons); o----o indicates values in the contralateral glands on the ganglionectomized side (From Häggendal and Dahlström, 1971 b)

retained ³H-NA were found 2—3 days after reserpine. Thereafter a period of
supranormal retention occurred and the maximum values were observed around
day 4 after reserpine. Then the recovery of ³H-NA declined to normal or somewhat
subnormal values after about one week (Fig. 2) (Häggendal and Dahlström,
1971 b, c). The shape of this curve is very like the shape of the curve in Fig. 1,
showing the axonal down-transport of new granules after reserpine per unit
of time.

On the ganglionectomized side the ³H-NA values obtained were lower than on
the intact side. The ³H-NA levels increased also on this side, but the removal of
the ganglion caused a delay in the recovery. The differences in retention between
the two sides was greatest around the 4th day, i.e. during the period when supranormal amounts of amine granules were transported down in the adrenergic
axons per unit of time.

The observation that axotomy markedly delayed the recovery of the ³H-NA
retention capacity in the salivary gland, together with the finding that the largest
difference between the two sides were present around day 4 after reserpine strongly
indicate that the recovery of the ³H-NA retention capacity in adrenergic nerve
terminals after reserpine is dependent on the axoplasmic transport of some
factor(s). The close relation between the recovery of ³H-NA retention and the
pattern of axoplasmic transport of NA granules after reserpine may indicate that
the amine granules represent a factor of great importance for this recovery.

In the spinal cord of reserpine-pretreated rats Andén and Lundborg (1970)
have observed that the recovery of ³H-NA retention (following administration of
³H-DOPA) in the part of cord caudal to a transection, performed 50 h beforehand,
occurred later than in the cranial part of the cord. These authors discuss this
observation to support the hypothesis that axonal transport of new amine granules
is of importance for recovery of ³H-NA retention capacity after reserpine.

C. Adrenergic Transmission and Transport of Granules

After reserpine the transmission is blocked, due to lack of transmitter substance
(for review see Andén *et al.*, 1969) and probably also due to lack of functioning
amine granules. Recovery of transmission starts about 36 h after reserpine and
appears to be normalized 2—3 days after the injection (for references see Andén
et al., 1969). At this time the levels of endogenous NA are very small. Häggendal
and Lindqvist (1963, 1964) have pointed out only very small amounts of transmitter substance appear to be necessary for maintaining a normal function, both in
the periphery and in the CNS. This has been confirmed by Andén, Magnusson
and Waldeck (1964), who in reserpine-pretreated rats stimulated adrenergic
nerves electrically and registrated mechanically the response of the stimulation.

The onset of recovery of transmission after reserpine, and the time needed for
normalization of this function appear to occur in parallel with the recovery and
normalization of the capacity of the terminals to retain ³H-NA. The recovery of
transmission may thus also be dependent on the axonal transport of amine
granules. Experiments are in progress in our laboratories to investigate the effect
of inhibition of transport of amine granules on the recovery of adrenergic transmission after reserpine.

D. Possible Differences in Properties between New and Old Granules

The studies concerning the recovery after reserpine of endogenous NA support the figures calculated for the life-span of amine granules regarding their capacity to store endogenous NA (about 4 weeks, e.g. Dahlström and Häggendal, 1970). During the process of NA recovery in the nerve terminals a *drop* in the NA levels was observed at 4 weeks (cf. Häggendal and Dahlström, 1971a). The most reasonable explanation for this drop seems at present to be the following: During the first week after reserpine supranormal amounts of new granules reach the nerve terminals. Then the amounts decline to normal and even subnormal levels (Fig. 1). At about 4 weeks after reserpine supranormal amounts of granules disintegrate, due to their limited life-span of 4 weeks. At this period after reserpine, the amounts of granules transported to the terminals are too small to compensate for the loss of the large amounts of granules which disintergrate. Therefore a drop in the NA level occurs. Normal NA levels were found 6 weeks after reserpine.

The recovery of ^{3}H-NA retention capacity, on the other hand, proceeded to normal levels within only a few days. This may imply that the young granules have a particularly high capacity for storing exogenous NA (cf. Dahlström and Häggendal, 1966b), and that the granules lose this capacity with increasing age in the terminals. A comparison between Fig. 2 and Fig. 1 may illustrate this point. In Fig. 2 it can be observed that in the glands with the intact adrenergic innervation the following occurred: a) a rapid *increase to normal* of the capacity to retain ^{3}H-NA, b) a following *supranormal* capacity of retention and c) a subsequent *decline* of this capacity. These events seem to be a reflection of the down-transport of new granules in the axons, which is indicated in Fig. 1. These observations seem to indicate that predominantly the young amine granules are involved in ^{3}H-NA retention in the nerve terminals.

Since transmission recovers in parallel to the ^{3}H-NA retention recovery it may be suggested that the young amine granules are of greater importance for transmission than the old granules. (see discussion in Häggendal and Dahlström, 1971b).

IV. Studies in Non-reserpinized Animals

In order to further investigate the role of axoplasmic transport for the function of the adrenergic nerve terminals, some experiments have been performed on normal, non-reserpinized rats.

Axotomy and Nerve Terminal Degeneration

It is well known that degeneration of peripheral adrenergic nerve terminals occurs about one day after axotomy. No, or very little, endogenous NA have been found in denervated tissues after this time, and the nerve terminals have disappeared (for reference see e.g. Iversen, 1967).

This degeneration of the terminals is probably due to interruption of the supply of material from the cell bodies, i.e. inhibition of the axoplasmic flow. In

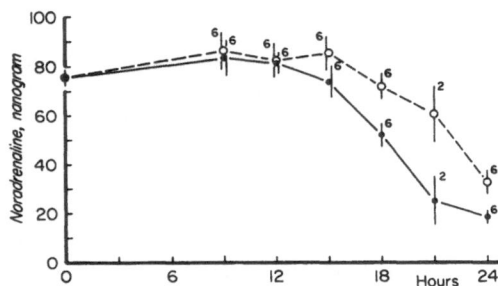

Fig. 3. The amounts of NA (ng/muscle) in rat gastrocnemic muscles at different times after axotomy of the sciatic nerves. ●——● indicates the values after axotomy at a low level; ○– – –○ shows the values after axotomy at a level 3 cm proximal to the level on the contra-lateral side. Vertical bars indicate S.E.M. and numerals numbers of observations

order to study if the transport of granules in particular has some importance in this relation the following experiment was performed.

The sciatic nerves of rats were sectioned at a high level on one side and at a low level on the contralateral side. The distance between the two levels was about 3 cm. At different time intervals after this operation the rats were killed and the gastrocnemic muscles (receiving all or most of their adrenergic vasoconstrictor nerves from the sciatic nerve) were removed bilaterally and assayed for NA. The results are shown in Fig. 3. The disappearance of NA occurred earlier in the muscles after a low section of the sciatic nerve than after a high section. The difference in time for the onset of the NA decrease appeared to be about 3 h.

The results indicate that the length of the nerve distal to the cut is of import-ance for the onset of degeneration of the adrenergic nerves, and that some sub-stance which is transported distally in the axons is of importance for the mainten-ance of the terminals. The time difference of 3 h observed between the two sides with a 3 cm level difference for the sciatic nerve transections may indicate that the substance of importance is transported at about 10 mm/h. In adrenergic nerves of rat the fastest transport rates have so far been found for the amine granules. In the sciatic nerve of the rat the amine granules have been calculated to travel at a rate of about 5 mm/h in the nerve part proximal to a ligation (cf. Dahlström and Häggendal, 1966). There is probably only a small if any difference in the rate of fast axonal transport between intact and ligated nerves, and in the nerves proximal or distal to a ligation, as suggested by the results obtained by Ochs and Ranish (1969). Therefore, it seems reasonable to assume that the rate of transport of amine granules in the nerve distal to the cut is in the order of about 5 mm/h. This rate is in the same order of magnitude as the rate of the substance, discussed to be of importance for the maintenance of the adrenergic nerves. Thus, it is possible that the axonal transport of amine granules is of importance for the maintenance and function of the nerve terminals. Of course, it cannot be excluded that some other, yet unidentified "nutrition factor" which is transported as fast as or faster than the amine granules, is of importance for preventing nerve terminal degeneration.

References

Andén, N. E., Carlsson, A., Häggendal, J.: Adrenergic mechanisms. Ann. Rev. Pharmacol. **9**, 119—134 (1969).
— Lundborg, P.: Recovery of the amine uptake-storage mechanism in nerve granules after reserpine treatment: inhibition by axotomy. J. Pharm. Pharmacol. **22**, 233—235 (1970).
— Magnusson, T., Waldeck, B.: Correlation between noradrenaline uptake and adrenergic nerve function after reserpine treatment. Life Sci. **3**, 19—25 (1964).
Banks, P., Magnall, D., Mayor, D.: The redistribution of cytochrome oxidase, noradrenaline and adenosine triphosphate in adrenergic nerves constricted at two points. J. Physiol. (Lond.) **200**, 745—762 (1969).
Carlsson, A.: Drugs which block the storage of 5-hydroxytryptamine and related amines. In: Handbuch der experimentellen Pharmakologie, S. 529—592. Eds. O. Eichler and A. Farah. Berlin-Heidelberg-New York: Springer 1965.
Dahlström, A.: The effect of reserpine and tetrabenazine on the accumulation of noradrenaline in the rat sciatic nerve after ligation. Acta physiol. scand. **69**, 167—179 (1967).
— Fuxe, K.: Evidence for the existence of monoamine-containing neurons in the central nervous system. II. Experimentally induced changes in the intraneuronal amine levels of bulbo-spinal neuron systems. Acta physiol. Scand. **64**, suppl. 247, 1—36 (1965).
— Häggendal, J.: Studies on the transport and life-span of amine storage granules in a peripheral adrenergic neuron system. Acta physiol. scand. **67**, 278—288 (1966a).
— — Recovery of noradrenaline levels after reserpine compared with the life-span of amine storage granules in rat and rabbit. J. Pharm. Pharmacol. **18**, 750—751 (1966b).
— — Recovery of nordrenaline in adrenergic axons of rat sciatic nerves after reserpine treatment. J. Pharm. Pharmacol. **21**, 633—638 (1969).
— — Axonal transport of amine storage granules in sympathetic adrenergic neurons. In: Biochemistry of simple neuronal models, Vol. 2, pp. 65—93. Eds. E. Costa and E. Giacobini, Advances in biochemical psychopharmacology. New York: Raven Press 1970.
Euler, U. S. v., Hillarp, N. Å.: Evidence for the presence of noradrenaline in submicroscopic structures of adrenergic axons. Nature (Lond.) **177**, 44—45 (1956).
Geffen, L. B., Ostberg, A.: Distribution of granular vesicles in normal and constricted sympathetic neurons. J. Physiol. (Lond.) **204**, 583—592 (1969).
Häggendal, J.: An improved method for fluorimetric determination of small amounts of adrenaline and noradrenaline in plasma and tissue. Acta physiol. scand. **59**, 242—254 (1963).
— Dahlström, A.: Uptake and retention of ^{3}H-noradrenaline in adrenergic nerve terminals after reserpine and axotomy. Europ. J. Pharmacol. **10**, 411—415 (1970).
— — The recovery of noradrenaline in adrenergic nerve terminals of the rat after reserpine treatment. J. Pharm. Pharmacol. **23**, 81—89 (1971a).
— — The functional role of the amine storage granules of the sympatho-adrenal system. Symposium on: Subcellular organization and function of endocrine tissues, April 1970. Bristol (in press) (1971b).
— — The effect of axotomy on the uptake retention of ^{3}H-noradrenaline in adrenergic nerve terminals of rat salivary glands after reserpine treatment. (In preparation) (1971c).
— Lindqvist, M.: Behaviour and monoamine levels during long-term administration of reserpine to rabbits. Acta physiol. scand. **57**, 431—436 (1963).
— — Disclosure of labile monoamine fractions in brain and their correlation to behaviour. Acta physiol. scand. **60**, 350—357 (1964).
— Malmfors, T.: The effect of nerve stimulation on catecholamines taken up in adrenergic nerves after reserpine pre-treatment. Acta physiol. scand. **75**, 33—38 (1969).
Hökfelt, T.: In vitro studies on central and peripheral monoamine neurons at the ultra structural level. Z. Zellforsch. **91**, 1—74 (1968).
— Distribution of noradrenaline storage particles in peripheral adrenergic neurons as revealed by electron microscopy. Acta physiol. scand. **76**, 427—440 (1969).
Iversen, L. L.: The uptake and storage of noradrenaline in sympathetic nerves. Cambridge: Univ. Press 1967.

Jonsson, G., Hamberger, B., Malmfors, T., Sachs, Ch.: Uptake and accumulation of ^{3}H-nor-adrenaline in adrenergic nerves of the rat iris. Effect of reserpine, monoamine oxidase and tyrosine hydroxylase inhibition. Europ. J. Pharmacol. 8, 58—72 (1969).
Laduron, P., Belpaire, F.: Transport of noradrenaline and dopamine-β-hydroxylase in sympathetic nerves. Life Sci. 7, 1—7 (1968).
Livett, B. G., Geffen, L. B., Austin, L.: Proximo-distal transport of ^{14}C-noradrenaline and protein in sympathetic nerves. J. Neurochem. 15, 931—939 (1968).
Ochs, S., Ranish, N.: Characteristics of the fast transport systems in mammalian nerve fibres. J. Neurochem. 1, 247—261 (1969).
Stjärne, L.: Studies of catecholamine uptake, storage and release mechanisms. Acta physiol. scand. 69, Suppl. 228 (1964).

Dr. Jan Häggendal
Dept. of Pharmacology
University of Göteborg
Göteborg, Sweden

Acta neuropath. (Berl.) Suppl. V, 249—256 (1971)
© by Springer-Verlag 1971

Axonal Transport of Proteins
in the Hypothalamo-Neurohypophysial System of the Rat *

A. Norström and J. Sjöstrand

Institute of Neurobiology, University of Göteborg, Sweden

Summary. Axonal transport of proteins in the hypothalamo-neurohypophysial system of the rat was studied after a local injection of (^{35}S)cysteine into the region of the supraoptic nucleus (SON). The migration of labelled proteins was followed by measuring the specific radio-activity of the proteins in various parts of the hypothalamo-neurohypophysial tract. Between 2 and 4 h after the isotope injection there was a sharp increase in the protein-bound specific radioactivity of the posterior pituitary lobe, demonstrating that a rapid transport of (^{35}S) labelled proteins had occurred from the SON to the neurohypophysis with a transport rate of approximately 60 mm/day. Fractionation of the neurohypophysial proteins by polyacrylamide gel electrophoresis revealed that a predominant part of the radioactivity of the soluble proteins was recovered in a single protein fraction. This protein component with properties of a neuro-physin is involved in the neurohypophysial response to osmotic stress since it disappeared from the posterior lobe following dehydration of the rat.

Colchicine injected into the subarachnoidal space before a local injection of (^{35}S) cysteine inhibited the rapid transport of radiolabelled constituents. As revealed by electron-microscopy colchicine only slightly affected the neurotubuli and neurofilaments of SON neurons.

The protein-bound radioactivity of the neurohypophysis was followed up to 30 days after isotope injection. Between 6 and 9 days an increase of protein radio-labelling was observed demonstrating an arrival of slowly migrating proteins at this time interval (0.5—1 mm/day). Osmotic stress and lactation did not increase the rate of axonal transport of neurohypophysial proteins. However, the labelled material was eliminated from the neural lobe at an increased rate upon stimulation.

Key-Words: Neurosecretion — Neurohypophysis — Axonal Transport.

Introduction

It is now a well-established concept that the magnocellular hypothalamic nuclei, the supraoptic nucleus (SON) and the paraventricular nucleus (PVN) are responsible for the synthesis of the hormones of the neurohypophysis. The hormones, vasopressin and oxytocin, become bound to carrier proteins, neurophysins and, held within neurosecretory granules, they are transported from the site of synthesis to the terminals in the neural lobe, where the storage and release occur. (Bargmann, 1949; Scharrer and Scharrer, 1954).

The present communication is a review of our studies during the preceeding year on axonal transport in the neurohypophysial system of the rat. The presence of two phases of axonal transport is described. One neurohypophysial protein constituent, transported at a rapid rate, is shown to have properties of a rat

* The present study was supported by grants from the Nathhorst Foundation, from the Swedish National Cancer Society (265-B70-02x) and from the University of Göteborg. We are indebted to Mrs. Marie-Louise Eskilsson and Miss Barbro Lilja for their excellent technical assistance. We are grateful to Miss Gull Grönstedt for careful secreterial work. We express our gratitude to Dr. H.-A. Hansson for his help with the electron microscopy.

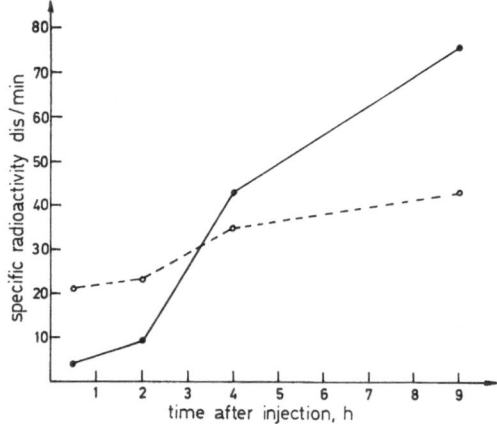

Fig. 1. Accumulation of radiolabelled proteins in the neurohypophysis after a local injection of (^{35}S) cysteine into the SON region. Solid and dashed lines represent specific radioactivity (dis/min/µg protein) in the TCA precipitate and in the TCA supernatant respectively. From Norström and Sjöstrand (1971)

neurophysin. The effects of colchicine treatment and functional stimulation on transport and release of neurosecretory material are discussed.

Results and Discussion

(^{35}S) cysteine was stereotactically injected without anaesthesia into the SON region using a chromatographic needle attached to a volume calibrated teflon tube. Details of this procedure have been described elsewhere (Norström, 1971). At various time intervals after isotope injection, the animals were sacrificed by decapitation. The SON region, the hypophysial stalk and the neurohypophysis were isolated, and protein amount and radioactivity were determined. The proteins were analyzed using disc electrophoresis on polyacrylamide gels (Ornstein, 1964; Davis, 1964) and the radioactivity in the protein bands was measured. For details see Norström and Sjöstrand (1971).

In Fig. 1 the specific radioactivity of the TCA precipitate and TCA soluble material in the neurohypophysis are presented for various time intervals after isotope injection. A change was found in the distribution of TCA precipitable radioactivity along the hypothalamo-neurohypophysial tract, with a marked increase in radiolabel occurring in the neurohypophysis with time. Up to 2 h after isotope injection no appreciable amount of TCA precipitable radioactivity was observed. Between 2 and 4 h after injection there was a marked increase in the specific radioactivity of the TCA-precipitated material, and a further increase was observed up to 9 h after isotope injection. The radioactivity profile of the TCA supernatant for the most part coincided with that of the TCA precipitate.

When separating neurohypophysial proteins by gel electrophoresis and determining the radioactivity in the various protein components, one fraction, fraction A, was found to contain more than 90 % of the radioactivity which had entered into

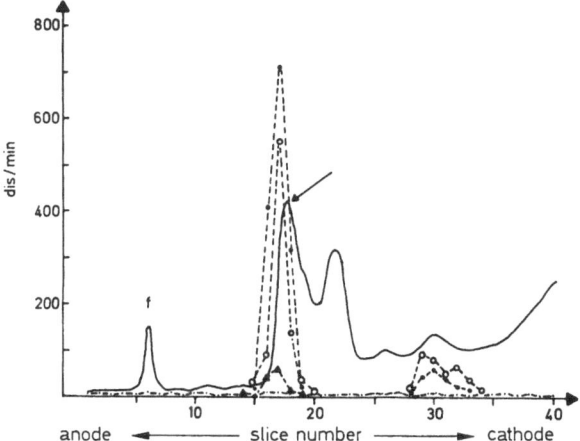

Fig. 2. Gel electrophoresis of proteins from the neurohypophysis at various time intervals after a local injection of (^{35}S) cystein into the SON region. Front band (f) and fraction A (arrow) are indicated. The intensity of the stain absorbed by the protein in each band was measured by transmission densitometry with a Vitatron Automatic Densitometer and integrating Recorder. From Norström and Sjöstrand (1971) ———— optical density; –·–·–·– radioactivity 60 min after ^{35}S cysteine injection; ▲- - - -▲ radioactivity 2 h after ^{35}S cysteine injection; o- - - -o radioactivity 4 h after ^{35}S cysteine injection; •- - - -• radioactivity 9 h after ^{35}S cysteine injection.

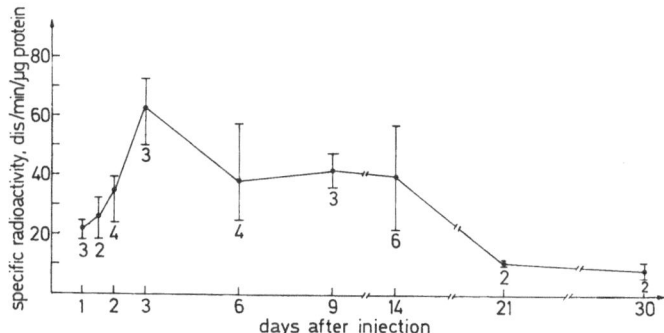

Fig. 3. Specific radioactivity of TCA precipitated material of the neurohypophysis at various time intervals after injection of (^{35}S) cysteine into the SON region

the gel (Fig. 2). No appreciable radioactivity was recovered until 2 h after isotope injection. In accordance with the marked increase of radiolabel in TCA precipitated material observed between 2 and 4 h after injection of (^{35}S) cysteine, a tenfold increase of incorporated isotope was found in fraction A during the same time interval. Thus, the accumulation of labelled material in the neural lobe 2 h after the injection of (^{35}S) cysteine into the SON region demonstrates the arrival of newly synthetized products at this time. Estimating the distance of the supra-optic-neurohypophysial tract to be 4 mm, a transport rate of at least 60 mm/day was calculated for the rapidly migrating proteins. These findings are consistent with the recent demonstration of a similar transport rate for the neurohypophysial hormones (Pickering and Jones, 1970).

In another experimental series the TCA precipitable radioactivity in the neurohypophysis was followed up to 30 days after injection of (^{35}S) cysteine into the SON region. The protein-bound radioactivity increased up to 72 h after isotope injection (Fig. 3). A decrease was then observed until the 6th day, after which a slight increase was observed. From the 14th to the 30th day there was a decline in TCA precipitable radioactivity. The fact that the radioactivity of the neural lobe slightly increased between 6 and 14 days after isotope injection, makes it probable that the turnover of the rapidly migrating proteins is balanced by the arrival to the neurohypophysis of more slowly migrating proteins, with a transport rate of 0.5—1 mm per day, at this time. In order to determine whether fraction A possessed the properties of a neurophysin, rats were deprived of water for 6 days. In agreement with earlier reports (Rennels, 1966; Friesen and Astwood, 1967) we found that after dehydration, the fast migrating fraction A disappeared or was considerably reduced. Upon rehydration fraction A reappeared within 24 h, and by 3 days conditions returned to normal. On the basis of these findings it was postulated that fraction A was involved in the response to osmotic stress. Electrophoretic separation of hydrochloric acid-extracted neural lobe protein on starch gel demonstrated that the highly labelled protein component had properties comparable to those of one of the porcine neurophysins (Norström, Sjöstrand, Livett, Uttenthal and Hope, 1971). Furthermore, the use of immunotechniques demonstrated that this fraction cross-reacted with a cross-species reactive anti-neurophysin serum. Thus it can reasonably be deduced that fraction A represents a rat neurophysin.

Effect of Colchicine on Axoplasmic Transport of Neurosecretory Material

The mechanism responsible for the axoplasmic transport of proteins is not yet known. It has been suggested that the neurotubuli take part in the transport of axonal constituents (Schmitt, 1968). Colchicine, which combines with and may induce the depolymerization of neurotubuli (for references see Schmitt, 1968,), has been shown to interfere with axonal flow (Kreutzberg, 1969; Dahlström, 1968; Karlsson and Sjöstrand, 1969; Sjöstrand et al., 1970; James et al., 1970). In order to investigate the effect of colchicine on the neurohypophysial system, the drug was injected into the subarachnoidal space in the region of the SON. The effect was studied by electron microscopy and by measuring the distribution of labelled proteins along the neurohypophysial tract after a local injection of (^{35}S) cysteine into the SON region. When 40—180 μg colchicine in distilled water had been given in 2—3 daily subarachnoidal injections, the TCA precipitable radioactivity decreased in all parts of the neurohypophysial tract as compared to controls. 24 h after isotope injection protein radiolabelling was considerably reduced in the hypophysial stalk and in the neurohypophysis of colchicine treated animals, i.e. 40% and 10% of control values, respectively. When neurohypophysial proteins were separated by polyacrylamide gel electrophoresis, an obvious change was observed in the radioactivity profile, i.e. hardly any radiolabel was recovered in neural lobe proteins from colchicine-treated animals (Fig. 4). The reduction in

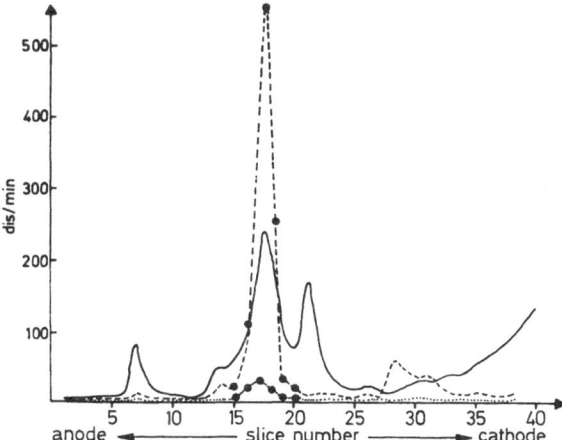

Fig. 4. Gel electrophoretical separation of neurohypophysial proteins 4 h after a local injection of (^{35}S) cysteine into the SON region. 40—180 µg colchicine was injected subarachnoidally 24 h before the isotope injection. From Norström *et al.* (1971) ———— optical density; - - - - - - radioactivity, control; ———— radioactivity, colchicine

radioactivity of the TCA-precipitable proteins of the neurohypophysis and the lack of specific protein radiolabelling, as revealed by gel electrophoresis in experimental animals, demonstrated that colchicine induces an inhibition of the rapid protein transport.

Following colchicine treatment the SON neurons showed ultrastructural changes characteristic of very actively synthetizing cells. The chromatin was dispersed, and the nucleolus was enlarged in the eccentrically situated nucleus. The granular endoplasmic reticulum was short and branching, and was distended by filamentous material. An increased number of free ribosomes and enlarged Golgi complexes were observed. An increased number of Herring bodies were found in the infundibulum. They were filled with neurosecretory granules, varying in number and density, as well as with microvesicles, mitochondria, lysosomes, some profiles of endoplasmic reticulum and numerous neurofilaments which were sometimes aggregated in strands. The axons and axon terminals in the neurohypophysis were characterized by being heavily loaded with microvesicles and neurosecretory vesicles with a core of apparently increased osmiophilia. Mitochondria were often arranged along dilatated, usually central, profiles of endoplasmic reticulum. A moderately increased number of neurofilaments and an unchanged number of intact neurotubuli were observed. Thus, the heavy accumulation of neurofilaments in strands, as described to occur in the cell bodies of motor neurons after colchicine treatment, was not observed in the neurosecretory neurons (Wiśniewsky and Terry, 1968).

The approximately fivefold increase in Herring bodies at the infundibular level may represent an ultrastructural manifestation of a blockage of axoplasmic transport. The increased number of heavily osmiophilic neurosecretory vesicles

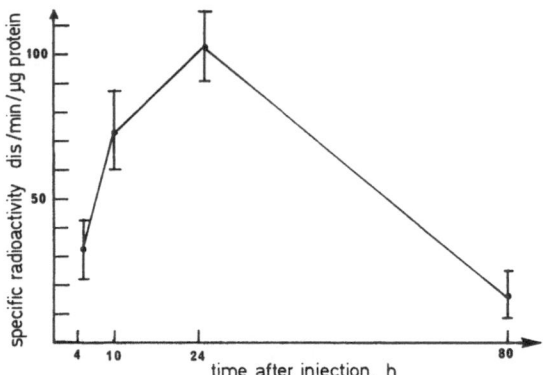

Fig. 5. Distribution of the specific radioactivity of the TCA precipitated material of the neuro-hypophysis. The rats were given 2% NaCl instead of drinking water for 9 days. The isotope was injected 4, 10, 24 and 80 h prior to sacrifice. Mean value of two animals together with the range at each time

in the dilatated nerve terminals of colchicine-treated animals may indicate that the drug interferes with the release mechanism.

Effect of Functional Stimulation on Transport and Turnover of Neurohypophysial Proteins

Rats were given 1 or 2% saline instead of drinking water. The animals were killed after varying periods of stimulation and at various time intervals after isotope injection. Salt loading did not increase the rate of axoplasmic transport of neurohypophysial proteins, i.e. radiolabelled proteins did not accumulate in the neural lobe until 2 h after injection of (^{35}S) cysteine into the SON region. The increase in neurohypophysial protein-bound radioactivity proceeded up to 24 h, as in control animals (Fig. 5). At 80 h after isotope injection neural lobe radioactivity was considerably reduced and at this time interval no radioactivity was recovered in fraction A, which was considerably reduced in amount (Fig. 6). Thus ingestion of 2% saline considerably increased the rate of release of labelled material from the neurohypophysis. 1% saline did not induce so rapid and marked changes as did 2% saline. However, the radioactivity that was recovered in TCA precipitated proteins was significantly lower in experimental than in control animals 6 and 14 days after isotope injection and ingestion of 1% saline for 20 and 28 days respectively (Norström and Sjöstrand, in preparation).

Investigating the effect of lactation on turn-over of neurohypophysial proteins, (^{35}S) cysteine was injected in the region of the SON and PVN of lactating rats. No radioactivity was recovered in the neural lobe until 2 h after isotope injection, thus supporting the view that stimulation does not increase the rate of transport. The radiolabelling pattern of neurohypophysial proteins of lactating rats did not differ from that of control female or male rats. Lactation increased the turnover rate of neurohypophysial proteins, as revealed by measuring the TCA precipitable radioactivity at various time intervals following isotope injection. Thus, after

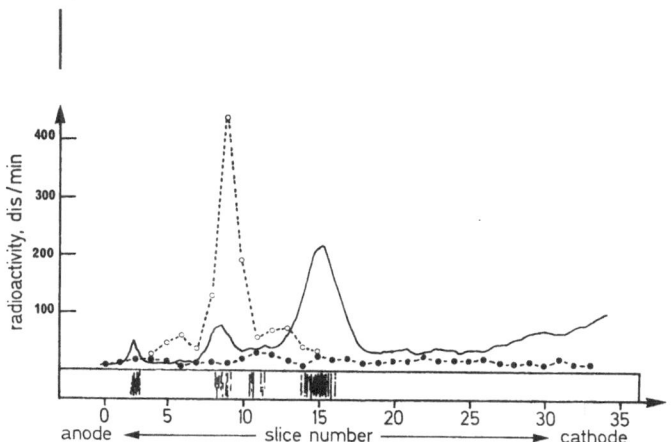

Fig. 6. Polyacrylamide gel disc electrophoresis of neurohypophysial proteins 9 days after in-jection of (^{35}S) cysteine into the SON region. ——— Optical density, rat given 1% NaCl 14 d, 2% NaCl 7 d; —·—·— radioactivity, rat given 1% NaCl 14 d, 2% NaCl 7 d; –o–o–o– radio-activity control

22 days of lactation and suckling and 16 days following (^{35}S) cysteine injection the neural lobe protein-bound radioactivity was reduced approximately 50% in comparison to control values (Norström and Sjöstrand, in preparation).

Reference

Bargmann, W.: Über die neurosekretorische Verknüpfung von Hypothalamus und Neuro-hypophyse. Z. Zellforsch. **34**, 610—634 (1949).

Dahlström, A.: Effect of colchicine on transport of amine storage granules in sympathetic nerves of rat. Europ. J. Pharmacol. **5**, 111—113 (1968).

Davis, B. J.: Disc electrophoresis. II. Method and application to human serum protein. Ann. N. Y. Acad. Sci. **121**, 404—427 (1964).

Friesen, H. G., Astwood, E. B.: Changes in neurohypophysial proteins induced by dehydration and ingestion of saline. Endocrinology **80**, 278—287 (1967).

James, K. A. C., Bray, J. J., Morgan, I. G., Austin, L.: The effect of colchicine on the transport of axonal protein in the chicken. Biochem. J. **117**, 767—771 (1970).

Karlsson, J.-O., Sjöstrand, J.: The effect of colchicine on axonal transport of protein in the optic nerve and tract of the rabbit. Brain Res. **13**, 617—619 (1969).

Kreutzberg, G. W.: Neuronal dynamics and axonal flow. IV. Blockage of intraaxonal enzyme transport by colchicine. Proc. nat. Acad. Sci. (Wash.) **62**, 722—728 (1969).

Norström, A.: A functional study of the hypothalamo-neurohypophysial system of the rat with the use of a newly developed method for localized administration of labelled pre-cursors. Brain Res. **28**, 131—142 (1971).

— Hansson, H.-A., Sjöstrand, J.: Effects of colchicine on axonal transport and ultrastructure of the hypothalamo-neurohypophysial system of the rat. Z. Zellforsch. **113**, 271—293 (1971).

— Sjöstrand, J.: Axonal transport of proteins in the hypothalamo-neurohypophysial system of the rat. J. Neurochem. **18**, 29—40 (1971).

— — Livett, B., Uttenthal, O., Hope, D. B.: Characterization of neurohypophysial proteins of the rat. Biochem. J. (in press) (1971 b).

Ornstein, L.: Disc electrophoresis I. Background and theory. Ann. N. Y. Acad. Sci. **121**, 321—349 (1964).

Pickering, B. T., Jones, C. W.: The biosynthesis and intraneuronal transport of neurohypophysial hormones: preliminary studies in the rat. Mem. Soc. Endocr. (in press) (1971).

Scharrer, E., Scharrer, B.: Hormones produced by neurosecretory cells. Recent Progr. Hormone Res. **101**, 183—240 (1954).

Schmitt, F. O.: Fibrous proteins-neuronal organelles. Proc. nat. Acad. Sci. (Wash.) **60**, 1092—1101 (1968).

Sjöstrand, J., Frizell, M., Hasselgren, P.-O.: Effects of colchicine on axonal transport in peripheral nerves. J. Neurochem. (in press).

Wiśniewsky, H., Terry, R. D.: Experimental colchicine encephalopathy. I. Induction of neurofibrillary degeneration. Lab. Invest. **17**, 577—587 (1967).

Dr. Anders Norström
Institute of Neurobiology
Medicinaregatan 5
Fack
S 400 33 Göteborg 33
Sweden

Acta neuropath. (Berl.) Suppl. V, 257—266 (1971)
© by Springer-Verlag 1971

Axonal Transport in the Goldfish Visual System *

J. S. ELAM **, E. A. NEALE ***, and B. W. AGRANOFF

Mental Health Research Institute, University of Michigan, Ann Arbor, Michigan/U.S.A.

Summary. Intraocular injection of either ^{3}H-proline or ^{3}H-asparagine produced highly specific labelling of the rapidly transported protein of the goldfish optic nerve. These amino acids are therefore ecxellent specific markers of rapid axonal flow. Studies on the accumulation of transported protein in the tectum show rapid transport to be a temperature dependent process occurring at the rate of 70—100 mm per day at 23°. Transported protein was found to be widely distributed among particulate subcellular fractions including synaptosomes, mitochondria and myelin, but not nuclei and ribosomes.

Rapidly transported protein can also be labelled by intraocular injection of ^{35}SO$_4$. Roughly half of the transported protein-bound sulfate label is isolated in two sulfated mucopolysaccharides, chondroitin sulfate and heparan sulfate. The rate of transport of the sulfated mucopolysaccharides appears to be identical to that of total rapidly transported protein.

Key-Words: Protein — Axonal Transport — Organelles, Axoplasmic — Synaptosomes — Electron Microscopy.

Introduction

On the basis of present evidence [2,10,12,18] for review see [11] it appears that rapidly transported axonal proteins are carried into the nerve endings and by implication are likely to be utilized in some aspect of synaptic function. It then seems advantageous to study these proteins in the nerve terminal region where factors such as rates of accumulation, rates of turnover, subcellular distribution and possible transsynaptic migration might be examined. However, in mammals studies of this sort are frequently hampered by the diffuse anatomical distribution of most nerve terminals.

In the fish optic tract this problem is greatly diminished since the retinal ganglion neurons terminate in a discrete region of the contralateral optic tectum, a brain area which is readily dissected. In studies on goldfish, McEwen and Grafstein [14] demonstrated that labelled rapidly transported protein accumulates in the contralateral optic tectum following intraocular injection of ^{3}H-leucine into one eye. However, a complication in their studies was the substantial amount of background labelling due to incorporation of ^{3}H-leucine brought to the brain by the blood. This systemic labelling is manifested as radioactivity in the ipsilateral tectum and the measurement of transported radioactivity is the difference Left (dpm/μg protein)—Right (dpm/μg protein). In confirmatory experiments conducted in our laboratory [6], about 50 % of the contralateral tectal radioactivity was in non-transported protein.

---
* This study was supported by grants from the National Science Foundation and the National Institute of Mental Health.
** Interdisciplinary fellow, National Institute of Mental Health.
*** Supported by Michigan Memorial Phoenix Project.

J. S. Elam, E. A. Neale, and B. W. Agranoff:

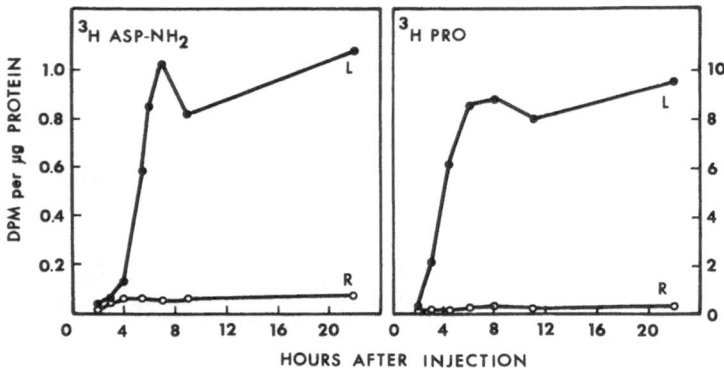

Fig. 1. Labelling of protein in the left and right optic tectum with intraocular injection of ³H-asparagine (0.52 μCi, 0.41 nmoles) or ³H-proline (2.5 μCi, 0.31 nmoles). Groups of 4—5 tecta were processed together for each time point. *L* left tectum; *R* right tectum [6]

Studies with Other Amino Acids

In order to further characterize the rapidly transported protein, it would be advantageous to reduce the level of background labelling. This is particularly true of studies on the subcellular distribution of the radioactivity, where comparison of fractions from separate left and right tectal homogenates is both tedious and highly subject to experimental error. One method for specifically labelling the transported proteins was found to be the use of certain other tritiated amino acid precursors in place of leucine [6]. From 0.2—0.5 nmoles of 19 different tritiated amino acids were injected into the right eye and tectal labelling was measured after 6 h. While most of the amino acids were similar to or only slightly superior to leucine in labelling the transported protein, we found that proline and asparagine were more efficiently incorporated into transported protein yet produced very little background labelling in the brain. The kinetics of transport of protein labelled with these amino acids are seen in Fig. 1. As was seen in experiments with ³H-leucine, there is a delay of 2—4 h in the arrival of labelled transported protein at the tectum and a rapid accumulation in the subsequent 4—5 h. Unlike the leucine experiments, however, the right tectal specific activity remains low at all time points. The physiological significance of the lower amount of systemic labelling has not been determined, but in the case of proline it is probably related to the fact that a very small fraction of the injected radioactivity enters the TCA-soluble pool of the brain [6].

Fish injected intraocularly with ³H-proline, unlike those given ³H-leucine [6,14], showed a 2—4 fold left to right difference in tectal TCA-soluble radioactivity. However, since the absolute amounts of radioactivity were small relative to the amount incorporated ($< 5\%$) and since the difference in TCA-soluble radioactivity appeared slightly later than the difference in protein radioactivity, it is unlikely that the TCA-soluble material served as precursor for a significant portion of the left tectal labelling.

Kinetics and Subcellular Distribution

Having obtained a system for specifically labelling rapidly transported protein, experiments were undertaken to further characterize the rate of transport and subcellular locus of these molecules. In experiments in which groups of fish were kept at 10°, 16° or 23° for 2 days, then injected with ^{3}H-proline, both the extent of labelling and the time of arrival of transported protein strongly depend upon the temperature of the fish [6]. Based on time of arrival of radioactivity at the tectum, the kinetics seen for 23° indicate a transport rate in our fish of 50 mm per day. McEwen and Grafstein [14] reported a rate of 40 mm per day at 20°. However, these estimates do not take into account the time required for incorporation of isotope into protein and possible subsequent steps prior to entering the axon. To clarify this point, individual fish were injected in the right eye and the portion of the right optic nerve rostral to the optic chiasm was removed at various times and analyzed for radioactivity in protein [6]. It was found that a band of radioactivity passes through the anterior portion of the nerve prior to arrival in the tectum and that this band does not leave the eye for up to 2 h after injection. This indicates that the rate of transport in the nerve *per se* is on the order of 70—100 mm/day.

Additional studies have been directed toward ascertaining the subcellular distribution of the rapidly transported proteins. Teflon-on-glass-produced tectal homogenates (8 h after injection of labeled proline) in 0.25 M sucrose were fractionated into conventional crude nuclear, crude mitochondrial, microsomal and soluble fractions by centrifugations of 750 × g (10 min), 11,000 × g (20 min) and 105,000 × g (60 min) respectively. The crude mitochondrial fraction was subdivided into fractions of myelin, synaptosomes, mixed synaptosomes and mitochondria and purified mitochondria by means of a discontinuous sucrose gradient as described by Von Hungen *et al.* [13]. The expected composition of the fractions was confirmed by assay of chemical and enzymatic markers including DNA for nuclei [16], cerebroside for myelin [6], acetylcholinesterase for synaptosomes [8], succinate-INT-reductase for mitochondria [17] and RNA for microsomes [16]. An independent check on the purity of the synaptosomal and mitochondrial fractions was made by electron microscopy (Fig. 2). The synaptosomal pellet is essentially devoid of free mitochondria. The mitochondrial pellet is seen to contain a number of synaptosomal profiles through approximately a third of its thickness, while the remaining two-thirds of the fraction appears relatively free of synaptosomes.

The distribution of label in a typical fractionation is shown in Fig. 3. Similar patterns were obtained using asparagine-labelled tectum. The data is plotted as dpm per μg protein vs μg protein, so that the area of a given rectangle is proportional to the total dpm in that fraction. It is apparent that right tectal radioactivity remains relatively low in all fractions and can in most cases be ignored in quantitating the results. The left tectal radioactivity appears to be largely particulate, in agreement with results obtained in numerous other studies [14,15,18]. It might however be argued that the radioactive protein is soluble *in vivo*, but adheres artifactually *in vitro* to particles during homogenization. Two lines of evidence argue against this hypothesis. The first is a "mixing" experiment in which labelled

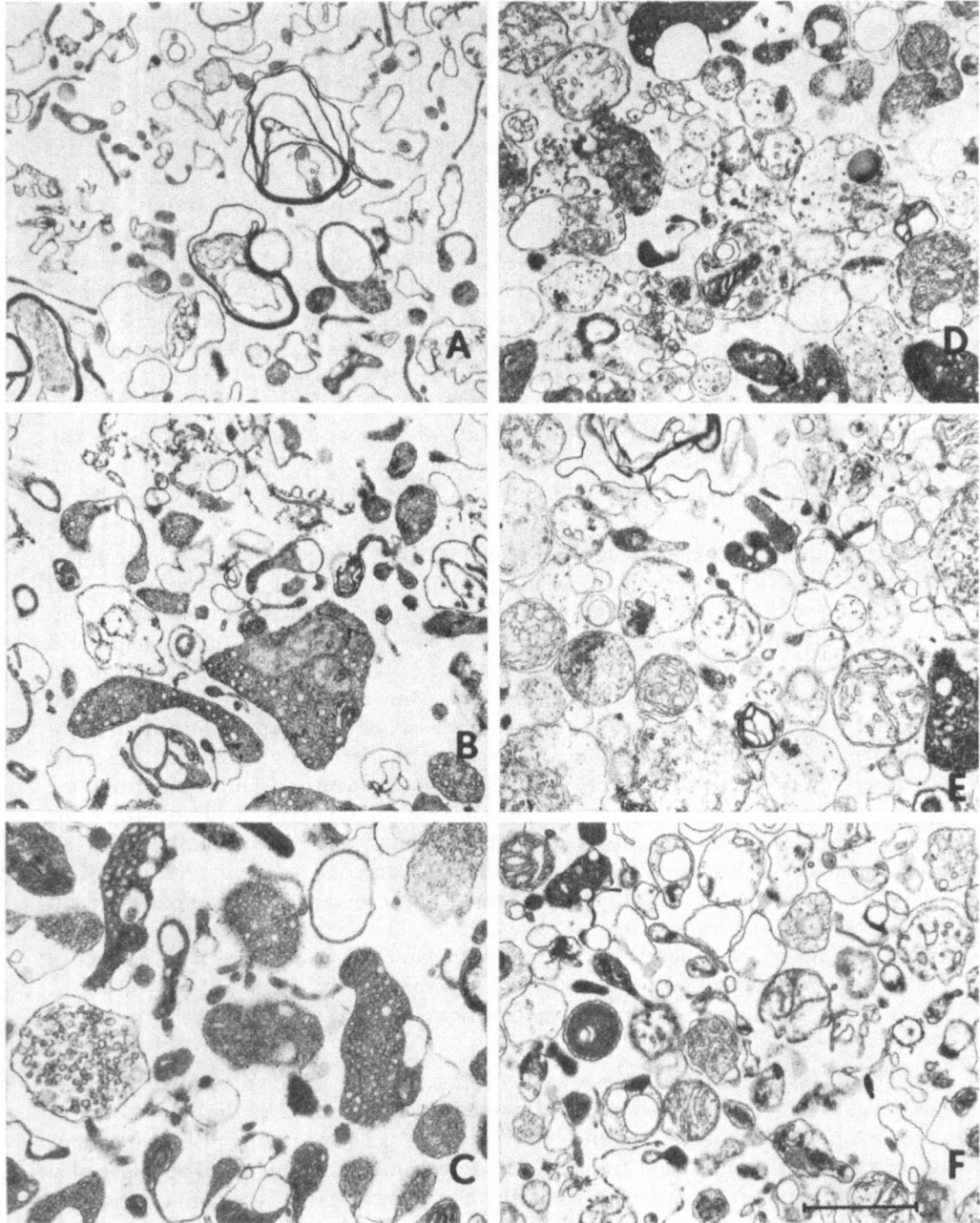

Fig. 2. Representative views of consecutive thirds through the thickness of pellets prepared according to Cotman and Flansburg [4] from the synaptosomal (A, B, C) and mitochondrial (D, E, F) fractions. Glutaraldehyde and osmium fixation. ×15,000

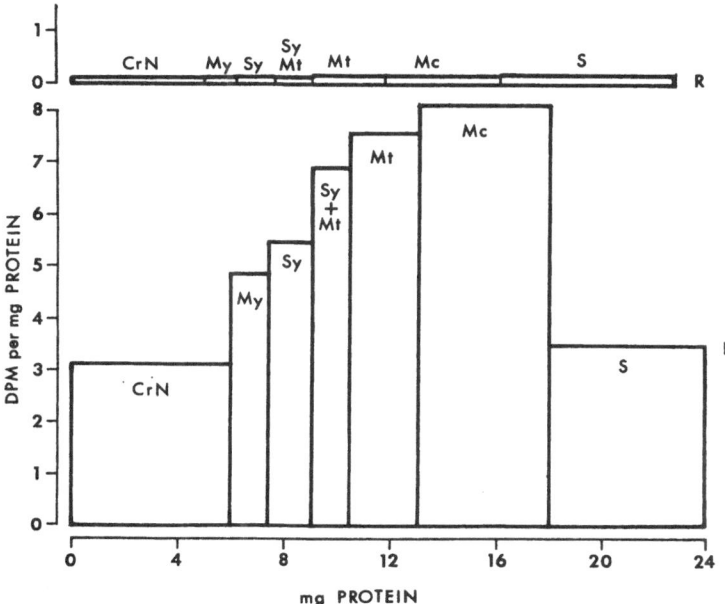

Fig. 3. Labelling of subcellular fractions of left and right tecta following injection of ³H-proline (2.5 μCi, 0.31 nmoles). Tecta from 40 fish were pooled and fractionated as described in the text. The area of each rectangle is proportional to the radioactivity in that fraction. *L* left tectum; *R* right tectum; *CrN* crude nuclear; *My* myelin; *Sy* synaptosomes; *Mt* mitochondria; *Mc* microsomes; *S* soluble [6]

100,000 × g soluble fraction was added back to a 10-fold excess (in protein) of unlabeled homogenate [6]. Following refractionation, 86% of the radioactivity was recovered again in the soluble fraction, indicating that labelled protein did not adhere to particulates *in vitro*. Secondly, labelled proteins non-covalently bound to subcellular particles would be expected to be released by relatively mild treatments with urea or detergent. However, as the data in Table 1 shows, the tectal particulate material remaining after treatment with increasing concentrations of either Triton or urea maintains a nearly constant specific radioactivity, even up to 70% solubilization. It therefore appears that artifactual binding of labelled protein by subcellular fractions does not complicate the experimental results.

Further examination of Fig. 3 reveals that a large fraction of the transported radioactivity is recovered in fractions other than synaptosomes. Barring transsynaptic movement, which does not appear to occur to an appreciable extent in this system [10], the results are most compatible with the view that many synaptosomes are ruptured in the process of isolation. It would then be expected that their components (mitochondria, membranes, etc.) will migrate with analogous structures derived from rupture of neuronal and glial cell bodies. In support of this view, examination of the microsomal fraction by electron microscopy revealed the presence of large numbers of collapsed synaptosomes and "synaptosomal

Table 1. *Equal volumes of proline labelled tectal homogenate were adjusted to the stated concentrations of Triton × 100 or urea and centrifuged at 100,000 × g for 1 h. Pellets were washed with 0.25 M sucrose and assayed for protein and radioactivity.* % *protein unsolubilized = (protein in 100,000 × g pellet from treated homogenate/protein in 100,000 × g pellet from untreated homogenate)* × 100

% Triton	% Protein unsolubilized	Specific activity of unsolubilized protein
0	100	14.8
0.003	94.0	14.4
0.006	80.1	15.1
0.013	76.0	12.3
0.063	44.5	11.3
0.13	28.6	13.6

Molarity of urea	% Protein unsolubilized	Specific activity of unsolubilized protein
0	100	13.8
0.5	97.5	10.1
1	91.8	14.3
2	86.6	13.8
3	82.1	14.0
4	68.7	14.3

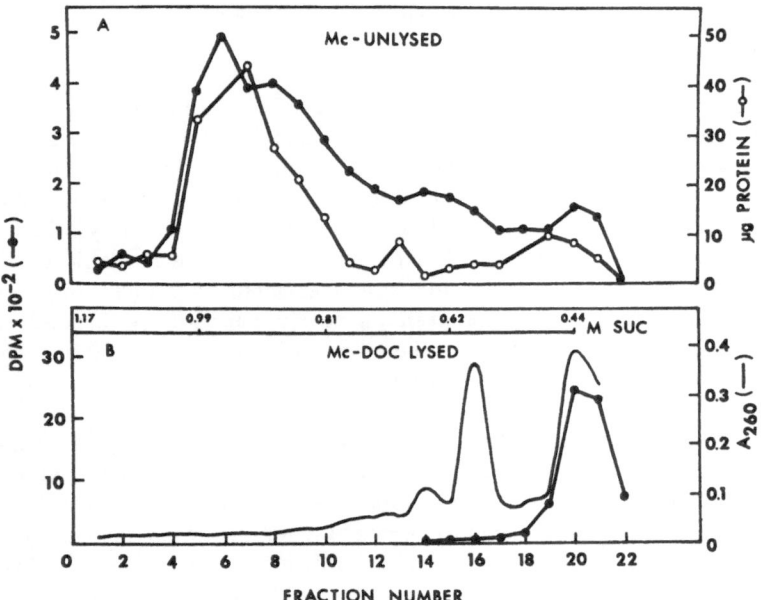

Fig. 4. Distribution of microsomal radioactivity and protein on a 15—40% sucrose gradient before (A) and after (B) lysis with 0.5% deoxycholate. Centrifugation was at 170,000 × g (SW-40 rotor) for 90 min

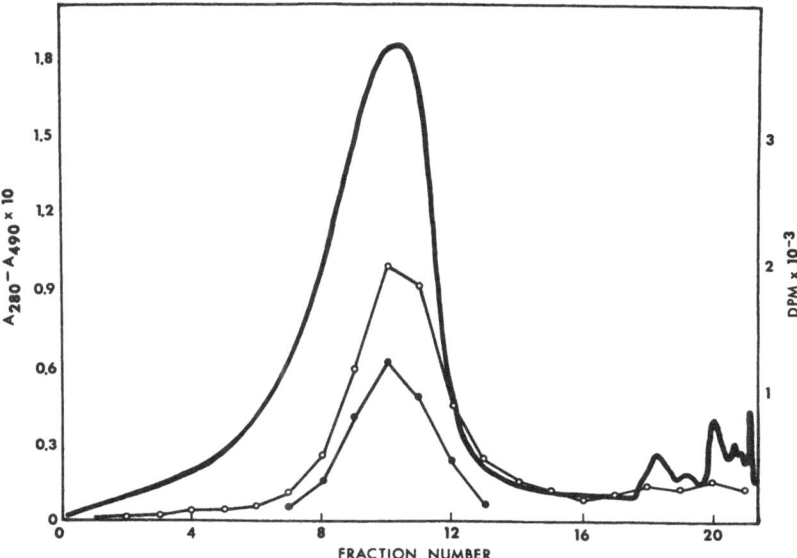

Fig. 5. Recentrifugation of the mitochondrial fraction (see Fig. 3) in a 0.8—2.0 M sucrose gradient (SW-40 rotor, 130,000×g, 1 h). o–o–o dpm, •–•–• OD 490 mμ (succinate-INT-reductase), —— OD 280 mμ

ghosts". Further, recentrifugation of the microsomal fraction on a continuous sucrose gradient revealed a broad peak in the region of 0.8—1.0 M sucrose (Fig. 4A), a density range characteristic of damaged synaptosomes [20]. The apparent low recovery of undamaged synaptosomes may be characteristic of our methods or reflect the properties of goldfish tectum. The observations should nevertheless serve as a note of caution in interpreting synaptosomal recoveries generally, since much higher estimates of yield have been reported [3]. Centrifugation of deoxy-cholate-treated microsomal fraction on an identical gradient (Fig. 4B) shows that essentially all of the radioactivity is associated with membranes and not ribosomes. This would appear to support the hypothesis that ribosomes are absent in nerve endings and that little or no postsynaptic labelling is occurring.

The apparent labelling of mitochondria (Fig. 3) is of interest in view of the conclusion from some studies [1, 19] that mitochondria are a component only of slow transport. It would seem likely that the amount of synaptosomal contamination observed (Fig. 2) is not in itself sufficient to account for the extensive labelling of the mitochondrial fraction. Further, when mitochondria were recentrifuged on a continuous 0.8 to 2.0 M sucrose gradient, there was essential comigration of the radioactivity and the mitochondrial enzymatic marker, succinate-INT-reduc-tase (Fig. 5). We have also tested the possibility that mitochondria are labelled by exchange of radioactivity with other labelled particulates during isolation [6]. When labelled myelin (0.4 mg protein), synaptosomes (0.6 mg protein) and micro-somes (0.6 mg protein) were each added to unlabelled homogenate (14 mg protein) and refractionated, none transferred more than 3% of its radioactivity to the

Table 2*. *Radioactivity in optic tectum 12 h following intraocular injection of* $Na_2{}^{35}SO_4$. *Combined tectal hemispheres (300 mg wet weight) were homogenized in 20 vol of chloroform-methanol (1:1), centrifuged and the pellet washed with an additional 20 vol of solvent. The pellet was washed three times with 20 vol of methanol-water (90:10) 1 mM in sodium sulfate. The residue was treated overnight at 60° with 1.2 mg of a protease from Streptomyces griseus (Type IV, Sigma Chemical) in 4 ml of 0.14 M This (pH 8) and centrifuged to remove a small amount of unsolubilized material. The supernatant was stirred 1 h with 1 ml of 2°/₀ cetylpyridinium bromide (CPB). The resultant precipitate was washed in 1ml of 0.05°/₀ CPB, dissolved in 1 ml of 60°/₀ n-propanol and precipitated overnight with 4 ml of EtOH containing 5°/₀ potassium acetate. The precipitate was washed with 1 ml of the EtOH-acetate and dissolved in 0.8 ml of water to which 0.2 ml of 50°/₀ TCA was added. After 30 min at 0°, the resulting precipitate (nucleic acids) was recovered and the SAP reprecipitated with 4 ml of EtOH-acetate and redissolved in 0.1 ml of water. Determination of radioactivity was achieved by liquid scintillation counting with the aid of an internal* ^{35}S *standard*

Fraction	Radioactivity (cpm)	
	Left tectum	Right tectum
1. Chloroform-methanol extracts	5,781	4,619
2. Methanol-water washes	23,470	24,270
3. Protease supernatant	86,000	5,320
4. Protease residue	773	49
5. CPB supernatant	33,900	2,800
6. CPB precipitate	30,100	2,010
7. TCA precipitate	314	5
8. Final EtOH precipitate	31,380	1,580

* From Elam, Goldberg, Radin and Agranoff: Science **170**, 458 (1970).

mitochondria. Thus labelling of mitochondria appears to be genuine and indicates the rapid axonal transport of either whole mitochondria or proteins which are metabolically incorporated into mitochondria at the nerve endings. It might be noted that Barondes [1] also observed an appreciable amount of rapid labelling of nerve ending mitochondria from mouse brain, but attributed it to either local incorporation or contamination. It appears unlikely that either of these factors can account for our results. The possibility exists that mitochondria migrate at more than one rate.

The labelling of myelin (Fig. 3) was undiminished by repeated hypo-osmotic washes and resedimentation on 0.8 M sucrose. This opens the possibility that some myelin protein may have a neuronal origin. The label in the crude nuclear fraction is apparently in non-nuclear material, since nuclei spun through 2 M sucrose showed less than $1/_3$ the specific activity of the crude fraction.

Experiments with $^{35}SO_4$

We shall review briefly the results of recent experiments which have employed Na_2 $^{35}SO_4$ as a marker of rapidly transported protein in the goldfish optic tract [7]. It was found that when carrier-free Na_2 $^{35}SO_4$ was injected into the right eye, the distribution of label in the left and right optic tectum after 12 h indicated rapid axonal flow of labelled material (Table 2). The small left/right difference in radioactivity of the chloroform-methanol and methanol-water washes indicates the absence of rapidly transported sulfolipids and/or free sulfate. However, the large

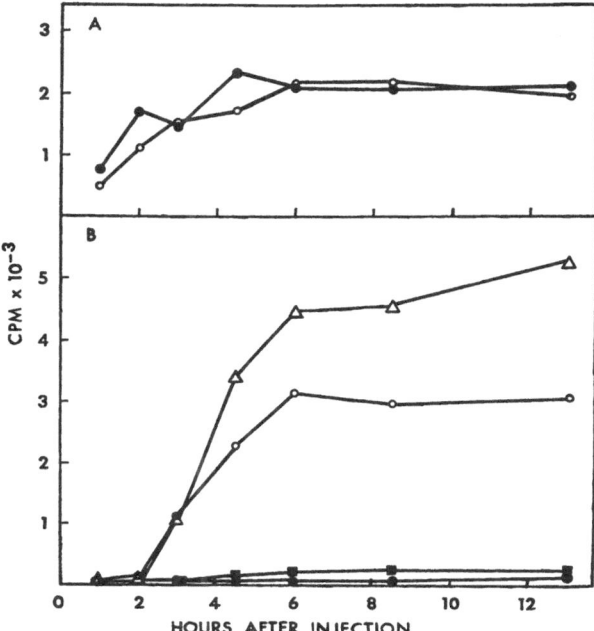

Fig. 6. Appearance of radioactivity into left and right tectal fractions following injection of ³H-proline and Na₂ ³⁵SO₄ into the right eye. *A* combined chloroform-methanol and methanol-water washes (Fraction 1 + 2). o–o–o ³⁵S in left tectum; •–•–• ³⁵S in right tectum. *B* supernatant following protease digestion (Fraction 3). ▵–▵–▵ ³H in the left tectum; ▪–▪–▪ ³H in the right tectum; o–o–o ³⁵S in the left tectum; •–•–• ³⁵S in the right tectum [7]

left to right difference in the protease digest is suggestive of transport of sulfated mucopolysaccharide proteins. Substantiating evidence for such transport is provided by the solubility characteristics of about $1/2$ the labelled material; precipitability in cetylpyridinium bromide and ethanol and solubility in 10% TCA, all of which are characteristic of sulfated mucopolysaccharides. Further evidence was provided by electrophoresis of the material isolated in fraction 8. Three bands appeared. The fastest comigrated with standard chondroitin sulfate and contained 29% of the radioactivity. The middle band migrated slightly slower than standard heparan sulfate and contained the remainder of the radioactivity. The unlabelled lower band comigrated with hyaluronic acid, a non-sulfated compound. Additional studies on susceptibility to hyaluronidase and degree of N-sulfation appeared to confirm the presence of labelled chondroitin sulfate and heparan sulfate. The portion of the transported radioactivity which was non-precipitable in cetylpyridinium bromide was shown to be 75% non-dialyzable and to have low mobility toward the anode on high voltage electrophoresis. These properties suggest sulfated glycopeptide, although further characterization was not performed. The kinetics of transport of protein doubly labelled with ³⁵SO₄ and ³H-proline are seen in Fig. 6. It is apparent from comparison of arrival of the two isotopes in the tectum that sulfated mucopolysaccharide proteins are transported at essentially the same rate as the total rapidly transported protein. In addition, the absence of an excess of label in the combined chloroform-methanol methanol-water fraction at early time points precludes the possibility that sulfated mucopolysaccharides are labelled by a rapidly transported pool of free sulfate or phosphoadenosine phosphosulfate.

Evidence for transport of sulfated mucopolysaccharide proteins is of interest in a number of respects. Their migration in a nerve tract suggests that they are produced by neurons. While glial production of mucopolysaccharide has been demonstrated in cell culture [5] evidence for their production in neurons has been fragmentary. In the present study the possibility that they are secreted by glial cells and transported extra-axonally has not been excluded. The high anionic charge of sulfated mucopolysaccharides raises the possibility that they may serve a special function in the transport of specific cations to the synapse. Interestingly, defects in sulfated mucopolysaccharide metabolism have been found in diseases such as Hurler's syndrome, where mental retardation is a characteristic factor [9].

Acknowledgements. The authors are indebted to Mrs. Pat Petiet and Mrs. Marianne Andrews for valuable technical assistance.

References

1. Barondes, S.: J. Neurochem. **13**, 721—727 (1966).
2. — J. Neurochem. **15**, 343—350 (1968).
3. Clementi, F., Whittaker, V. P., Sheridan, M. N.: Z. Zellforsch. **72**, 126—138 (1966).
4. Cotman, C. W., Flansburg, D. A.: Brain Res. **22**, 152—156 (1970).
5. Dorfman, A., Ho, P.-L.: Proc. nat. Acad. Sci. (Wash.) **66**, 495—499 (1970).
6. Elam, J. S., Agranoff, B. W.: J. Neurochem. **18**, 375—387 (1971).
7. — Goldberg, J. M., Radin, N. S., Agranoff, B. W.: Science **170**, 458—460 (1970).
8. Ellman, G. L., Courtney, D., Andres, V., Featherstone, R. M.: Biochem. Pharmacol. **7**, 88—95 (1961).
9. Fratantoni, J. C., Hall, C. W., Neufeld, E. F.: Proc. nat. Acad. Sci. (Wash.) **64**, 360—366 (1968).
10. Grafstein, B.: Science **157**, 196—198 (1967).
11. — Advanc. Biochem. Psychopharmacol. **1**, 11—25 (1969).
12. Hendrickson, A.: Science **165**, 194—196 (1969).
13. Hungen, K., von, Mahler, H. R., Moore, W. J.: J. biol. Chem. **243**, 1415—1423 (1968).
14. McEwen, B. S., Grafstein, B.: J. Cell Biol. **38**, 494—508 (1968).
15. Ochs, S., Sabri, M. I., Johnson, J.: Science **163**, 686—687 (1969).
16. Santen, R. J., Agranoff, B. W.: Biochim. biophys. Acta (Amst.) **72**, 251—262 (1963).
17. Sellinger, O. Z., Hiatt, R. A.: Brain Res. **7**, 191—200 (1968).
18. Sjöstrand, J., Karlsson, J. O.: J. Neurochem. **16**, 833—844 (1969).
19. Weiss, P., Pillai, A. L.: Proc. nat. Acad. Sci. (Wash.) **54**, 48—56 (1965).
20. Whittaker, V. P., Michaelson, I. A., Kirkland, R. J. A.: Biochem. J. **90**, 293—303 (1964).

Bernard. W. Agranoff
Mental Health Research Institute
University of Michigan
Ann Arbor, Michigan 48104, U.S.A.

(Monographien aus dem Gesamtgebiete der Psychiatrie / Psychiatry Series, Band 3)

A.E. Adams
Informationstheorie und Psychopathologie des Gedächtnisses

Methodische Beiträge zur experimentellen und klinischen Beurteilung mnestischer Leistungen

Von Dr. med. Alfred E. Adams, Privatdozent für Neurologie und Psychiatrie, Oberarzt der Neurologischen Klinik Köln-Merheim

Mit 12 Abbildungen
IX, 124 Seiten. 1971
Gebunden DM 48,—
US $ 13.20

Die Bezieher des „Archiv für Psychiatrie und Nervenkrankheiten", der „Zeitschrift für Neurologie/Journal of Neurology" und des „Zentralblatt für die gesamte Neurologie und Psychiatrie" erhalten die „Monographien" zu einem gegenüber dem Ladenpreis um 10 % ermäßigten Vorzugspreis.

Diese Arbeit ist eine Einführung in klinisch wichtige Methoden und Ergebnisse der modernen Informationstheorie. Es wird eine informationstheoretisch ausgerichtete Psychopathologie des Gedächtnisses unter Berücksichtigung aktueller hirnpathologischer, neurophysiologischer und experimentalpsychologischer Tatsachen dargestellt. Mnestische Störungen entstehen vornehmlich durch Läsionen definierter Leistungsstrukturen des Gehirns. Die hypothetischen Hirn-Engramme des Gedächtnisses sind jedoch fragwürdig und wurden bisher in den Nervensystemen des Menschen oder des höheren Vertebraten nicht nachgewiesen. Mit neuen Ergebnissen wird gegen unbewiesene Hypothesen argumentiert.

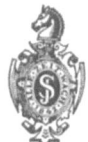

SPRINGER-VERLAG
BERLIN · HEIDELBERG · NEW YORK

A.Wackenheim · J.P.Braun

Angiography of the Mesencephalon

Normal and Pathological Findings

By **A. Wackenheim,** Professor, Head of the Neuroradiological Dept., C.H.U. Strasbourg, and Dr. **J. P. Braun,**
Head of the Neuroradiological Dept., C.H.R. Colmar

With 128 figures
XI, 154 pages. 1970
Cloth DM 98,–
US $ 27.00

In this monograph the authors deal with the practical interpretation of angiography in the mid-brain area, using for
this purpose x-rays of the arteries, capillaries and veins
exclusively. After a thorough review of the literature, the
authors consider the various criteria of normal roentgen
diagnosis on the basis of normal angiography and anatomical preparations. The second part of the book is devot-
ed to the roentgenological changes seen in the arteries,
capillaries (capillarography) and veins in pathological
conditions. These include tumours of the pineal region,
tumours of the posterior thalamus and cerebral peduncles,
meningiomas of the tentorium, aneurysms and arterio-
venous malformations, and active hydrocephalus.

■ **Prospectus
on request**

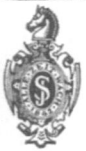

**Springer-Verlag
Berlin · Heidelberg · New York**